# PRINCIPLES OF
# MANUAL MEDICINE

*Editor:* Timothy S. Satterfield
*Associate Editor:* Linda Napora
*Copy Editor:* Anne Schwartz
*Design:* Dan Pfisterer
*Illustration Planning:* Lorraine Wrzosek
*Production:* Anne G. Seitz

Copyright © 1989
Williams & Wilkins
428 East Preston Street
Baltimore, Maryland 21202, USA

Accurate indications, adverse reactions, and dosage schedules for drugs are provided in this book, but it is possible that they may change. The reader is urged to review the package information data of the manufacturers of the medications mentioned.

*Printed in the United States of America*

Library of Congress Cataloging-in-Publication Data

Greenman, P. E., 1928–
    Principles of manual medicine/Philip E. Greenman.
        p.    cm.
    Includes bibliographies and index.
    ISBN 0-683-03556-8
    1. Manipulation (Therapeutics) 2. Medicine, Physical. I. Title.
    [DNLM: 1. Manipulation, Orthopedic. 2. Physical Medicine. WB
460 G814p]
RM724.G74 1989
615.8'2—dc19
DNLM/DLC
                                                            88-21588
                                                               CIP

                                                          91   92
                               2   3   4   5   6   7   8   9   10

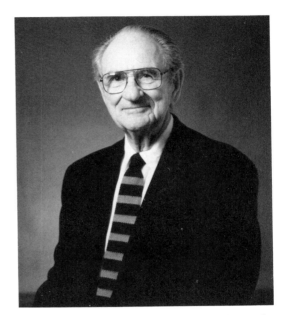

To E. DeVer Tucker, D.O., friend, colleague, and mentor who for over sixty years has served his patients, his profession, and his community—a skilled physician who is loved by his patients, respected by his colleagues, and who epitomizes a model of excellence for all osteopathic students.

# PREFACE

Manual medicine, or the therapeutic application of the hands in patient care, is as old as medicine itself. It can be found in ancient civilizations and in modern times throughout the world. Many concepts and theoretical models are used to explain various systems of manual medicine; terminology is not uniform. Many different educational systems and institutions have contributed to the teaching of this art.

In the past 100 years there has been increasing interest in the field, both in the orthodox medical community and with the development of osteopathic medicine and chiropractic within the United States. Although there may be many intraprofessional philosophical and political differences, the principles underlying structural diagnosis and manual medicine therapeutic interventions are quite similar.

In 1977, the North American Academy of Manipulative Medicine opened its membership to persons in the osteopathic medical profession with the interest to expand the educational opportunities for medical practitioners who had no previous experience. In 1978, the first offering of the course Principles of Manual Medicine was jointly sponsored by NAAMM and Michigan State University and its colleges of Osteopathic Medicine and Human Medicine. This initiated the development of a

series of courses currently offered. The original faculty included both M.D. and D.O. physicians noted for their experience and teaching capability in the field.

The 1970s also witnessed changes in the field of manual medicine within the osteopathic profession. The Educational Council of Osteopathic Principles was organized and developed at this time and continues to standardize teaching/learning opportunities, terminology, and concepts and principles. This decade also saw the development and implementation of new therapeutic systems such as muscle energy technique and counter strain procedures.

*Principles of Manual Medicine* is designed to support the educational series in manual medicine offered by Michigan State University and cosponsored by the North American Academy of Manipulative Medicine. It provides the basic concepts, principles, and technique procedures included therein. It is not meant to be comprehensive but to provide the learner with basic principles that structure the course series. Beginning students in many professions will find these basic principles of assistance in understanding their field and in integrating the differing literatures currently available. In Section I, the principles and concepts of the field of manual medicine are addressed. In Section II are found the specific technique procedures for the entire musculoskeletal system using the approaches of high-velocity, low-amplitude (mobilization with impulse technique), and muscle energy technique. This volume is not intended to be an exhaustive treatise of the field but to provide learners with the principles necessary to develop and utilize procedures that benefit their patients.

Philip E. Greenman, D.O., F.A.A.O.

# ACKNOWLEDGMENTS

Although this book is presented by a single author, acknowledgments must be given to many people who have contributed to its development. Particularly, I wish to acknowledge the contribution of the mentors with whom I was privileged to study. The list reads like a Who's Who of osteopathic medicine and includes C.G. Beckwith, D.O.; G. Cathie, D.O.; D. Heilig, D.O.; P.E. Kimberly, D.O.; P.T. Lloyd, D.O.; F.L. Mitchell, Sr., D.O.; R.M. Tilley, D.O.; and P.T. Wilson, D.O.

I also with to acknowledge the contributions of my colleagues at Michigan State University including M.C. Beal, D.O.; B. Briner, D.O.; L. Brumm, D.O.; J. Goodridge, D.O.; W. Johnston, D.O.; F. Mitchell, D.O.; and R. Ward, D.O.

Special acknowledgment goes to J. McM. Mennell, M.D., and J.F. Bourdillon, M.D., for their leadership in the North American Academy of Manipulative Medicine and their support in the development of the educational series at Michigan State University. They have served as faculty members from the beginning and have contributed to the ecumenical movement within the field of manual medicine.

To M.S. Magen, D.O., Dean, Michigan State University, College of Osteopathic Medicine, goes special appreciation for the continued support and opportunities provided. His inaugural efforts in the development of linkage to the manual medicine community worldwide are appreciated.

To Bruce Miles, Ph.D., go many thanks for the photographic and graphics assistance, and to A. Summitt go my thanks for much of the artwork. Thanks are extended to models, J.P. Greenman, D. Neff, and M. Seffinger.

Special appreciation is extended to D. Thullen and K. Bongard for their efforts for secretarial support.

Special acknowledgment also goes to R. Fred Becker, Ed., for use of prints 1.1 through 1.6 from his book, *The Anatomical Basis of Medical Practice,* Williams & Wilkins, Baltimore, 1971.

Last but not least my everlasting thanks to my wife for her support and understanding throughout the many months included in this effort.

# CONTENTS

SECTION II.    TECHNIQUE PROCEDURES

*Section* **1**  *PRINCIPLES AND CONCEPTS*

# 1

# STRUCTURAL DIAGNOSIS AND MANIPULATIVE MEDICINE

## HISTORY

Manual medicine is as old as the science and art of medicine itself. There is strong evidence of the use of manual medicine procedures in ancient Thailand, as shown in statuary at least 4,000 years old. The use of the hands in treatment of injury and disease was practiced by the ancient Egyptians. Even Hippocrates, the father of modern medicine, was known to use manual medicine procedures, particularly traction and leverage techniques, in the treatment of spinal deformity. The writings of such notable historical figures in medicine as Galen, Celisies, and Oribasius refer to the use of manipulative procedures. There is a void in the reported use of manual medicine procedures corresponding to the approximate time of the split of physicians and barbersurgeons. As physicians became less involved in patient contact, and as direct hands-on patient care became the province of the barber-surgeons, the role of manual medicine in the healing art seems to have declined. This period also represents the time of the plagues and perhaps physicians were reticent to come in close personal contact with their patients.

The 19th century found a renaissance of interest in this field. Early in the 19th century Doctor Edward Harrison, a 1784 graduate of Edinburgh University, developed a sizable reputation in London utilizing manual medicine procedures. Like many other proponents of manual medicine in the 19th century, he became alienated from his colleagues by his continued use of these procedures. The 19th century was a popular period for "bone-setters" both in England and in the United States. The work of Mr. Hutton, a skilled and famous bonesetter, led such eminent physicians as James Paget and Wharton Hood to report in such prestigious medical journals as the *British Medical Journal* and *Lancet* that the medical community should pay attention to the successes of the unorthodox practitioners of bonesetting. In the United States the Sweet family practiced skilled bonesetting in the New England region of Rhode Island and Connecticut. It has also been reported that some of the descendants of the Sweet family emigrated West in the mid-19th century. Sir Herbert Barker was a well known British bonesetter who practiced well into the first quarter of the 20th century and was of such eminence that he was knighted by the crown.

The 19th century was also a time of turmoil and controversy in medical practice. Medical history of the day is replete with many nonorthodox systems of healing. Two individuals who would profoundly influence the field of manual medicine were products of this period of medical turmoil. Andrew Taylor Still, M.D., was a medical physician trained in the preceptor fashion of the day, and D.D. Palmer was a grocer turned self-educated manipulative practitioner. Still (1828–1917) first proposed his philosophy and practice of osteopathy in 1874. His disenchantment with the medical practice of the day led to his formulation of a new medical philosophy which he termed osteopathic medicine. He appeared to have been a great synthesizer of medical thought and built his new philosophy on both ancient medical truths and current medical successes, while being most vocal in denouncing what he viewed as poor medical practice, primarily the inappropriate use of medications then in current use.

Still's strong position against the drug therapy of his day was not well received by his medical colleagues and is certainly not supported by contemporary osteopathic physicians. However, he was not alone in expressing concern about the abuse of drug therapy. In 1861 Oliver Wendell Holmes said, "If all of the MATERIA MEDICA were thrown into the oceans, it will be all the better for mankind, and worse for the fishes"—and, Sir William Osler, one of Still's contemporaries, stated, "One of the first duties of the physician is to educate the masses not to take medicine. Man has an inborn craving for medicine. Heroic dosing for several generations has given his tissues a thirst for drugs. The desire to take medicine is one feature which distinguishes man, the animal, from his fellow creatures."

Still's new philosophy of medicine in essence consisted of the following:

1.  The unity of the body.
2.  The healing power of nature. He held that the body had within itself all those things necessary for the maintenance of health and recovery from disease. The role of the physician was to enhance this capacity.
3.  The somatic component of disease. He felt that the musculoskeletal system was an integral part of the total body and alterations within the musculoskeletal system affected total

body health and the ability of the body to recover from injury and disease.
4.  Structure-function interrelationship. The interrelationship of structure-function had been espoused by Virchow early in the 19th century and Still applied this principle within his concept of total body integration. He strongly felt that structure governed function and function influenced structure.
5.  The use of manipulative therapy. This became an integral part of Still's philosophy because he believed that restoration of the body's maximal functional capacity would enhance the level of wellness and assist in recovery from injury and disease.

Still's attempt to interest his medical colleagues in these concepts was rebuffed, particularly when he took them to Baker University in Kansas. As he became more clinically successful, and nationally and internationally well known, many individuals came to study with him and learn the new science of osteopathy. This led to the establishment in 1892 of the first college of osteopathic medicine at Kirksville, Missouri. In 1986 there were 15 colleges of osteopathic medicine in the United States graduating almost 2,000 students per year. Osteopathy in other parts of the world, particularly in the United Kingdom and in the Commonwealth countries of Australia and New Zealand, is a school of practice limited to structural diagnosis and manipulative therapy, although strongly espousing some of the fundamental concepts and principles of Still. Osteopathic medicine in the United States has from its inception, and continues to be, a total school of medicine and surgery while retaining the basis of osteopathic principles and concepts and continuing the use of structural diagnosis and manipulative therapy in total patient care.

Daniel David Palmer (1845–1913) was, like Still, a product of the midwestern portion of the United States in the mid-19th century. While not schooled in medicine, he was known to practice as a magnetic healer and became a self-educated manipulative therapist. There continues to be controversy as to whether Palmer was ever a patient or student of Still's at Kirksville, Missouri but it is known that Palmer and Still met in Clinton, Iowa early in the 20th century. D.D. Palmer moved about the country a great deal and founded his first college in 1896. The early colleges were at Davenport, Iowa and in Oklahoma City, Oklahoma.

While D.D. Palmer is given credit for the origin of chiropractic, it was his son Bartlett Joshua Palmer (1881-1961) who gave the chiropractic profession its momentum. Palmer's original concepts were that the cause of disease was a variation in the expression of normal neural function. He believed in the "innate intelligence" of the brain and central nervous system and felt that alterations in the spinal column (subluxations) altered neural function, causing disease. Removal of the subluxation by chiropractic adjustment was viewed to be the treatment. Chiropractic has never professed to be a total school of medicine and does not teach surgery or the use of medication beyond vitamins and simple analgesics. There remains a split within the chiropractic profession between the "straights" who continue to espouse and adhere to the original concepts of Palmer and the "mixers" who believe in a broadened scope of chiropractic that includes other therapeutic interventions such as physiotherapy, electrotherapy, diet, and vitamins.

In the mid-1970s the Council on Chiropractic Education (CCE) petitioned the United States Department of Education for recognition as the accrediting agency for chiropractic education. The CCE was strongly influenced by the colleges with a "mixer" orientation which has led to increased educational requirements both prior to and during chiropractic education. Chiropractic is practiced throughout the world, but the vast majority of chiropractic training continues to be in the United States. The late 1970s found increased recognition of chiropractic in both Australia and New Zealand and their registries are participants in the health programs in these countries.

The 20th century has found renewed interest in manual medicine in the traditional medical profession. In the first part of the 20th century the elder Mennell (James) and the elder Cyriax (Edgar) brought joint manipulation recognition within the London medical community. The younger Mennell (John) has continued the work of his father and contributed extensively to the manual medicine literature and to its teaching worldwide. He was one of the founding members of the North American Academy of Manipulative Medicine and was instrumental in opening the membership in NAAMM to osteopathic physicians in 1977. He has strongly advocated the expanded role of appropriately trained physical therapists to work with the medical profession in providing joint manipulation in patient care. The younger Cyriax (James) is well known for his textbooks in the field and also fostered the expanded education and scope of physical therapists. He incorporated manual medicine procedures in the practice of "orthopedic medicine" and founded the Society for Orthopedic Medicine. In his later years James Cyriax came to believe that manipulation restored function to derangements of the intervertebral discs and spoke less and less about specific arthrodial joint effects. He had no use for "osteopaths" or other manipulating groups and the influence of his dynamic personality will be felt long after his death in 1985.

## THE PRACTICE OF MANUAL MEDICINE

Manual medicine should not be viewed in isolation nor separate from "regular medicine", and clearly is not the panacea for all ills of mankind. Manual medicine considers the functional capacity of the human organism, and its practitioners are as interested in the dynamic processes of disease as those who look at the disease process from the static perspective of laboratory data, tissue pathology, and the results of autopsy. Manual medicine focuses upon the musculoskeletal system which comprises over 60% of the human organism and through which evaluation of the other organ systems must be made. Structural diagnosis not only evaluates the musculoskeletal system for its particular diseases and dysfunctions, but also can be utilized to evaluate the somatic manifestations of disease and derangement of the internal viscera. Manipulative procedures are used primarily to increase mobility in restricted areas of musculoskeletal function and to reduce pain. Some practitioners focus upon the concept of pain relief, while others are more interested in the influence of increased mobility in restricted areas of the musculoskeletal system. When appropriately utilized, manipulative procedures have been noted to be clinically effective in reducing pain within the musculoskeletal system, increasing the level of wellness of the patient, and in helping patients with a myriad of disease processes.

## GOAL OF MANIPULATION

In 1983 a 6-day workshop was held in Fischingen, Switzerland, which included approximately 35 experts in manual medicine from throughout the world. They represented many different countries and schools of manual medicine with considerable diversity in clinical experience. The proceedings of this workshop (Dvorak J, Dvorak V. Schneider W. (eds): *Manual Medicine 1984*, Heidelberg, Springer-Verlag, 1985) represents the state of the art of manual medicine of the day. That workshop reached a consensus on the goal of manipulation.

> The goal of manipulation is to restore maximal, pain-free movement of the musculoskeletal system in postural balance.

This definition is comprehensive but specific and is well worth consideration by all students in the field.

## ROLE OF THE MUSCULOSKELETAL SYSTEM IN HEALTH AND DISEASE

It is indeed unfortunate that much medical thinking and teaching looks at the musculoskeletal system only as the coat rack on which the other organ systems are held, and as an organ system which is susceptible to its own unique injuries and disease processes. The field of manual medicine looks at the musculoskeletal system in a much broader context, particularly as an integral and interrelated part of the total human organism. While most physicians would accept the concept of integration of the total body including the musculoskeletal system, specific and usable concepts of how that integration occurs and its relationship in structural diagnosis and manipulative therapy seem limited.

There are five basic concepts which this author has found useful. Since the hand is an integral part of the practice of manual medicine, and includes five digits, it is easy to recall one concept for each digit in the palpating hand. These concepts are:

1. Holistic man
2. Neurologic man
3. Circulatory man
4. Energy-spending man
5. Self-regulating man

(The use of the term "man" is in the context of Homo sapiens and does not reflect only masculine gender.)

The concept of *holistic man* emphasizes that the musculoskeletal system deserves thoughtful and complete evaluation, wherever and whenever the patient is seen, irrespective of the nature of the presenting complaint. It is just as inappropriate to avoid evaluating the cardiovascular system in a patient presenting with a primary musculoskeletal complaint as it is to avoid evaluation of the musculoskeletal system in a patient presenting with acute chest pain thought to be cardiac in origin. The concept is one of a sick patient who needs to be evaluated. The musculoskeletal system comprises most of the human body and alterations within it influence the rest of the human organism; diseases within the internal organs manifest themselves in alterations in the musculoskeletal system, frequently in the form of pain. It is indeed fortunate that holistic concepts have gained increasing popularity in the medical community recently, but the concept expressed here is one that speaks to the integration of the total human organism rather than a summation of parts. We must all remember that our role as health professionals is to treat patients and not to treat disease.

The concept of *neurologic man* speaks to the simple fact that man has the most highly developed and sophisticated nervous system in the animal kingdom. All functions of the body are under some form of control by the nervous system. A patient is constantly responding to stimuli from the internal and external body environment through complex mechanisms within the central and peripheral nervous systems. As freshmen in medical school, we all studied the anatomy and physiology of the nervous system. Let us briefly review a segment of the spinal cord (Fig. 1.1). On the left side are depicted the

classic somaticosomatic reflex pathways with efferent impulses coming from skin, muscle, joint and tendon. Afferent stimuli from the nociceptors, mechanoreceptors, and proprioceptors, all feed in through the dorsal root and ultimately synapse, either directly or through a series of interneurons, with an anterior horncell from which an efferent fiber extends to the skeletal muscle. It is through multiple permutations of the central reflex arc that we respond to external stimuli including injury, orient our bodies in space, and accomplish many of the physical activities of daily living. The right hand side of the figure represents the classical viscerovisceral reflex arc wherein afferents from the visceral sensory system synapse in the intermediolateral cell column and then to the sympathetic lateral chain ganglion or collateral ganglia to synapse with a post ganglionic motor fiber to the target end organ viscera. Note that the skin viscera are also receivers of efferent stimulation from the lateral chain ganglion. These sympathetic reflex pathways innervate the pilomotor activity of the skin, the vasomotor tone of the vascular tree, and the secre-

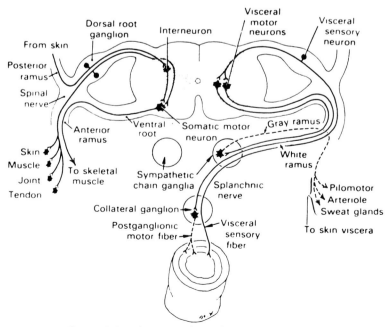

**Figure 1.1.** Cross-section spinal cord segment.

tomotor activity of the sweat glands. Alteration in the sympathetic nervous system activity to the skin viscera results in palpatory changes which are identifiable by structural diagnostic means. While this figure separates these two pathways, they are in fact interrelated so that somatic afferents influence visceral efferents and visceral afferents can manifest themselves in somatic efferents. This figure represents the spinal cord in horizontal section and it must be recalled that ascending and descending pathways from spinal cord segment to spinal cord segment, as well as from the higher centers of the brain, are occurring as well.

Another neurolgical concept worth recalling is that of the autonomic nervous system. The ANS is made up of two divisions,

the parasympathetic and sympathetic. The parasympathetic division includes cranial nerves III, VII, VIII, IX, X and the S2, 3, and 4 levels of the spinal cord. The largest and most extensive nerve of the parasympathetic division is the vagus. The vagus innervates all of the viscera from the root of the neck to the midportion of the descending colon and all glands and smooth muscle of these organs. The vagus nerve (Fig. 1.2) is the primary driving force of the cardiovascular, pulmonary, and gastrointestinal systems, and has an extensive distribution. Many pharmaceutical agents alter parasympathetic nervous activity, particularly that of the vagus.

The sympathetic division of the autonomic nervous system (Fig. 1.3) is repre-

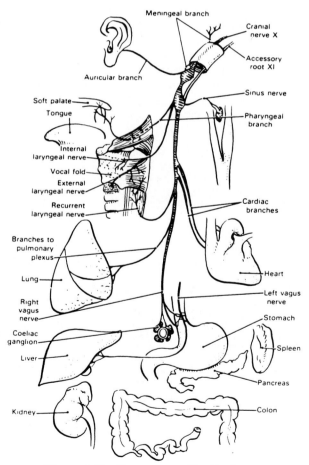

**Figure 1.2.**   Vagus nerve distribution.

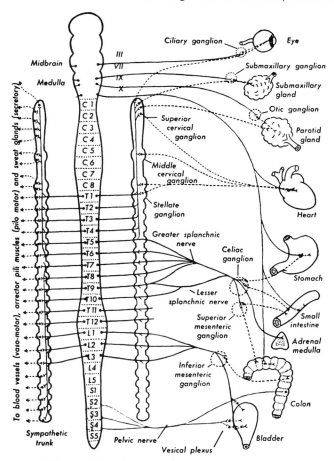

**Figure 1.3.** Autonomic nervous system.

sented by preganglionic neurons originating in the spinal cord from T1 to L2, and the lateral chain ganglion including the superior, middle, and inferior cervical ganglia, the thoracolumbar ganglia from T1 to L2, and the collateral ganglia. Sympathetic fibers innervate all of the internal viscera as do the parasympathetic division but are organized differently. The sympathetic division is organized segmentally. It is interesting to note that all of the viscera above the diaphragm receive their sympathetic innervation from preganglionic fibers above T4 and T5, and all of the viscera below the diaphragm receive their sympathetic innervation preganglionic fibers from below T5. It is through this segmental organization that the relationships of cer-

tain parts of the musculoskeletal system and certain internal viscera are correlated. Remember that the musculoskeletal system receives only sympathetic division innervation and receives no parasympathetic innervation. Control of all glandular and vascular activity in the musculoskeletal system is mediated through the sympathetic division of the ANS.

Remember that all these reflex mechanisms are constantly under the local and central modifying control of excitation and inhibition. Conscious and subconscious control mechanisms from the brain constantly modify activity throughout the nervous system, responding to stimuli. The nervous system is intimately related to another control systems, the endocrine system, and it is useful to think in terms of neuroendocrine control. Recent advances in the knowledge of neurotransmitters, endorphins, enkephalins, and materials such as substance P, have both enlightened us as to the detail of many of the mechanisms previously not understood, and also begin to provide answers for some of the mechanisms through which biomechanical alteration of the musculoskeletal system can alter bodily function.

Emphasis has been placed upon the reflex and neural transmission activities of the nervous system, but the nervous system has a powerful trophic function as well. Highly complex protein and lipid substances are transported antegrade and retrograde along neurons and crossover the synapse of the neuron to the target end organ. Alteration in neurotrophin transmission can be detrimental to the health of the target end organ.

The third concept is that of *circulatory man*. The concept can be simply described as the maintenance of an appropriate cellular milieu for each and every cell of the body (Fig. 1.4). Picture a cell, a group of cells making up a tissue, or a group of tissues making up an organ, resting in the middle of the "cellular milieu". That cell is dependent for its function, whatever its function is,

upon the delivery of oxygen, glucose, and all other substances necessary for its metabolism being supplied by the arterial side of the circulation. The arterial system has a powerful pump, the myocardium of the heart, to propel blood forward. Cardiac pumping function is intimately controlled by the central nervous system, particularly the autonomic nervous system, through the cardiac plexus. The vascular tree receives its vasomotor tone control through the sympathetic division of the autonomic nervous system. Anything that interferes with sympathetic autonomic nervous system outflow, segmentally mediated, can influence vasomotor tone to a target end organ.

The arteries are also encased in the fascial compartments of the body and are subject to compressive and torsional stress which can interfere with the delivery of arterial blood flow to the target organ cell. Once the cell has received its nutrients and proceeded through its normal metabolism, the end products must be removed. The low pressure circulatory systems, the venous and the lymphatic systems, are responsible for the transport of metabolic waste products. Both the venous and lymphatic systems are much thinner walled than the arteries and they lack the driving force of the pump-

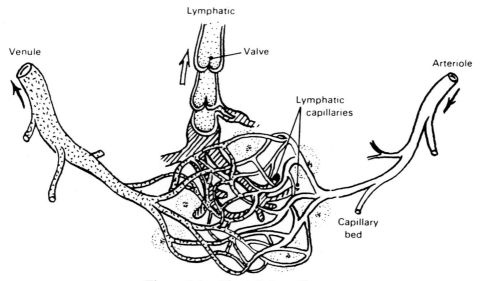

**Figure 1.4.**    The cellular milieu.

ing action of the heart, depending instead on the musculoskeletal system for their propelling action. The large muscles of the extremities contribute greatly to this activity but the major pump of the low pressure systems is the diaphragm (Fig. 1.5).

The diaphragm has an extensive attachment to the musculoskeletal system including the upper lumbar vertebra, the lower six ribs, the xiphoid process of the sternum, and through myofascial connections with the lower extremities, the psoas and quad-

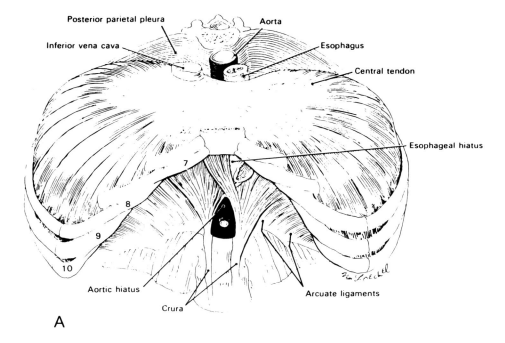

A

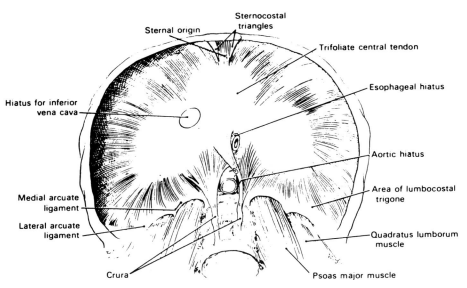

B

**Figure 1.5.** Thoracoabdominal diaphragm.

ratus lumborum muscles. The activity of the diaphragm modulates the negative intra-thoracic pressure which provides a sucking action upon venous and lymphatic return through the vena cava and the cisterna chyli. Because of the extensive attachment of the diaphragm with the musculoskeletal system, and from its innervation via the phrenic nerve from the cervical spine, alter-ations in the musculoskeletal system at a number of levels can alter diaphragmatic function and, consequently venous and lym-phatic return. Congestion of metabolic end products in the cellular milieu interferes with the health of the cell and its recovery from disease or injury. It should be pointed out that the foramen for the inferior vena cava is at the apex of the dome of the dia-phragm. There is some evidence that dia-phragmatic excursion has a direct squeezing and propelling activity upon the inferior vena cava.

Another circulatory concept related to musculoskeletal function concerns the lym-phatic system (Fig. 1.6), and the location where it empties into the venous system. The lymph from the right side of the head, right side of the neck, and right upper ex-tremity enters into the right subclavian vein at the thoracic inlet just behind the anterior end of the first rib and the medial end of the clavicle. The lymph from all of the rest of the body empties into the left subclavian vein at the thoracic inlet behind the anterior extremity of the left first rib and the medial end of the left clavicle. Alteration in the bio-mechanics of the thoracic inlet, particularly its fascial continuity, can affect the thin walled lymph vessels as they empty into the venous system. Maximal function of the musculoskeletal system is an important fac-tor in the efficiency of the circulatory sys-tem and the maintenance of a normal cellu-lar milieu throughout the body.

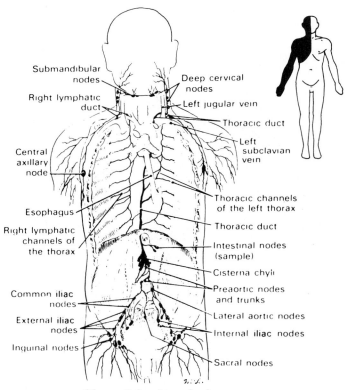

**Figure 1.6.**   Lymphatic system.

The fourth concept is that of *energy-spending man* primarily through the musculoskeletal system. The musculoskeletal system not only comprises over sixty percent of the human organism but also is the major expender of body energy. Any increase in activity of the musculoskeletal system calls upon the internal viscera to develop and deliver energy to sustain that physical activity. The greater the musculoskeletal activity, the greater the demand. If dysfunction alters the efficiency of the musculoskeletal system, there is an increase in demand for energy, not only for increased activity, but for normal activity as well. If we have a patient with a comprised cardiovascular and pulmonary system, who has chronic congestive heart failure, any increase in demand for energy delivery to the musculoskeletal system can be detrimental. For example, a well compensated chronic congestive heart failure patient who happens to sprain an ankle and attempts to continue normal activity, might well have a rapid deterioration of the compensation because of the increased energy demand by the altered gait of the sprained ankle. Obviously, it would make more sense to treat the altered musculoskeletal system by attending to the ankle sprain, than to increase the dosage of medications controlling the congestive heart failure. Restriction of one major joint in a lower extremity can increase the energy expenditure of normal walking by as much as 40% and, if two major joints are restricted in the same extremity, as much as 300%. Multiple minor restrictions of movement of the musculoskeletal system, particularly in the maintenance of normal gait, can also have a detrimental effect upon total body function.

The fifth concept is that of *self-regulating man*. There are literally thousands of self-regulating mechanisms operative within the body all of the time. These homeostatic mechanisms are essential for the maintenance of health, and if altered by disease or injury, need to be restored. All physicians are dependent upon these self-regulating mechanisms within the patient for successful treatment. The goal of the physician should be to enhance all of the body's self-regulating mechanisms to assist in the recovery from disease. Physicians should not interfere with self-regulating mechanisms more than absolutely necessary during the treatment process. All things that are done to, or placed within the human body, alter these mechanisms in some fashion. When any foreign substance is given to a patient, the beneficial, as well as the detrimental potential of the substance, must be considered. As modern pharmacology grows by leaps and bounds with ever-more potent pharmacological effects, we must all recognize the potential for iatrogenic disease. Many patients are on multiple medications, particularly in the hospital environment, and the actions and interactions of each must be clearly understood to avoid iatrogenic problems. Only physicians cause iatrogenic disease. It has been reported that one in seven hospital days in the United States is due to adverse reaction to pharmacological intervention.

## THE MANIPULABLE LESION

Manual medicine deals with the identification of the manipulable lesion and the appropriate use of a manual medicine procedure to resolve the condition. The field of manual medicine has suffered from multiple, divergent, and sometimes confusing definitions of the entity ameanable to manipulative intervention. It has been called the "osteopathic lesion", "chiropractic subluxation", "joint blockage", "loss of joint play", "joint dysfunction", and many others. Currently the acceptable term for this entity is somatic dysfunction. It is defined as:

> *Somatic dysfunction*: Impaired or altered function of related components of the somatic (body framework) system; skeletal, arthrodial, and myofascial structures; and related vascular, lymphatic, and neural elements. (Hospital Adaption of the International Classification of Disease, ed 2. 1973.)

Notice that the emphasis is on *altered function* of the musculoskeletal system, not a disease state or pain syndrome. Obviously, if a somatic dysfunction is present which alters vascular, lymphatic, and neural function, a myriad of symptoms might well be present including painful conditions and disease entities. The diagnosis of somatic dysfunction can accompany many other diagnoses, or can be present as an independent entity. The art of structural diagnosis is to define the presence of somatic dysfunction(s) and determine any significance to the patient's complaint or disease process presenting at the time. If significant, it should be treated by manual medicine intervention just as other diagnostic findings might also need appropriate treatment.

## DIAGNOSTIC TRIAD FOR SOMATIC DYSFUNCTION

The diagnostic criteria for identification of a somatic dysfunction can be expressed by the mnemonic ART. *A* stands for asymmetry of related parts of the musculoskeletal system, either structural or functional. Examples are altered shoulder height, height of iliac crest, and contour and function of the thoracic cage, usually identified by palpation and observation. *R* stands for range of motion of a joint, several joints, or region of the musculoskeletal system. The range of motion could be abnormal either by being increased (hypermobility) or restricted (hypomobility). The usual finding in somatic dysfuction is restricted mobility, identified by observation and palpation using both active and passive patient cooperation. *T* stands for tissue texture abnormality of the soft tissues of the musculoskeletal system (skin, fascia, muscle, ligament, etc.). Tissue texture abnormalities are identified by observation and a number of different palpatory tests. Utilizing these three criteria, one attempts to identify the presence of somatic dysfunctions, their location, whether they are acute or chronic, and particularly whether or not they are significant for the state of the patient's wellness or illness at that moment in time. In addition to the diagnostic value, changes in these criteria can be of prognostic value in monitoring the response of the patient, not only to manipulative treatment directed towards the somatic dysfunction, but also to other therapeutic interventions.

# 2

# PRINCIPLES OF STRUCTURAL DIAGNOSIS

Structural diagnosis in manual medicine is specifically directed toward evaluation of the musculoskeletal system with the goal of identification of the presence and significance of somatic dysfunction(s). It is a component part of the physical examination of the total patient. Most of the evaluation of the internal viscera takes place by evaluation of these structures through the musculoskeletal system. Therefore, it is easy to examine the musculoskeletal system while evaluating the internal viscera of the neck, chest, abdomen, and pelvic regions. Structural diagnosis utilizes the traditional physical diagnostic methods of observation, palpation, percussion, and auscultation. Of these, observation and palpation are the most useful. Structural diagnosis of the musculoskeletal system should never be done in isolation and should always be done within the context of a total history and physical evaluation of the patient.

The diagnostic entity sought by structural diagnosis is somatic dysfunction. It is defined as follows:

*Somatic dysfunction:* impaired or altered function of related components of the somatic (body framework) system; skeletal, arthrodial, and myofascial structures; and related vascular, lymphatic, and neural elements. (HICDA, ed 2, 1973.)

The three classical diagnostic criteria for somatic dysfunction can be identified with the mnemonic ART as follows:

A —a symmetry: asymmetry of related parts of the musculoskeletal system either structural or functional. Examples might be the height of each shoulder by observation, height of iliac crest by palpation, and contour and function of the thoracic cage both by observation and palpation. Asymmetry is usually discerned by observation and palpation.

R —range-of-motion abnormality: alteration in range of motion of a joint, several joints, or region of the musculoskeletal system is sought. The alteration may be either restricted or increased mobility. Restricted motion is the most common component of somatic dysfunction. Range-of-motion abnormality is determined by observation and palpation, using both active and passive patient cooperation.

T —tissue texture abnormality (TTA): alteration in the characteristics of the soft tissues of the musculoskeletal system (skin, fascia, muscle, ligament) is ascertained by observation and palpation. Percussion is also used in identifying areas of altered tissue texture. A large number of descriptors are used in the literature to express the quality of the abnormal feel of the tissue.

In structural diagnosis it is important for the physician to maximize the coordinated use of the palpating hands and the observing eyes. When using vision for observation, it is important to know which eye is dominant so that it can be appropriately placed in relation to the patient for accuracy in visual discrimination. Since most structural diagnosis uses hand-eye coordination with the arms extended, it is best to test for the dominant eye at arm's length distance (Fig. 2.1). The test is as follows:

1. Extend both arms and form a small circle with the thumb and index finger of each hand.
2. With both eyes open, sight through the circle formed by the thumbs and fingers at an object at the other end of the room. Make the circle as small as possible.
3. Close your left eye only. If the object is still seen through the circle, you are right-eyed dominant. If the object is no longer seen through the circle, you are left-eyed dominant.
4. Repeat the procedure closing the right eye and note the difference.

When looking for symmetry or asymmetry, it is important that the dominant eye be located midway between the two anatomical parts being observed and/or palpated. For example, when palpating each acromian process to identify the level of the shoulders, the dominant eye should be in the midsagittal plane of the patient, equidistant from each palpating hand. In other words, the dominant eye should be on the midline of the two anatomical parts being compared. With a patient supine on the examining table, a right-eyed-dominant examiner should stand on the right side of the patient and a left-eyed-dominant examiner should stand on the left side of the patient. Remember that the hands and eyes should be on the same reference plane when one is attempting to determine if paired anatomical parts are symmetrically placed. For example, when evaluating the height of the shoulders by palpating the two acromian processes and visualizing a level against the horizontal plane, the eyes should be on the same horizontal plane as the palpating hands. When palpating the two iliac crests to identify if they are level against the horizontal plane, the eyes should be at the level of the iliacs crests in the same plane as the palpating hands. Whenever possible the eyes should be in the plane against which anatomical landmarks are being compared for symmetry or asymmetry.

All physicians utilize palpation in physical examination of the abdomen for masses, normal organs for size and position, point of maximum impulse of the heart, tactile fremitus of the lungs, and pulsations of the peripheral vessels. Palpation is also used to identify masses, normal and abnormal lymph nodes, and other changes of the tissues. In structural diagnosis palpation requires serious consideration and practice to develop high-level diagnostic skill. Palpatory skill affects:

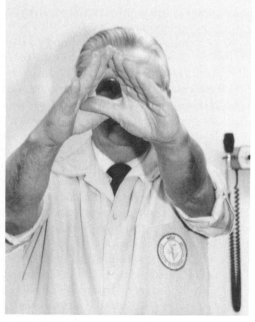

**Figure 2.1.** Test for dominant eye.

1. The ability to detect tissue texture abnormality.
2. The ability to detect asymmetry of position, both visual and tactile.
3. The ability to detect differences of movement in total range, quality of movement during the range, and quality of sensation at the end of the range of movement.
4. The ability to sense position in space of both the patient and examiner.
5. The ability to detect change in palpatory findings, both improvement and worsening, over time.

It is important to develop coordinated and symmetrical use of the hands so that they may be linked with the visual sense. In developing palpatory skill, one must be aware that different parts of the hands are valuable for different tests. For example, the palms of the hands are best suited for use in the stereognostic sense of contour; the dorsum of the hands are more sensitive to temperature variations; the fingerpads are best for fine discrimination of textural differences, finite skin contour, etc.; and the tips of the fingers, particularly the thumbs, are useful as pressure probes for the assessment of differences in depth.

Three stages in the development and perception of palpatory sense have been described. These stages are:

1. Reception
2. Transmission
3. Interpretation

The proprioceptors and mechanoreceptors of the hand receive stimulation from the tissues being palpated. This is the reception phase. These impulses are then transmitted through the peripheral and central nervous system to the brain where they are analyzed and interpreted. During the palpation process, care must be exercised to assure efficiency of reception, transmission, and interpretation. Care must be taken of the examiner's hands to protect these sensitive diagnostic instruments. Avoidance of injury abuse is essential, hands should be clean,

and nails an appropriate length. During the palpation process the operator should be relaxed and comfortable to avoid extraneous interference with the transmission of the palpatory impulse. In order to accurately assess and interpret the palpatory findings, it is essential that the physician concentrate on the act of palpation, the tissue being palpated, and the response of the palpating fingers and hands. All extraneous sensory stimuli should be reduced as much as possible. Probably the most common mistake in palpation is the lack of concentration by the examiner.

Tissue palpation can be further divided into light touch and deep touch. In light touch the amount of pressure is very slight and the examiner attempts to assess tissue change both actively and passively. By simply laying hands on the tissue passively, the examiner is able to make tactile observation of the quality of the tissues under the palpating hand. By moving the lightly applied hand in an active fashion, scanning information of multiple areas of the body can be ascertained, both normal and apparently abnormal. Deep touch is the use of additional pressure to palpate deeper into the layers of the tissue of the musculoskeletal system. Compression is palpation through multiple layers of tissue and shear is a movement of tissue between layers. Combinations of active and passive palpation and light and deep touch are used throughout the palpatory diagnostic process.

It is useful to develop appropriate terms to describe the changes in the anatomy being palpated and evaluated. The use of paired descriptors such as superficial-deep, compressible-rigid, moist-dry, warm-cold, painful-nonpainful, circumscribed-diffuse, rough-smooth, among others, are most useful. It is best to define in anatomical and physiological terms both normal and abnormal palpatory clues. Secondly, it is useful to define areas of altered palpatory sense by describing the state of the tissue change as either acute, sub-acute, or chronic in nature. Thirdly, it is useful to develop a scale to measure the severity of the altered tissue textures being palpated. Are the tissues normal, or are there changes that could be identified as mild, moderate, or severe? A zero, 1+, 2+, 3+, scale is useful in diagnosing the severity of the problem and in monitoring response to therapeutic intervention over time. Try to use descriptive language that a colleague can comprehend.

## LAYER PALPATION

The following describes a practice session which has been found helpful in learning skill in layer palpation of the tissues of the musculoskeletal system. Two individuals sit across from each other with their arms placed on a narrow table (Fig. 2.2). Each individual's right hand is the examining instrument and the left forearm is the part for the partner to examine. Starting with the left palm on the table, each individual places the right hand (palms and fingers) over the forearm just distal to the elbow.

1. The right hand gently makes contact with the skin. No motion is introduced by the operator's right hand. The operator "thinks" skin. How thick is it? How warm or cold is it? How rough or smooth is it? The left forearm is now supinated and the examiner's right hand is placed on the volar surface of the forearm in the same fashion. Again analysis of the skin is made and com-

parison made between the dorsal and volar aspects (Fig. 2.3). Which is the thickest? Which is the smoothest? Which is the warmest? It is interesting to note the ability to identify significant difference between skin of one area and another by concentration on skin alone.

2. With the right hand firmly in contact with the skin, slight movement of the skin is made, both longitudinally and horizontally, to evaluate the subcutaneous fascia. You now concentrate upon the second layer, the subcutaneous fascia. How thick is the layer? How loose is it? It is within this layer that many of the tissue texture abnormalities associated with somatic dysfunction are found.

3. Within the subcutaneous fascia layer are found the vessels, arteries, and veins. Palpate these structures for their identification and description.

4. Gently increase the pressure until you sense the deep fascia layer which envelops the underlying structures. Think deep fascia. It can be described as smooth, firm, and continuous. By palpating the deep fascia layer, and moving the hand gently horizontally across the forearm, you can identify areas of thickening which form fascial compartments between bundles of muscle. The ability to define these enveloping layers of deep fascia is helpful, not only in separating one muscle from another, but as a means of

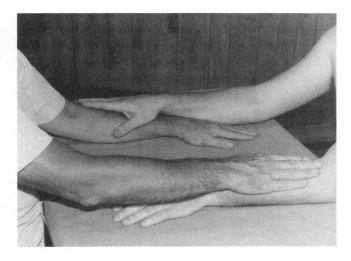

**Figure 2.2.** Layer palpation dorsal forearm.

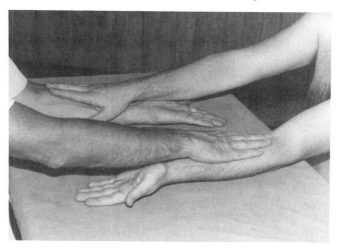

**Figure 2.3.** Layer palpation volar forearm.

getting deeper into underlying structures between muscle.

5. Palpating through the deep fascia, you now concentrate on the underlying muscle and, through concentration, identify individual fibers and the direction in which the fibers run. While palpating muscle, both individuals slowly open and close their left hands, energizing the muscles of the forearm. Your right hand is now palpating contracting and relaxing muscle. Next, squeeze the left hand as hard as possible and palpate muscle during that activity. You are now palpating "hypertonic" muscle. This is the most common tissue texture abnormality feel at the muscle level in areas of somatic dysfunction.

6. While palpating at the muscle level, slowly course down the forearm until you first feel change in tissue and the loss of ability to discern muscle fiber. You have now contacted the musculotendinous junction, a point in muscle which is vulnerable to injury (Fig. 2.4).

7. Continue to course down toward the wrist, beyond the musculotendinous junction, and palpate a smooth, round, firm structure called a tendon. Note the transition from muscle through musculotendinous junction to tendon.

8. Follow the tendon distally until you palpate a structure which binds the tendons at the wrist. Palpate that structure (Fig. 2.5). It is the transverse carpal ligament. What

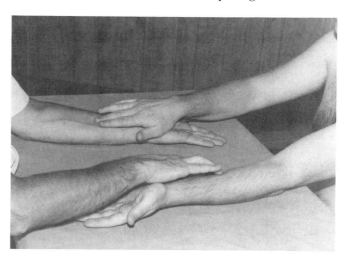

**Figure 2.4.** Palpation musculo-tendinous junction.

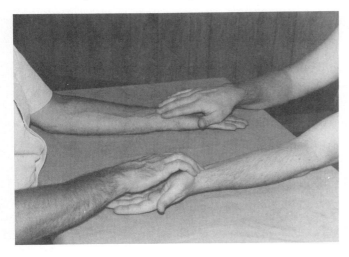

**Figure 2.5.** Palpation transcarpal ligament.

are its characteristics? What direction does its fibers course? How thick is it? How firm is it? Ligaments throughout the body feel quite similar.

9.  Now return your palpating right hand to the elbow with your middle finger overlying the dimple of the elbow in the dorsal side and your thumb opposite it on the ventral side to palpate the radial head (Fig. 2.6). Stay on bone, and think bone. How hard it is? Is there any "life" in it?

10.  Now move just proximal with your palpating thumb and index finger until you fall into the joint space. Underlying your palpating fingers is a structure which you should not be able to feel, namely, the joint capsule. Palpable joint capsules are present in pathological joints and are not usually found in somatic dysfunction. In fact, some individuals feel that a palpable joint capsule, with the limited exception of the knee joint, is a contraindication to direct-action manipulation therapy.

You have now palpated skin, subcutaneous fascia, blood vessels, deep fascia, muscle, musculotendinous junction, tendon, ligament, bone and joint space. After utilizing the forearm as the model, these same structures are palpable throughout the body. Practice and experience can enhance your capability as a structural diagnostician.

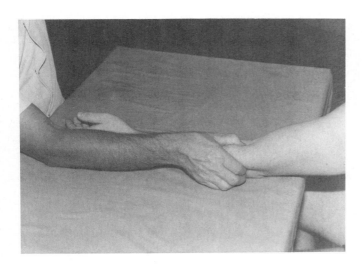

**Figure 2.6.** Palpation radial head.

The development of a high level of palpation skill requires considerable practice, and is accumulated over time if a concentrated effort is made. It is also important to avoid the three most common errors in palpation, namely:

1. Lack of concentration
2. Too much pressure
3. Too much movement

As stated earlier, the most common error is the lack of concentration on the task at hand. The beginner frequently attempts to gain information rapidly and presses much too hard. Remember, the harder you press, the more stimulation you provide to your own mechanoreceptors increasing the amount of sensory impulse being transmitted. The beginner is also prone to use too much movement in searching for anatomical landmarks and in identifying layers of tissue. We call this the "jiggling hands syndrome". One must remember that the more motion exerted by the hands, the more stimulation there is to the afferent system to be transmitted and interpreted by the nervous system. Therefore, concentrate, don't push too hard, and don't move too much.

### MOTION SENSE

In identifying areas of somatic dysfunction by defining alterations in the diagnostic triad of asymmetry, altered range of motion, and tissue texture abnormality, a combination of observation and palpation is used. In palpation both static and dynamic dimensions are present. Statically we look for levels of paired anatomical parts to identify asymmetry. Both by static and dynamic palpation we look for alteration in tissue texture abnormality. In palpating tissues without movement the examiner is interested in such things as skin temperature, smoothness, thickness, and other qualifiers of the state of the tissue. In dynamic palpation one evaluates, by both compression and shear movement within the tissue, the thickness of the tissue, the amount of normal tissue tone and a sense of which tissues are abnormal. It is within the evaluation of the range of motion that the palpatory sense becomes highly refined. Since restoration of the maximal normal amount of motion possible in the tissue is the desired end point, it is essential that we be able to identify normal and abnormal ranges of motion within both soft tissue and arthrodial structures.

Motion sense is an essential component of the palpatory art in structural diagnosis. The examiner attempts to identify whether there is normal mobility, restricted movement (hypomobility), or too much movement (hypermobility). In motion testing, the examiner may put a region or part of the body through both active and passive movement to ascertain how that part complies with the motion demand placed upon it. Information is sought as to whether the mobility is abnormal in a regional sense or confined to one segment. A wide variety of techniques can be utilized, both actively and passively, to test for motion.

It is essential that good contact be made with the examiner's hand(s) on the part(s) being palpated. As the part is taken through range of motion, either actively or passively, the examiner is interested in three elements, 1)range of movement; 2)quality of movement during the range; and 3)"endfeel". In determining range of movement, one is interested in the quantity of movement. Is it normal, restricted, or increased in range? Secondly, how does it feel during the movement throughout the range. Is it smooth? Is it "sticky" or "jerky" or "too loose"? There are a number of alterations in movement feel during the range that can be of assistance to the examiner in determining what factors might be altering the range of movement. Thirdly, what is the feel at the end point of the range of movement? Is there symmetry to the range, and does each extreme of the range of movement feel the same? If there is alteration in the endfeel, what are the qualities of the end point? Is it hard? Is it soft? Is it spongy? Is it jerky? There are a wide variety of characteristic endfeels which experience will teach the examiner. The quality of the endfeel is most helpful in determining what the cause of the restrictive movement might be, and what type of manipulative therapy might be most effective.

Manual medicine procedures are used to overcome restrictions of movement. Techniques which increase mobility should not be used in the presence of hypermobility. Hypermobility is present when there is an increase in the range of movement, a loose feeling throughout the range of movement, and loss of normal tissue resiliency at the endfeel. Hypermobility might very well be normal in certain highly trained athletes, such as gymnasts and acrobats, but in most individuals it must be considered abnormal. In the vertebral complex it is not uncommon to find relative hypermobility of one vertebral motion segment adjacent to a vertebral motion segment that is restricted. This has been described as "compensatory hypermobility" and has been explained as the body's attempt to maintain mobility of the total mechanism in the presence of restricted mobility of a part of the vertebral axis. It is not infrequent to find that hypermobile segments are the areas of symptomotology. As such, they gain a great deal of attention from the examiner. Care must be exercised not to provide manual medicine procedures which increase the relative hypermobility of these segments, rather than appropriately applying mobilizing techniques to the segment(s) with restricted mobility. Hypermobility can be taken to the stage that can best be described as instability. Instability occurs when the integrity of the tissues supporting the joint structure cannot maintain appropriate functional apposition of the moving parts so the relative stability of the motion unit is lost. The dividing line between hypermobility and instability is not always definite and good objective measures to quantify instability are still not available. Nonetheless, the skilled clinician must develop some sense of normal motion, hypomobility, hypermobility, and instability of anatomical structures within the musculoskeletal system. It is for this reason

that the development of a motion sense is worth the effort.

One must also develop the skill of motion sense to identify change in the range of motion, quality of movement during a range, and the endfeel following a manual medicine intervention. It is useful in prognosis as well as diagnosis. It should be possible to identify change in range of motion, and its quality, if a manual medicine intervention has been successful. Retesting the range of motion available is always the last step in any manual medicine therapeutic intervention.

Motion sense is an essential component of the palpatory art in structural diagnosis. As in any art form, practice is the major requirement for mastery.

## SCREENING EXAMINATION

The screening examination is designed to evaluate the total musculoskeletal system as part of the examination of the patient. It answers the question, "is there a problem within the musculoskeletal system that deserves additional evaluation?" While different formats for a screening examination can be used, the following ten-step procedure is one that can be accomplished rapidly and still be comprehensive in scope.

Step one starts with the analysis of the gait. In multiple directions, observations are made of the length of the stride, swing of the arm, heel to toe strike of the foot, tilt of the pelvis and adaptation of the shoulder girdle (Fig. 2.7). Gait analysis provides rapid evaluation of the integrated activities of the motor system. Observation of the static posture is made from the front (Fig. 2.8) to evaluate weight distribution, carriage of the head, level of the shoulders, and placement of the feet. Observation from the back evaluates head carriage, distribution of weight, levels of the shoulders, and foot placement (Fig. 2.9). Observation from the side is made for evaluation of posture against the plumb line, the position of the knees in extension, analysis of the AP curves, and ob-

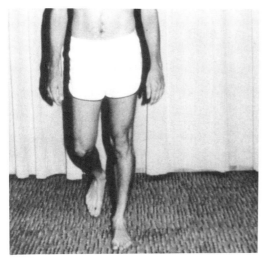

**Figure 2.7.**   Gait analysis.

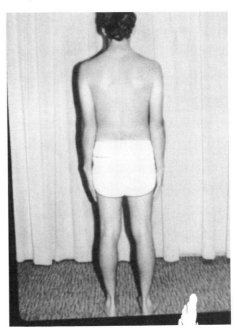

**Figure 2.9.**   Observation of sta   osture dorsal surface.

servation of the abdomen (Fig. 2.10). Similar evaluation is made with the opposite lateral stance posture. In addition, symmetry of left to right is evaluated. In the standing posture palpatory analysis is made of the medial arch and the inversion-eversion, pro-

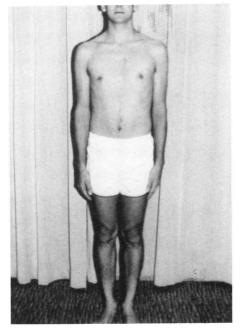

**Figure 2.8.**   Observation of static posture ventral surface.

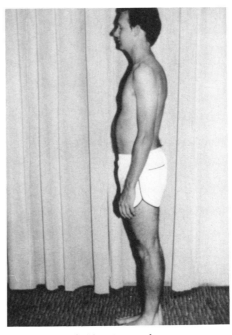

**Figure 2.10.**   Lateral posture.

nation-supination of the feet. Combining palpation and observation, analysis is made of the level of the shoulders, particularly at the acromioclavicular joint (Fig. 2.11). The hands are placed upon the most superior aspect of both iliac crests observing levels across the horizontal plane (Fig 2.12). The hands and eyes should be at the same horizontal plane level. Similar analysis of the height of the greater trochanter of each femur is made to evaluate the relative length of the lower extremities (Fig. 2.13).

Step two includes some dynamic testing of trunk mobility in lateral flexion. Sidebending to the left (Fig. 2.14) without rotation of the trunk is introduced and compared with sidebending to the right (Fig. 2.15). The ease of attaining fingertip motion against the lateral leg and the amount of induced thoraco-lumbar curvature is observed. This test gives information on the adaptation of the vertebral column in weight-bearing side-bending mechanics.

Step three attempts to evaluate functional mobility. The standing flexion test starts with the patient standing with feet approximately acetabular distance apart and weight equally distributed. The examiner places the thumbs on the inferior slope of the posterior superior iliac spine (Fig. 2.16). Instruction is given to the patient to bend

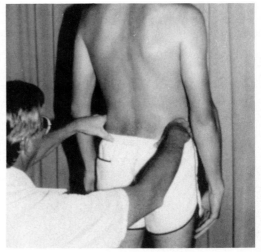

**Figure 2.12.** Observation of iliac crest height.

forward as far as possible without flexing the knees (Fig. 2.17). The physician follows the relative excursion of each posterior superior iliac spine (PSIS). The one that travels the greatest distance in the cephalic and ventral direction is identified as positive. The PSIS that has the greatest excursion is paradoxically on the side of greatest restriction within the osseous pelvis. This is identified as a positive standing flexion test.

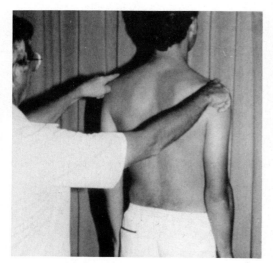

**Figure 2.11.** Observation of shoulder level.

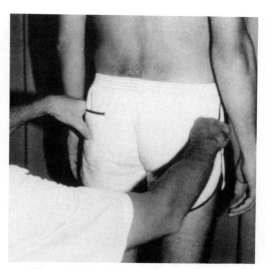

**Figure 2.13.** Observation of greater trochanteric height.

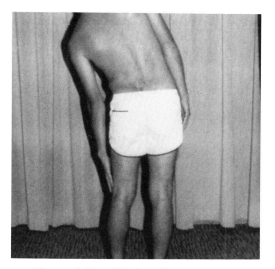

**Figure 2.14.** Sidebending trunk left.

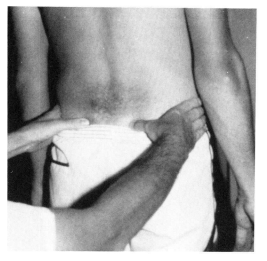

**Figure 2.16.** Palpation posterior/superior iliac spine.

Observation is also made of the behavior of the thoracolumbar spine during forward bending. Observation is made of the presence or absence of segmental rhythm, and the appearance of prominence of either side of the vertebral column.

Step four attempts to find the presence or absence of altered vertebral and pelvic mechanics without weight bearing (Fig. 2.18). The seated flexion test starts with the patient seated on a stool with the weight equally distributed on the two ischial tuberosities, the feet flat on the floor, and the knees apart. With the examiner palpating and following the movement of the posterior superior iliac spines, the instruction to the patient is to forward bend as far as comfortably possible (Fig. 2.19). Once again the posterior superior iliac spine that moves the furthest in the cephalic and ventral direction is called the "positive side" and is indicative of restricted mobility on that side of the

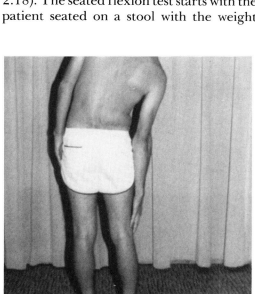

**Figure 2.15.** Sidebending trunk right.

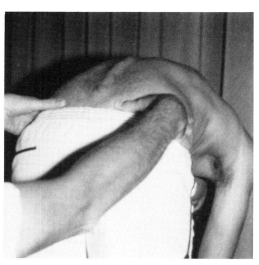

**Figure 2.17.** Standing forward flexion test.

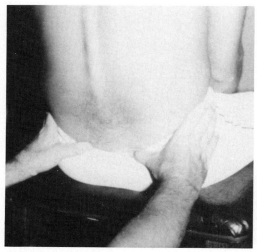

**Figure 2.18.** Palpation posterior/superior iliac spine.

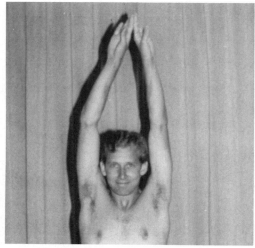

**Figure 2.20.** Screening test upper extremities.

hemipelvis in the seated position. Again analysis is made of vertebral segmental mobility and the introduction of lateral prominence in the vertebral axis.

Step five evaluates the upper extremities (Fig. 2.20). With the patient seated, instructions are given to fully abduct both extremities in the coronal plane, reach to the ceiling, and turn the backs of the hands together. To accomplish this maneuver the sternoclavicular, acromoclavicular, gleno-

humeral, elbow, and wrist joints all participate (Fig. 2.21). Asymmetry indicates that additional evaluation is necessary.

Step six evaluates the capacity of the trunk to rotate in the seated position. With the patient sitting tall, with normal vertebral curves in place, the examiner introduces right rotation (Fig. 2.22) and then rotation to the left (Fig. 2.23). Evaluation is made of range, quality of movement during the range, and quality of the endfeel.

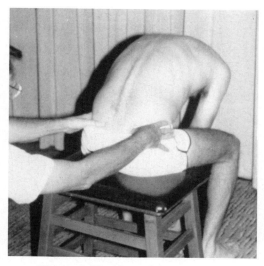

**Figure 2.19.** Seated flexion test.

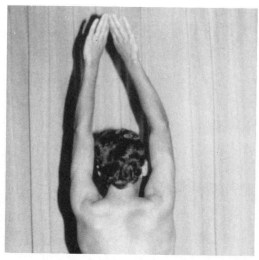

**Figure 2.21.** Screening test upper extremities.

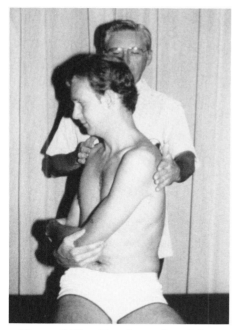

**Figure 2.22.** Trunk rotation right.

Step seven evaluates the capacity of the trunk to sidebend in the seated position. With the patient sitting in an upright position, the physician introduces left side bending and evaluates compliance of the trunk (Fig. 2.24). Right side bending is then introduced and again evaluation is made of the quality of thoracic and lumbar movement to this challenge (Fig. 2.25).

Step eight evaluates the passive movement of the head. With the patient sitting upright, the examiner introduces backwards bending which should continue to 90° from the vertical (Fig. 2.26). Forward bending is then introduced, approximately 45° from the vertical is the normal extent of movement (Fig. 2.27). Cervical rotation is introduced to the right, (Fig. 2.28) and then to the left to evaluate range, quality, and endfeel (Fig. 2.29). Sidebending to the right (Fig. 2.30) is then introduced and is followed with side bending movement to the left (Fig. 2.31). Analysis of symmetry, or lack of same, is made.

Step nine evaluates the respiratory movements of the thoracic cage in both in-

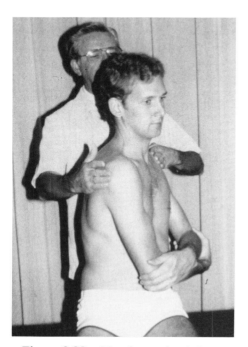

**Figure 2.23.** Trunk rotation left.

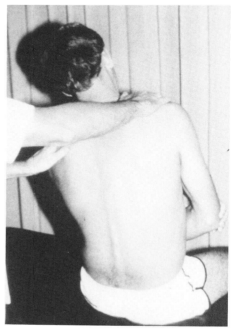

**Figure 2.24.** Trunk sidebending left.

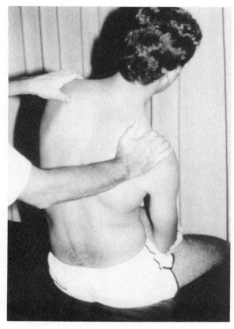

**Figure 2.25.** Trunk sidebending right.

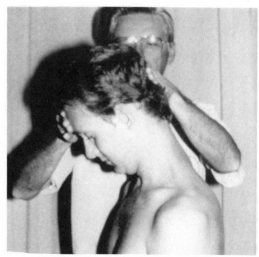

**Figure 2.27.** Cervical forward bending.

halation and exhalation. It begins in the upper thoracic region and continues to the middle thoracic region (Fig. 2.32). Symmetry of inhalation or exhalation is evaluated as well as total excursion. The lower rib cage completes the evaluation, and analysis of lateral rib cage function if primarily made at this level (Fig. 2.33).

Step ten evaluates multiple elements of the lower extremities. Starting with the Patrick test, flexion, abduction and external rotation of the hip joint with flexion of the knee is evaluated (Fig. 2.34). Symmetrical length of the hamstring is evaluated by monitoring the opposite anterior superior iliac spine, and elevating the extended leg until first motion is perceived (Fig. 2.35). The opposite leg is then evaluated in a similar fashion with the endpoint being the first posterior rotation of the pelvis. Evaluation

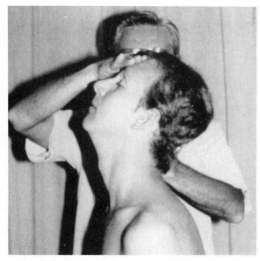

**Figure 2.26.** Cervical backward bending.

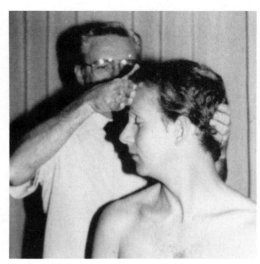

**Figure 2.28.** Right cervical rotation.

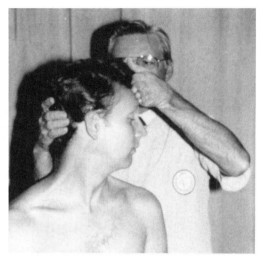

**Figure 2.29.** Left cervical rotation.

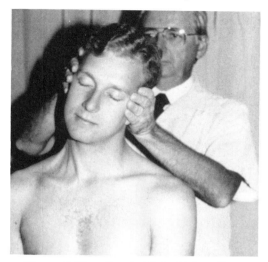

**Figure 2.31.** Cervical left sidebending.

of other joints of the lower extremity is made by the Squat test (Fig. 2.36). With the patient standing by the side of the table, so that one hand can stabilize the body, the patient squats down as far as possible while keeping the back straight and attempting to keep the heels on the floor. The movement requires flexion of the hip, flexion of the knees, dorsiflexion of the ankles, and stability of the feet. Inability to perform this test suggest further evaluation of the lower extremity.

## SCANNING EXAMINATION

Once an area of the musculoskeletal system has been identified during the screening examination as being of sufficient abnormality for further investigation, a scanning procedure of that region is initiated. The scanning examination is designed to answer the question what part of the region, and what tissues within the region, are significantly dysfunctional? The object is to locate the areas which might account for the abnormal

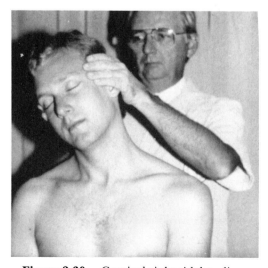

**Figure 2.30.** Cervical right sidebending.

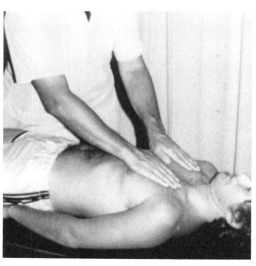

**Figure 2.32.** Respiratory rib motion upper group.

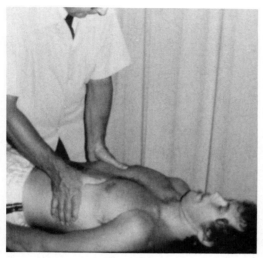

**Figure 2.33.** Respiratory rib motion lower group.

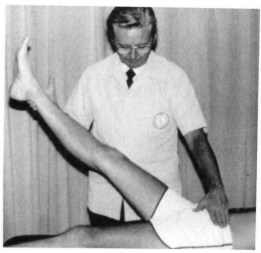

**Figure 2.35.** Straight leg raising for hamstring length.

finding. Utilizing the analogy of a microscope, we have gone from low power (the screening examination) to high power (scanning examination). More definitive evaluation of soft tissue can be accomplished with active and passive light and deep touch.

Thumbs or fingers can be used as a pressure probe searching for areas of tenderness or more specific signs of tissue texture change. Multiple variations of motion scanning can be introduced to look for alterations in symmetry of range, quality of movement, and sensations at endfeel. Respiratory effort might be utilized to evaluate the response of the region to inhalation and exhalation efforts. Responses within the region to de-

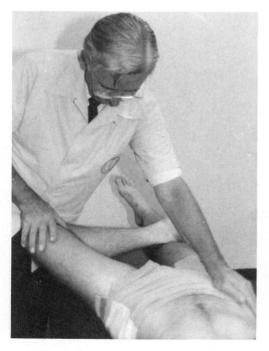

**Figure 2.34.** Patrick test hip joint.

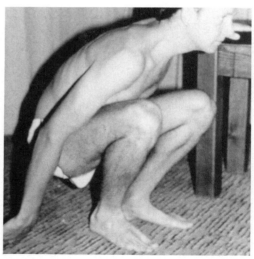

**Figure 2.36.** Lower extremities screening squat test.

mands placed upon it from more remote areas of the musculoskeletal system are frequently useful in better defining the area requiring specific attention.

One valuable diagnostic test for scanning procedures is the skin-rolling test. In this examination a fold of skin is grasped between the thumb and index finger and rolled as if one were rolling a cigarette (Fig. 2.37). Skin rolling can be accomplished symmetrically on each side of the body, testing for normal pain-free laxity of the skin and subcutaneous fascia. A positive finding is that of tenderness and pain provocation in certain dermatonal levels of skin with tightness and loss of resiliency within the skin and subcutaneous fascia. Frequently, tender nodules will be palpated while accomplishing this test. They are interpreted to represent alteration in dermatomal innervation from dysfunctions within the vertebral axis. In the examination of the thoracic and lumbar regions of the spine it is recommended that the skin be rolled in the mid-line overlying the spinous processes and more laterally, coursing from below upward, comparing changes on one side to the other. While defined as a scanning procedure, skin rolling can be quite specific in defining specific segmental dysfunction because of the clinically observable dermatomal relationship to altered vertebral motion segment function.

## SEGMENTAL DEFINITION

The third element to the diagnostic process is segmental definition, used to identify the specific vertebral motion segment, or peripheral joint, that is dysfunctional. It is also used to determine the specific motion restriction that is involved. An attempt is made to identify the tissue(s) that are most involved in the dysfunctional segment.

One method of identifying the specific joint that is dysfunctional, and the motion that is lost, is to test for joint-play movements. This concept has been advocated for many years by Mennell. Joint-play movements are defined as being independent of the action of voluntary muscle and are found within synovial joints. The range of joint play is very small but very precise. Normal joint-play movement allows for easy, painless performance of voluntary movement. The amount of joint play is usually less than one-eighth of an inch in any one plane within a synovial joint. Mennell defines joint dysfunction as the loss of joint-play movement that cannot be recovered by the action of voluntary muscles. Once the precise system for identifying joint play is learned, very similar maneuvers can be utilized therapeutically in restoring anatomical and physiological function to the joint by restoring its normal joint play.

There are numerous diagnostic procedures that can specifically define within the

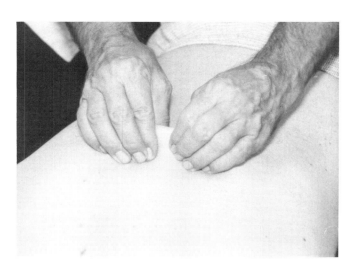

**Figure 2.37.**   Skin rolling.

vertebral motion segment, or within the synovial extremity joint, the specific dysfunction that is present. Subsequent chapters will deal with the methods most commonly used by this author. The primary goal is to determine which specific vertebral motion segment is dysfunctional, which joint within that vertebral motion segment is dysfunctional, the direction of altered motion(s), and some estimate of the tissue involved in the restricted motion. Primary emphasis is placed upon motion loss and its characteristics. Many diagnostic systems depend upon localization of pain or provocation of pain by certain motion introduc-

tions. In the opinion of this author, motion loss and its characteristics are more valuable diagnostic criteria than the presence of pain and the provocation of pain by movement. Pain and its provocation can be of assistance in diagnosis but they are not diagnostic in and of themselves.

These principles of structural diagnosis need to be studied extensively and mastered by the physician who wishes to be skilled in the field of manual medicine. An accurate and specific diagnosis is essential for successful results from manual medicine therapeutic interventions.

# 3

# BARRIER CONCEPTS IN STRUCTURAL DIAGNOSIS

Within the diagnostic triad of (*a*)asymmetry, (*b*)range of motion abnormality, and (*c*) tissue texture abnormality, perhaps the most significant is alteration in the range of joint and tissue movement. Loss of normal motion within the tissues of the musculoskeletal system, or one of its component parts, responds most favorably to appropriate manual medicine therapeutic intervention. To achieve the goal of manual medicine intervention and restore maximal, pain-free movement to a musculoskeletal system in postural balance, we must be able to identify both normal and abnormal movement. In the presence of altered movement of the hypomobility type, an appropriate manual medicine intervention might be the treatment of choice. We must strive to improve mobility of all of the tissues of the musculoskeletal system, bone, joint, muscle, ligament, fascia, and fluid, with the anticipated outcome of restoring normal physiological movement and maximum functional physiology as well.

In the musculoskeletal system there are inherent movements, voluntary movements, and involuntary movements. The inherent movement has been described by some authors as relating to the recurrent coiling and uncoiling of the brain and longitudinal movement of the spinal cord, together with a fluctuation of the cerebral spinal fluid. Inherent also is the movement of the musculoskeletal system in relation to respiration. It has been observed that during inhalation the curves within the vertebral column straighten and with exhalation the curves are increased. With inhalation the extremities rotate externally, and with exhalation, internally. The voluntary movements of the musculoskeletal system are active movements resulting from contraction of muscle from voluntary conscious control. The involuntary movements of the musculoskeletal system are described as passive movements. Passive movement is induced by an external force moving a part of the musculoskeletal system through an arc of motion. The joint-play movements described by Mennell are also involuntary movements. They are not a component of the normal active or passive range of movement but are essential for the accomplishment of normal active and passive movement.

In structural diagnosis we speak of both normal and abnormal barriers to joint and tissue motion. The examiner must be able to identify and characterize normal and abnormal range of movement and normal and abnormal barrier to movement in order to make an accurate diagnosis. Most joints have motion in multiple planes, but for descriptive purposes we describe barriers to movement within one plane of motion for one joint. The total range of motion (Fig.

**31**

3.1) from one extreme to the other is limited by the anatomical integrity of the joint and its supporting ligaments, muscles, and fascia. Exceeding the anatomical barrier causes fracture, dislocation, or violation of tissue such as ligamentous tear. Somewhere within the total range of movement is found a midline neutral point.

Within the total range of motion there is a range of passive movement available which the examiner can extraneously introduce (Fig. 3.2). The limits to this passive range of movement have been described by some as the elastic barrier. At this point all tension has been taken within the joint and its surrounding tissues. There is a small amount of potential space between the elastic barrier and the anatomical barrier described by Sandoz as the paraphysiological space. It is within this area that the high-velocity low-amplitude thrust appears to generate the popping sound which results from the maneuver.

The range of active movement (Fig. 3.3) is somewhat less than that available with passive movement, and the end point of the range is called the physiological barrier. The normal endfeel is due to resilience and tension within the muscle and fascial elements.

Frequently there is reduction in available active motion due primarily to myofascial shortening (Fig. 3.4). This is often seen with aging but it can occur at all ages. It is the stretching of this myofascial shortening

that all individuals, particularly athletes, should do as part of physical exercise. Stretching exercise to the muscles and fascia enhances the active motion range available and the efficiency of myofascial function.

When motion is lost within the range it can be described as major (Fig. 3.5) or minimal (Fig. 3.6). The barrier which prevents movement in the direction of motion lost is defined as the restrictive barrier. The amount of active motion available is limited on one side by the normal physiological barrier and on the opposite by the restrictive barrier. The goal of a manual medicine intervention would then be to move the restrictive barrier as far into the direction of motion loss as possible. Another clinically describable phenomena associated with motion loss is the shifting of the neutral point from midline to the middle of the available active range. This is described as the "pathological" neutral and is usually but not always in the midrange of active motion available.

Each of the barriers described have palpable findings which can be described as either normal or abnormal endfeel. Within a normal range of passive movement, the elastic barrier will have a normal sensation at the end point as a result of the passively induced tension within the joint and its surrounding structures. At the end of the range of active movement, the physiological barrier likewise has a characteristic feel which results from the voluntary increase in resistance due to the apposition of the joints

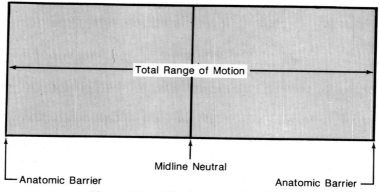

**Figure 3.1.**    Total range of motion.

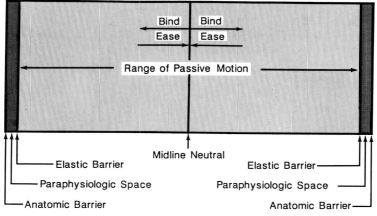

**Figure 3.2.**   Range of passive movement.

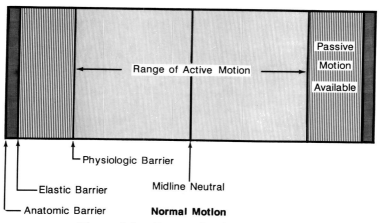

**Figure 3.3.**   Range of active movement.

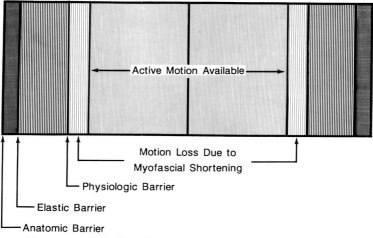

**Figure 3.4.**   Reduced range from myofascial shortening.

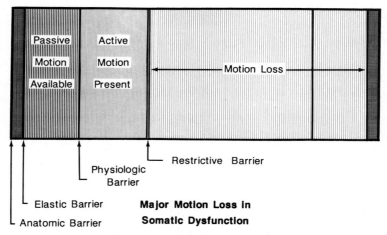

**Figure 3.5.** Major motion loss.

and the myofascial tension developed during voluntary muscular activity.

Let us return to the layer palpation exercise (Chap. 2) and begin at the point where one examiner was evaluating the joint space at the proximal radiohumeral joint (Fig. 3.7). While palpating this joint with the thumb placed anteriorly and the index finger placed posteriorly, have the subject actively introduce pronation and supination (Fig. 3.8). You will note that the range is not symmetrical in pronation and supination, and that the endfeel is not the same at the terminal range of pronation and supination. Which range is greater? Which

endfeel seems tighter? Now grasp the subject's hand and wrist and passively introduce pronation and supination while monitoring at the proximal radiohumeral joint (Fig. 3.9). Note that you are now receiving proprioceptive impulse from your palpating hand at the radiohumeral joint, as well as from your hand as it passively introduces, through the subject's hand and wrist, the pronation and supination effort (Fig. 3.10). Again look for total range of movement, the quality of movement during the range, and the endfeel. In supination and pronation, which has the greatest range? Which has the tighter or looser endfeel? How does this

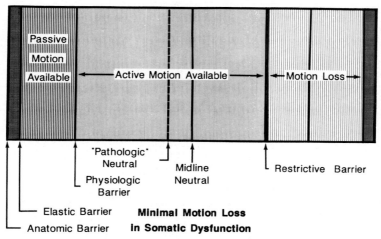

**Figure 3.6.** Minimal motion loss.

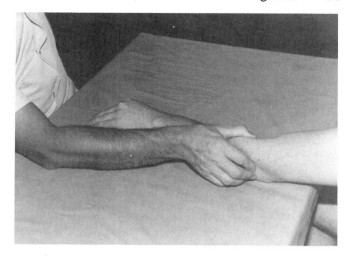

**Figure 3.7.**   Palpate radiohumeral joint.

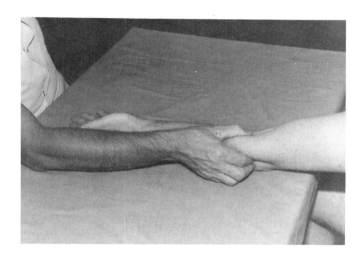

**Figure 3.8.**   Active pronation-supination.

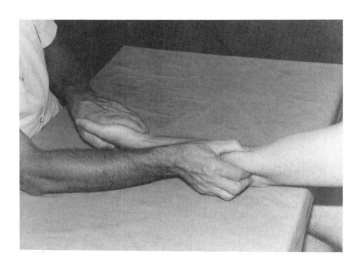

**Figure 3.9.**   Passive pronation-supination.

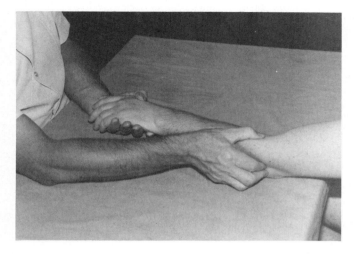

**Figure 3.10.**   Sensing hand of pronation-supination.

compare with the active movement? Now let us take it one step further. While passively introducing pronation and supination you should notice that tension increases the closer you get to the end points of the range. As you move in the opposite direction it appears to get somewhat easier or more free. See if you can, by decreasing increments of pronation and supination, find the point between the two extremes of movement wherein the joint feel is the most free. Even though pronation and supination is not a symmetrical range of movement at this joint, it is possible to find a point within the range that is the most free and could be described as the physiological neutral point.

We now have another concept of joint motion, the concept of "ease" and "bind" (Fig. 3.11). The more one moves in the direction of the neutral point, whether it be a midline neutral point in a normal range of motion, or a "pathological" neutral point somewhere within the range of altered motion, it becomes more free, or there is more "ease". Conversely, as one moves away from the neutral "free" point, one begins to sense a certain amount of "bind", or increase in resistance to the induced movement. Understanding this concept of ease and bind, and the ability to sense this phenomenon, are essential to mastering the functional (indirect) techniques (Chap. 10). In the elbow exercise which you just accomplished, the hand pal-

pating over the proximal radiohumeral joint was the "sensing hand", and your other hand, which introduced passive supination and pronation at the subject's hand, was the "motor hand".

### RESTRICTIVE BARRIERS

The restrictive barriers limit movement within the normal range of motion and have different palpatory characteristics than the normal physiological, elastic, and anatomical barriers. The restrictive barrier can be within the following tissues:

Skin
Fascia
Muscle, long and short
Ligament
Joint capsule and surfaces

Restrictive barriers can be found within one or more of these tissues and the number and type contribute to the palpable characteristics at the restrictive barrier. Different pathological changes within these tissues can give quite different endfeel sensations. For example, congestion and edema within the tissues will give a diffuse, boggy sensation quite like a sponge filled with water. Chronic fibrosis within these tissues will give a harder, more unyielding, rapidly ascending endfeel when compared to the more boggy, edematous sensation. A restrictive

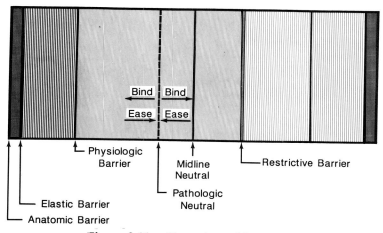

**Figure 3.11.**   Neutral ease-bind point.

barrier due to altered muscle physiology, whether it be spasm, hypertonus, or contracture, will give a more jerky and tightening type of endfeel than one due to edema or fibrosis. Do not forget that pain can be a restrictive barrier as well. If a movement is painful, it will result in restriction as the body attempts to compensate for relief of pain by reduction of movement. When examining ranges of movement, and particularly when looking for normal and abnormal barriers to movement, one should constantly keep in mind the potential for hypermobility. The classical feel of a hypermobile range of motion is one of looseness for a greater extent of the range than would be anticipated, and with a rapidly escalating, hard endfeel when one approaches the elastic and anatomical barriers.

Restrictive barriers may also be long or short. They may involve a single joint or spinal segment, or cross over more than one joint or series of spinal segments. It is important to identify the tissue or tissues involved in the restrictive barrier, their extent, and the functional pathology found within the tissues. Some types of manual medicine intervention are more appropriate for certain restrictive barriers than others.

In structural diagnosis, alteration of range of movement is an essential criterion for a diagnosis of somatic dysfunction. It is necessary to evaluate the total range of

movement, the quality of movement available during the range, and the feel at the end point of movement in order to make an accurate diagnosis of the restrictive barrier. Therapeutic intervention by manipulative means can be described as an approach to these pathological barriers. Multiple methods are available and different activating forces can be used toward the goal of restoring maximal physiological movement available within the anatomy of the joint(s) and tissue(s).

### Definitions

*1. Active motion*: movement of an articulation between the physiological barriers limited to the range produced voluntarily by the patient.

*2. Anatomical barrier*: the bone contour and/or soft tissues, especially ligaments, which serve as the final limit to motion in an articulation beyond which tissue damage occurs.

*3. Barrier*: an obstruction; a factor that tends to restrict free movement.

*4. Elastic barrier*: the resistance felt at the end of passive range of motion when the slack has been taken out.

*5. Motion*: movement, act, process, or instance of changing places.

*6. Paraphysiological space*: that sensation of a sudden "give" beyond the elastic barrier of resistance, usually accompanied by a "cracking" sound with a slight amount of movement beyond the usual physiological limit but within the anatomical barrier.

7. *Passive motion*: movement induced in an articulation by the operator. This includes the range of active motion as well as the movement between the physiological and anatomical barriers permitted by soft tissue resiliency which the patient cannot do voluntarily.

8. *Physiological barrier*: the soft tension accumulation which limits the voluntary motion of an articulation. Further motion toward the anatomical barrier can be induced passively.

9. *Restrictive barrier*: an impediment or obstacle to movement within the physiological limits of an articulation that reduces the active motion range.

# 4

# THE MANIPULATIVE PRESCRIPTION

In the practice of medicine it is essential that an accurate diagnosis be made prior to the institution of either curative or palliative therapy. When a therapeutic intervention is deemed to be indicated, particularly when utilizing pharmacotherapeutic agents, a specific and accurate prescription need be written. No self-respecting physician would make a diagnosis of throat infection and write a prescription for antibiotic.

DX—Throat infection
RX—Antibiotic

The physician would seek to identify the infectious agent, either bacterial or viral, causing the throat infection. When a specific infectious agent was identified, responsive to antibiotic therapy, a specific prescription would be written for the antibiotic agent. A prescription would identify the antibiotic to be utilized, the strength of each dose, the number of doses per day, and the duration of therapy.

In manual medicine it is all too common to find practitioners being more lax in their structural diagnosis and the prescription of the manual medicine therapeutic intervention to be applied. All too often a diagnosis is made of somatic dysfunction and manual medicine is the prescription, such as:

DX—Somatic dysfunction
RX—Manipulative therapy

In manual medicine it is just as important to know the location, nature, and type of somatic dysfunction before a specific manual medicine therapeutic intervention is prescribed. The same elements are needed for a manual medicine prescription as for a pharmaceutical agent. One wants to be specific about the type of manual medicine, the intensity, the frequency, and the total length of the treatment plan. Therefore, the manipulative prescription requires an accurate diagnosis of the somatic dysfunction to be treated, a specific description of the type of manipulative procedure, the intensity, and the frequency.

Manipulative therapeutic procedures are indicated for the diagnostic entity somatic dysfunction. As previously noted, somatic dysfunction is impaired or altered function of related components of the somatic (body framework) system: skeletal, arthrodial, and myofascial structures, and the related vascular, lymphatic and neural elements. There are many synonymous terms used to describe this entity including joint blockage, chiropractic subluxation, osteopathic lesion, loss of joint play, and minor intervertebral derangements. In defining somatic dysfunction, one employs the diagnostic triad of A—asymmetry of form or function of related parts of the musculoskeletal system; R—range of motion, primarily alteration of motion, looking at range, quality of motion during the range, and the "endfeel" at the limit of movement; and, *T*—tissue texture abnormality, alteration in the feel of the soft tissues, mainly in the form of muscle hypertonicity, and in skin and connective tissues, described as hot/cold, soft/hard, boggy, doughy, etc.

## CLINICAL GOALS FOR MANIPULATIVE TREATMENT

As previously stated, the goal of manipulation is the use of the hands in a patient-management process using instructions and maneuvers to achieve maximal, painless, movement of the musculoskeletal (motor) system in postural balance. In achieving this goal different types of therapeutic effects upon the patient can be sought. They can be classified as:

1. Circulatory effects
   A. Move body fluids
   B. Provide tonic effect

2. Neurologic effect—modify reflexes
   A. Somato-somatic
   B. Somato-visceral
   C. Viscero-somatic
   D. Viscero-visceral
   E. Viscero-somato-visceral
   F. Somato-viscero-somatic

3. Maintenance therapy for irreversible conditions

Depending upon the outcome desired, different models of manual medicine concepts in therapeutic applications need be considered by the clinician.

## MODELS AND MECHANISMS OF MANUAL MEDICINE INTERVENTION

Several different conceptual models can be utilized in determining the manual medicine approach to a patient. Five such models will be described, but it should be evident that when a manual medicine procedure is provided it has multiple effects and is mediated through a number of different mechanisms. The five models are:

1. Postural structural
2. Neurologic
3. Respiratory circulatory
4. Bioenergy
5. Psycho-behavioral

The *postural structural model* is probably the one most familiar to practitioners of manual medicine. In this model the patient is approached from a biomechanical orientation toward the musculoskeletal system. The osseous skeleton is viewed as a series of building blocks piled one on top of the other, starting with the bones of the foot and ending with the skull. The ligamentous and fascial structures are the tissues which connect the osseous framework, and the muscles are the prime movers of the bones of the skeleton, working across single and multiple joint structures. Alteration of the patient's musculoskeletal system is viewed from the alignment of the bones and joints, the balance of muscles as movers and stabilizers of the skeleton, the symmetry of tone of the ligaments, and the integrity of the continuous bands of fascia throughout. Alteration in joint apposition, alteration in muscle function either due to hypertonicity or weakness, tightness or laxity of ligament(s), and shortening or lengthening of fascia, are all considered when approaching a patient from this perspective. The manual medicine therapy would be directed toward restoring maximal motion to all joints, symmetry of length and strength to all muscles and ligaments, and symmetry of tension within fascial elements throughout the body. The goal is to restore maximal function of this musculoskeletal system in postural balance and the patient can be approached either starting at the feet and ending with the head, or vice versa, starting from the top and ending at the feet.

The most important element of the postural structural model in this author's experience has been the restoration of maximum pelvic mechanics in the walking cycle. The pelvis becomes the cornerstone of the postural structural model and influences from below or above must be considered to achieve symmetrical movement of the osseous pelvis during walking.

This model is most useful in approaching patients with pain resulting from either single instances of trauma, or microtrauma over time, due to postural imbalance from such entities as anatomical shortening of one leg, unilateral fallen arch, etc. This conceptual model includes much of the current biomechanical engineering research in the areas of joint mechanics; properties of ligaments, tendons, and fascia; and kinetics and kinematics.

The *neurological model* concerns influencing neural mechanisms through manual medicine intervention. One mechanism of action is through the autonomic nervous system. There is a large body of basic research into the influence of the somatic (motor) system on the function of the autonomic nervous system, primarily the sympathetic division. This basic research is consistent with clinical observations, but we need additional clinical research into the influence of alteration in the soma on bodily function and the potential mediation through the sympathetic division of the autonomic nervous system.

The concept is based upon the organization of the sympathetic nervous system. The preganglionic fibers take their origin from the spinal cord from T1 to L2. The lateral chain ganglia are paired and overlie the posterior thoracic and abdominal wall where synaptic junction occurs with postganglionic fibers. The lateral chain ganglia in the thoracic region are tightly bound by the fascia to the posterior chest wall and overlie the heads of the ribs. It is hypothesized that altered mechanics of the costovertebral articulations could mechanically influence the lateral chain ganglia. There are peripheral ganglia through which the sympathetic nervous system synapses with postganglionic fibers that are relatively adjacent to the organs being innervated.

The sympathetic nervous system is the sole source of autonomic nervous system activity to the musculoskeletal system itself. There is no parasympathetic innervation to the somatic tissues. The sympathetic nervous system has a wide range of influence on visceral function, endocrine organs, reticuloendothelial system, circulatory system, peripheral nervous system, central nervous system, and muscle. Korr has worked extensively on the function of the sympathetic nervous system and points out the wide diversity of influence that sympathetic hyperactivity has on target end organs. Many factors can affect sympathetic hypertonia, one of which is afferent impulses from segmentally related areas of soma. It would seem reasonable, therefore, to attempt to reduce aberrant afferent stimulus to hyperirritable sections of the sympathetic nervous system to reduce the hyperactivity on target end organs.

Since the sympathetic nervous system is organized segmentally, it can be used in a map-like fashion to look for both alterations of afferent stimulus, and areas which might be influenced through manual medicine intervention. All of the viscera and soma above the diaphragm receive their preganglionic sympathetic nervous system fibers from above cord level T4. All visceral and soma below the diaphragm receive preganglionic sympathetic nervous system fibers from T5 and below. Understanding this anatomy helps in relating identified somatic dysfunctions to the patient's problem, and can lead the physician to give appropriate manual medicine intervention to those areas of somatic dysfunction thought to contribute to increased somatic afferent stimulus to cord levels which might manifest themselves through increased sympathetic nervous system activity.

The parasympathetic nervous system takes its origin from the brain, brain stem, and sacral segments of the spinal cord. It does not have the segmental organization of the sympathetic division of the autonomic nervous system. However, the cranial nerves, including those with parasympathetic activity, exit from the skull through numerous foramina and penetrate the dura. These nerves are at risk for entrapment with alteration of craniomechanics and dural tension. Many times the clinical goal of craniosacral technique is to improve the function of cranial nerves as they exit the skull and sacrum. The autonomic nervous system neurologic model therefore leads the therapist toward a patient approach based upon the anatomy/physiology of the two divisions of the autonomic nervous system and how best to affect them through manual medicine means.

A second neurological model focuses more upon the interrelationships of the peripheral and central nervous systems, their reflex patterns, and their multiple pathways. This model is particularly useful in managing patients with pain syndromes, such as back pain. While controversy remains about the origin of back pain, much is known about the location and type of nociceptors and mechanoreceptors within the musculoskeletal system. The pain stimulus can originate in a number of tissues and then be transmitted by peripheral afferent neurons to the spinal cord for integration and organization. A segmental cord response occurs and transmission up and down the spinal cord affects other neuronal pools. Transmission to the higher centers can result in pain perception, and stimulatory and inhibitory activities within the brain, and subsequently through the cord, to other areas. Utilizing this model, the therapist focuses upon alterating noxious stimuli and afferent input from the areas of somatic dysfunction; reduction or removal of afferent impulse from areas not manifesting pain; and, ultimately, restoring the normal integrated function of the peripheral and central nervous systems.

A clear understanding of the anatomy and physiology of the musculoskeletal system and particularly the spine and paraspinal tissues is necessary to develop a therapeutic plan for removal of pain from the patient. Manual medicine approaches might be modified depending upon the type and location of dysfunctional pathology. If it is felt that muscle contraction and hypertonicity are primary factors in painful somatic afferent activity then a muscle energy procedure might be most beneficial. If it is felt that there is major restriction in a posterior facet joint, a mobilizing or thrusting procedure might be more efficacious.

The third concept within the neurologic model is that of neuroendocrine control. Since the late 1970s, there has been a rapidly expanding body of knowledge about the role of endorphins, enkephalins, and other neural peptides. These substances are not only active in the nervous system but also profoundly affect the immune system. There appears to be ample evidence that alteration in musculoskeltal activity influences their liberation and activity. It has been hypothesized that some of the beneficial effects of manipulative therapy might result from the release of endorphins and enkephalins with subsequent reduction in the perception of pain. Because of the influence of the substances in areas other than the central nervous system, other systemic effects may result from manual medicine procedures. This neuroendocrine mechanism might explain some of the general body tonic effects.

All of these neurological mechanisms are highly complex and have been only superficially dealt with here. They can be used, however, as conceptual models to approach a patient with a myriad of problems.

The *respiratory circulatory model* looks at a different dimension of the activity of the musculoskeletal system. In this model the patient is viewed from the perspective of blood and lymph flow. Skeletal muscles and the diaphragm are the pumps of the venous and lymphatic systems. The goal is restoring the functional capacity of the musculoskeletal system to assist return circulation and the work of respiration. The function of the diaphragm to modify the relative negative intrathoracic pressure to assist in inhalation and exhalation requires that the torso, including the thoracic cage and the abdomen, have the capacity to respond to these pressure gradient changes. Thus the thoracic spine and the rib cage must be functionally flexible, particularly the lower six ribs where the diaphragm attaches. The lumbar spine must be flexible enough to change its anterior curvature for breathing. The abdominal musculature should have symmetrical tone and length and the pelvic diaphragm should be balanced and non-restrictive.

The respiratory circulatory model looks at somatic dysfunction(s) and its influence upon fluid movement and ease of respiration, rather than neural entrapment or biomechanical alteration. Thus, some of the techniques that are applied are less segmentally specific and are more concerned with tissue tensions that might impede fluid flow. The guiding principle of this model is the progression from central to distal. The beginning point is usually in the thoracic cage, primarily at the thoracic inlet, so that the tissues of the thoracic cage are able to respond to respiratory effort and the pumping action of the diaphragm, to receive the fluids trapped in the peripheral tissues. Attention to the thoracic inlet also aids in the drainage of fluid from the head, neck and upper extremities. Recall that all of the lymph ultimately drains into the venous system at the thoracic inlet behind the anterior extremity of the first rib and the medial end of the clavicle. When the thoracic cage is functioning at maximal capacity, one progresses to the lumbar spine, pelvis, and lower extremities attempting to remove any potential obstruction to fluid flow that occurs in these tissues. The therapeutic goals of the respiratory circulatory model are to reduce the work of breathing and to enhance the pumping action of the diaphragm and extremity muscles to assist lymphatic and venous flow.

The *bioenergy model* is somewhat more ethereal than those preceding and focuses upon the inherent energy flow within the body. Some clinicians are skilled at both observing and feeling energy transmission, or the absence of same, from patients. We are all familiar with the phenomena of Kirlian photography which enables us to visualize radiant energy outside the anatomical limits of the body. This may be but one example of perceptible energy that emanates from the human organism. The bioenergy model focuses upon the maximization of normal energy flow within the human body and its response to its environment. Many clinicians have reported sensations of release of energy during manual medicine procedure that appear to emanate from the patient.

There is also the element of the transfer of energy from the therapeutic touch of the physician. Many of the ancient, oriental forms of healing have focused upon elements of "life force", "energy field", etc., and it is within this domain that a manual medicine practitioner can apply this conceptual model. The craniosacral manual medicine approach is one in which one of the major goals of treatment is to restore the normal inherent force of the central nervous system, including the brain, spinal cord, meninges, and cerebral spinal fluid, to maximize a symmetrical, smooth, normal rhythmic CRI (cranial rhythmic impulse).

The *psycho-behavioral model* views the patient from the perspective of enhancing the capacity to relate to both the internal and external. There are many racial, social, and economic factors which influence the patient's perception of such things as pain, health, illness, disease, disability, and death. The patient's ability or inability to cope with all the stresses of life may well manifest itself in a wide variety of symptoms and physical signs. The physician's ability to understand the patient's response to stress and coping mechanisms, and methods to assist the patient with this process, are important components of this conceptual model. "Therapeutic touch" is an integral part of the doctor-patient interaction in this model. The influence of manual medicine may be less a biomechanical, neurological, or circulatory effect than just an important caring function. Awareness of this model is also important in understanding the difficulty in clinical research within manual medicine because of the "placebo" effect of the "laying on of hands".

It is beyond the scope of this volume to do anything but highlight the various models that are available for consideration when employing a manual medicine intervention. It should be obvious that more than one model can be operative at the same intervention. It is strongly recommended, however, that the physician use some conceptual model before a manual medicine intervention. I support the contention of F.L. Mitchell, Jr. (personal communication) that manual medicine therapy is more than "a search and destroy mission of somatic dysfunction."

## THE MANUAL MEDICINE ARMAMENTARIUM

Manual medicine procedures can be classified as follows:

—Soft tissue procedures
—Articulatory procedures (mobilization without impulse)
—Specific joint mobilization

The *soft tissue procedures* are those in which manual application of force is directed toward influencing specific tissue(s) of the musculoskeletal system, or, by peripheral stimulation, enhancing some form of reflex mechanism which alters biological function. The direct procedures include massage, effleurage, kneading, stretching, friction rub, etc. These procedures can prepare the tissues for additional specific joint mobilization, or they can be a therapeutic end in themselves. The therapeutic goals are to overcome congestion, reduce muscle spasm, improve tissue mobility, enhance circulation, and to "tonify" the tissue. These procedures are some of the first learned and practiced by manual medicine physicians and can be used effectively in a variety of patient conditions.

A number of reflex mechanisms have been described which stimulate the peripheral tissues of the musculoskeletal system. These include acupuncture, reflex therapy, Chapman's reflexes, Travell's trigger points, etc. Some manual, mechanical, or electrical stimulus is applied to certain areas of the body to enhance a therapeutic re-

sponse. Some of these systems have been postulated on neurologic models, lymphatic models, neuroendocrine models and in some instances, without any explanation for the observable clinical phenomena. Suffice it to say, many of these peripheral stimulating therapeutic points are consistent across patients, observable by multiple examiners, and provide a predictable response.

The *articulatory procedures* (mobilization without impulse) are utilized extensively in physiotherapy. They consist primarily of putting the elements of the musculoskeletal system, particularly the articulations, through ranges of motion in some graded fashion, with the goal of enhancement of the quantity and quality of motion. These procedures are therapeutic extensions of the diagnostic process of evaluating range of motion. If there appears to be a restriction of motion in one direction, with some alteration in sense of ease of movement in that direction, a series of gentle, rhythmic, operator-directed efforts in the direction of motion restriction can be found therapeutically effective. These articulatory procedures are especially useful for their tonic and/or circulatory effect.

The *specific joint mobilization* procedures all have two common elements:

1) *Method*—the method of approaching the restricted barrier and
2) *Activating force*—the intrinsic or extrinsic forces(s) exerted.

Therefore, we speak of methods and activating forces.

The specific joint mobilization methods are:

1. *Direct method*—All direct procedures engage the restrictive barrier and by application of some force attempt to move the restrictive barrier closer to the normal physiological barrier to active movement.
2. *Exaggeration method*—This therapeutic effort applies a force against the normal physiological barrier in the direction opposite the motion

loss. The force is usually a high-velocity low-amplitude thrust and has been found to be quite successful. There are systems of manual medicine which only provide therapeutic force in the direction of pain-free movement, and it is within this exaggeration method that such therapy seems to be operative.

3. *Indirect method*—In these procedures the operator moves the segment away from the restrictive barrier into the range of "freedom" or "ease" of movement to a point of balanced tension ("floating" of the segment(s)). The segment can then be held in that position for 5 to 90 seconds to relax the tension in the tissues around the articulations so that enhanced mobility occurs. Procedures utilizing this method are termed (a) functional technique; (b) balance-and-hold technique; and, (c) release-by-positioning technique.

4. *Combined method*—Sometimes it is useful to use combinations of direct, exaggeration, and indirect methods in sequence to assist in the ultimate therapeutic outcome. Frequently a combined method series of procedures is more effective than multiple applications of the same method.

5. *Physiological response method*—These procedures apply patient positioning and movement in response to position direction to obtain a therapeutic result. A series of body positions may utilize nonneutral mechanics to restore neutral mechanics to the musculoskeletal system. Another example of a physiological method is the use of respiratory effort to affect mobility of vertebral segments within spinal curvatures. Inhalation effort enhances straightening of the curves and hence backward bending movement in the thoracic spine and forward bending in the cervical and lumbar spines; ex-halation effort causes just the reverse.

The activating forces can be categorized into extrinsic and intrinsic. The extrinsic forces are those which are applied from outside the patient's body directly to the patient. These can include:

1. Operator effort
   a. Guiding
   b. Springing
   c. Thrust
2. Adjunctive (such as straps, pads, traction, etc.)
3. Gravity—the weight of the body part and the patient position.

The intrinsic group are those forces which occur from within the patient's body and are utilized for their therapeutic effectiveness. They are classified as:

1. Inherent force—nature's tendency toward balance and homeostasis
2. Respiratory force
   a. Inhalation—straightens curves in vertebral column and externally rotates extremities
   b. Exhalation—enhances curves in vertebral column and internally rotates extremities
3. Muscle force of the patient
   a. Muscle cooperation
   b. Muscle energy, especially isometrics

It is possible to design multiple variations of activating forces and methods to achieve the desired clinical goal. The more skilled one becomes in using different methods and activating forces, the more successful one becomes as a manual medicine therapist.

## FACTORS INFLUENCING TYPE OF MANIPULATIVE PROCEDURES

In addition to a wide variety of types and styles of manual medicine procedures available and a number of different clinical goals, there are other factors which influence the type of manual medicine procedure instituted. These are:

1.  Age of patient:
2.  Acuteness or chronicity of problem;
3.  General physical condition of patient;
4.  Operator size and ability;
5.  Location (office, home, hospital, etc.);
6.  Effectiveness of previous and/or present therapy.

If one were prescribing a pharmaceutical agent the dosage would be adjusted to the age of the patient, so too in the use of manual medicine. Clearly one approaches an infant differently than a young adult. In an elderly debilitated patient one is much more careful and judicious in the use of some of the more forceful direct action types of technique. Osteoporosis in the female is not necessarily a contraindication to to manual medicine, but indirect procedures with intrinsic activating forces would be more appropriate.

The type of manual medicine procedure is also modified by the acuteness or chronicity of the problem. In acute conditions, inflammatory swelling and acute muscle spasm are frequently encountered. The physician might use the respiratory circulatory model to relieve the inflammatory congestion and perhaps some soft tissue procedure to reduce the amount of acute muscle spasm. In more chronic conditions with long-standing fibrosis in the ligaments, muscles, and fascia, a more direct action myofascial release or direct action high-velocity thrust procedure might be more appropriate. In the patient who is acutely ill, with reduced capacity to withstand aggressive and intensive therapy, a more conservative approach such as indirect technique might be more appropriate. Also remember that manual medicine procedures, particularly those using intrinsic activating forces, result in energy expenditure by the patient. Keep the therapeutic application within the physical capacity of the acutely ill patient. In

chronic conditions do not expect to overcome all of the difficulty with a single manual medicine intervention.

The operator's size, strength, and technical ability will also influence the type of procedure used. While strength is not necessarily the primary determinant of a successful procedure, the proper application of leverage usually is. Ability with and understanding of a number of manual medicine procedures makes a more effective clinician. With only one antibiotic available, the ability to treat infectious disease is clearly hampered. Likewise, with only one form of manual medicine therapy, you are clearly hampered as an effective manual medicine practitioner.

The physician should have the capacity to provide an effective manual medicine treatment irrespective of the location of the patient. While there are some procedures which are clearly more effective in the office setting with specific therapeutic tables, stools and other equipment, one should be able to devise an effective procedure anywhere. In a hospital bed or at home on a soft mattress, the capacity to utilize a high velocity, low amplitude thrust is clearly compromised. However, muscle energy activating forces and other intrinsic force techniques can be more appropriate in such locations.

Past therapy is also highly important in determining the type of procedure to be used. You must know if there has been a previous surgical intervention, manual medicine intervention, or pharmacotherapeutic treatment. If surgery has changed the anatomy, you might wish to modify the therapeutic procedure to meet the altered anatomy. Lack of response to previous manual medicine is not necessarily a reason not to employ a different form of manual medicine therapy. Previous medication, particularly muscle relaxants, tranquilizers, and anti-inflammatory agents, might clearly modify the type of procedure to be utilized. With long-standing steroid therapy, be aware of the potential for laxity of ligaments and softening of cancellous bone.

These are but a few of the factors which affect the choice of a manual medicine procedure. In addition there are three cardinal rules for any effective manual medicine procedure. They are

1. Control;
2. Balance;
3. Localization.

Control includes the physician's control of body position in relationship to the patient; control of the patient in a comfortable position; control of intrinsic or extrinsic forces; and control of the type of therapeutic intervention being applied. Balance of both patient and operator ensures that adequate patient relaxation can occur and the operator can engage the restrictive barrier in comfort. Localization refers to the adequate engagement of a restrictive barrier in a direct action procedure; the localization on the point of maximum ease in a balance-and-hold indirect procedure; the localization of a most pain-free position in a release by positioning procedure, etc.

## CONTRAINDICATIONS TO MANUAL MEDICINE PROCEDURES

Much has been written about absolute and relative contraindications to manual medicine procedures. This author holds the view that there are none, *if*, and it is a big *if*, there is an accurate diagnosis of somatic dysfunction that requires treatment to effect the overall management of the patient, and the manual medicine procedure is appropriate for that diagnosis and the physical condition of the patient. However, there are a number of conditions that require special precautions. Some of these are as follows:

1. The vertebral artery in the cervical spine;
2. Primary joint disease (e.g., rheumatoid arthritis, infectious arthritis, etc.);
3. Metabolic bone disease (e.g., osteoporosis, etc.);
4. Primary or metastatic malignant bone disease;
5. Genetic disorders (e.g., Down's syndrome), particularly in the cervical spine;
6. Hypermobility in the involved segments. This should clearly be avoided. One should look for restricted mobility elsewhere in the presence of hypermobility.

Following these principles a specific and appropriate manual medicine therapeutic prescription can be written for a diagnosis much as one does with traditional therapeutic interventions. Returning to our original example, the thinking physician identifies the infectious agent in a throat infection before deciding upon a therapeutic intervention. If, for example, the throat infection was due to a streptococcus, the physician might select ampicillin as the antibiotic of choice. With the specific infectious agent identified and an appropriate antibiotic chosen, then, adequate dosage on an appropriate schedule for a sufficient length of time would be ordered.

Diagnosis—Throat infection (streptoccocal)
RX—Ampicillin 250 mg q. 6 h, x 10 days

With an appropriate diagnosis of somatic dysfunction, an accurate manual medicine prescription can be written based upon the principles addressed above. One would choose the type of procedure and specify the method, the activating force, the dosage, the length of time of treatment, and the frequency of treatments. For example:

Diagnosis—Somatic dysfunction, T6, ERS, Rt
RX—Manual medicine, direct action muscle energy type to flexion, left rotation, and left sidebending
Reexamine in 48 hours.

The specific somatic dysfunction has been identified with its position and subsequent motion restriction. A direct procedure and an intrinsic activating force was chosen. It was anticipated that the effectiveness of the procedure would last 48 hours and therefore reexamination at that time was indicated.

As manual medicine practitioners, we should all prescribe our therapy as precisely as we prescribe any other therapeutic agent. It is hoped that these principles will assist in the appropriate use of manual medicine.

# 5

## CONCEPTS OF NORMAL VERTEBRAL MOTION

The vertebral column consists of 26 segments. There are usually 7 cervical segments, 12 thoracic segments and 5 lumbar segments. Anomalous development occurs in the spine and is most common in the lumbar region where four or six segments are occasionally found. The lumbar region is also the site of the greatest number of anomalous developmental changes, particularly in the shape of the transverse processes and apophyseal joints. The first and second cervical segments are uniquely atypical. The vertebra motion segment consists of two adjacent vertebrae and the intervening ligamentous structures (Fig. 5.1). The typical vertebra consists of two parts, the body and the posterior arch. The vertebral body articulates with the intervertebral disk above and below at the location of the vertebral end plate. The posterior arch consists of the two pedicles, two superior and two inferior apophyseal joints, two laminae, two transverse processes, and a single spinous process. Two adjacent vertebra are connected ventro dorsad by the anterior longitudinal ligament, the intervertebral disk with its central nucleus and surrounding annulus, the posterior longitudinal ligament, the articular capsules of the apophyseal joints, the ligamentum flavum, the interspinous ligament, and the supraspinous ligament.

In the cervical region we find the atypical atlas (C1) and axis (C2). The atlas (Fig. 5.2) does not have a vertebral body and consists primarily of a bony ring with two lateral masses. On the posterior aspect of the anterior arch is a small joint structure for articulation with the anterior aspect of the odontoid process of the axis. Each lateral mass consists primarily of the articular pillars. The shape of the superior apophyseal joints is concave ventrodorsad and laterally. The long axis of each superior apophyseal joint

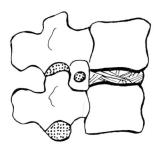

**Figure 5.1.** Vertebral motion segment.

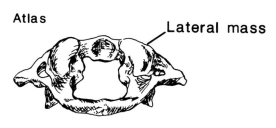

**Figure 5.2.** Atlas (C1).

projects from the lateral to medial dorso-ventrad. This results in an anterior wedging of the long axis of these joints. They articulate with the condyles of the occiput and their shape is a major determinant of the amount and type of motion available between the occiput and the atlas. The inferior apophyseal joints are quite flat but when the articular cartilage is attached become convex ventrodorsad and laterally. These inferior apophyseal joints articulate with the superior apophyseal joints of the axis. The transverse processes are quite long and are easily palpable in the space between the tip of the mastoid process of the temporal bone and the angle of the mandible.

The axis (C2) (Fig. 5.3) has atypical characteristics in its superior portion and more typical characteristics in its inferior portion. The vertebral body is surmounted by the odontoid process, developmentally the residuum of the body of the atlas. On the anterior aspect of the odontoid process is an articular facet for the posterior aspect of the anterior arch of the atlas; the posterior aspect has an articular facet for the transverse atlas ligament. The superior apophyseal joints are convex ventrodorsad and laterally. They are higher on the medial than lateral aspect and their contour resembles a pair of shoulders. The spinous process of C2 is quite long and is one of the more easily palpable spinous processes in the cervical region.

The typical cervical vertebrae, from the inferior surface of C2 down to the cervical thoracic junction have the following charac-teristics (Fig. 5.4). The vertebral body is relatively small in relation to the posterior arch. The superior surface is convex ventrodorsad and concave laterally, while the inferior surface is concave ventrodorsad and convex laterally. When two typical vertebral bodies are joined by the intervertebral disk, the shape is similar to a universal joint. At the posterolateral corner of each vertebral body is found a small synovial joint called the uncovertebral joint of Luschka. These joints are found only in the cervical region and are subject to degenerative change which occasionally encroaches upon the intervertebral canal posteriorly. The pedicles are quite short and serve as the roof and floor of the related intervertebral canal. The articular pillars are relatively large and are easily palpable on the posterolateral aspect of the neck. The apophyseal joints are relatively flat and face backward and upward at approximately a 45° angle. The shape and direction of the apophyseal joints and the universal joint characteristics between the vertebral bodies largely determine the type of movement available in the typical cervical spinal segments. The laminae are flat and the spinous processes are usually bifid with the exception on C7. The transverse processes are unique in this region having the intertransverse foramen for the passage of the vertebral artery on each side. The tips of the transverse processes are bifid and serve as attachments for the deep cervical muscles. They are quite tender to palpation and are not easily used in structural diagnosis of the cervical spine. The intervertebral canals on each side are ovoid in shape and are limited by the inferior margin of the pedicle above, the posterior aspect of the intervertebral disk and Luschka's joints in front, the superior aspect of the pedicle of the vertebral below, and by the anterior aspect of the apophyseal joints behind. The vertebral canal is relatively large and provides the space necessary for the large area of the spinal cord in the cervical region.

In the thoracic region (Fig. 5.5) the vertebral bodies become somewhat larger in

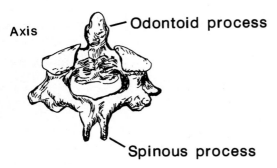

**Axis** — **Odontoid process**

**Spinous process**

**Figure 5.3.**    Axis (C2).

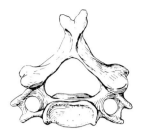

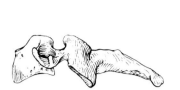

**Figure 5.4.** Typical cervical vertebra.

descent and have unique characteristics for articulation with the heads of the ribs. T1 has a uni-facet found posterolaterally for the articulation of the heads of rib one bilaterally. From the inferior surface of T1 down are found demi-facets, which together with the intervertebral disk, provide an articular fossa for the head of each rib. The apophyseal joints are vertical in orientation and the superior facets project backward and laterally. Theoretically this should provide a great deal of freedom of movement in multiple directions but the attachment of the ribs to the thoracic vertebra markedly restricts the available motion. The transverse processes have an articular facet on their anterior aspect for articulation with the tubercle of the rib. This forms the costotransverse articulation bilaterally. The transverse processes become progressively narrower in descent, with those at T1 being widest at their tips, and at T12 the narrowest. The laminae are shingled and continue to the spinous processes which are also shingled from above downward. The spinous processes are quite long and overlap each other, particularly in the mid to lower

region. The relation of the palpable tips of the spinous processes to the thoracic vertebral bodies is spoken of as "the rule of 3s" (Fig. 5.6). The spinous processes of T4 to 6 project one-half vertebra below that to which they are attached. The spinous processes of T7 to 9 are located a full vertebra lower than the vertebra to which they are attached. The spinous processes of T10 through 12 return to being palpable at the same level as the vertebral body to which they are attached.

In the lumbar region the vertebral bodies (Fig. 5.7) become even more massive and support a great deal of weight. The spinous processes project posteriorly in relation to the vertebral body to which they are attached and are broad, rounded, and easily palpable. The transverse processes project laterally with those attached to L3 being the broadest in range. The apophyseal joints have a concave/convex relationship between the superior and inferior apophyseal joints of adjacent vertebra which greatly restricts the amount of sidebending and rotation available. The plane of facet joints is usually considered a sagittal (yz) plane with

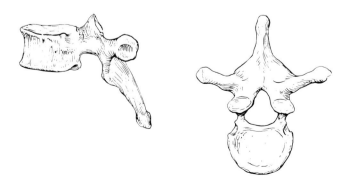

**Figure 5.5.** Thoracic vertebra.

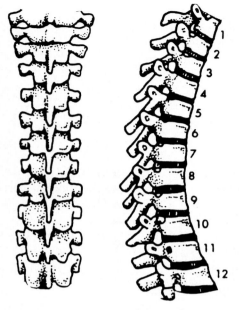

**Figure 5.6.**   Thoracic spine rule of threes.

the lumbosacral apophyseal joints considered closer to the coronal (xy) plane. However, in the lumbar region asymmetrical facing of the apophyseal joints is not uncommon.

The muscles overlying the vertebral column are many and layered. They can be described as follows:

Layer one: the trapezius, latissimus dorsi, and lumbodorsal fascia;
Layer two: the levator scapulae, the major and minor rhomboids;
Layer three: the erector spinae mass including the spinalis, semispinalis, longissimus, and iliocostalis;

Layer four: multifidi, rotatores, and intertransversarii.

The anteroposterior curves of the vertebral column develop over time. The primary curve at birth is convex posteriorly. The first secondary curve to develop is in the cervical region which becomes convex anteriorly when the infant begins to raise its head. The second curve develops in the lumbar region on assuming the biped stance. This is convex anteriorly. Appropriate alignment of the three curves of the vertebral axis is an essential component of good posture (Fig. 5.8).

### LAYER PALPATION

The palpation of these structures is an essential component of structural diagnosis. The following exercise in palpation might be useful in gaining familiarity with some of them for further use both diagnostically and therapeutically.

1.  Place the palms and palmer surfaces of the fingers overlying the posterior aspect of the thorax with each hand over the spine of the scapulae (Fig. 5.9). Palpate just the skin to sense skin characteristics and thickness. Now gently move your hands downward, in parallel, palpating for any changes in temperature, smoothness, thickness, or pliability.
2.  Return to starting position and gently move the skin over the subcutaneous fascia vertically, horizontally, and in rotary fashion.

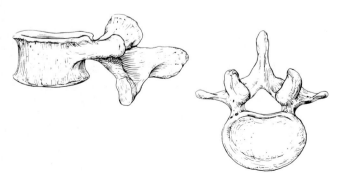

**Figure 5.7.**   Lumbar vertebra.

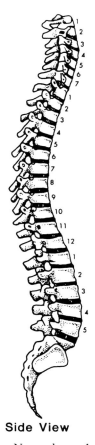

**Side View**

**Figure 5.8.** Normal vertebral curves.

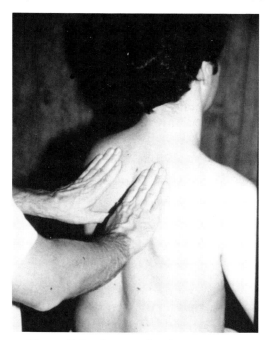

**Figure 5.9.** Layer palpation posterior thorax.

Gain a sense of the amount of skin movement over the subcutaneous tissues.

3. Using the thumb and index finger of each hand, pick up the skin and subcutaneous fascia and gently roll the skin over you thumbs by the action of your index fingers coming from below upward (Fig.5.10). Repeat starting medially and going laterally. Do this procedure symmetrically and bilaterally looking for differences in the thickness and pliability of the skin and also ascertaining if, and where, this procedure produces pain in the patient. The skin-rolling test can be quite valuable in identifying levels of somatic dysfunction.

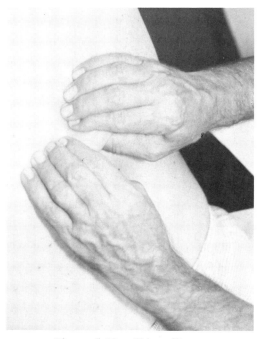

**Figure 5.10.** Skin rolling.

4. Place two to three fingers over the midline of the back palpating through skin and subcutaneous fascia down to the resistance structure below (Fig 5.11). Attempt to move the skin vertically and horizontally over the underlying tissues. Note the tightness of the skin attachment in this region compared to the more lateral regions.

5. Palpate through the skin and subcutaneous fascia down to the superspinous ligament. Particularly palpate at the interspace and note the difference in the quality of the feel of the superspinous ligament at the interspinous space when compared to the attachment to the tip of the spinous process. Palpate the spinous process through the skin, subcutaneous fascia, and superspinous ligament. Note the firm, resistant feel of the bony process.

6. Palpate through skin and subcutaneous fascia to the supraspinous

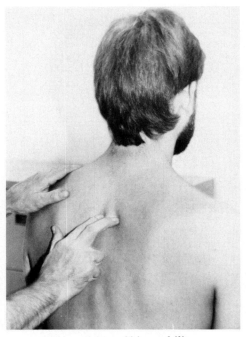

**Figure 5.11.** Skin mobility.

ligament at approximately two or three interspinous levels. Ask the patient to bend the head forward and backward on the trunk and palpate the changing dimension of the interspinous space with this maneuver. You are testing the forward- and backward-bending capability of the segments being palpated. With one finger in an interspace, palpate the inferior margin of the superior vertebra and the superior margin of the inferior forward-bending until the superior vertebra moves but the inferior does not. Repeat with backward-bending and again feel the superior vertebra move but not the inferior.

7. Palpate the area between the spine and the vertebral border of the scapula at approximately the level of the spine of the scapula. Palpate down through the skin and subcutaneous fascia to deep fascia overlying muscle. Now begin to think muscle and palpate the first layer of muscle encountered. What is the fiber direction of that layer of muscle? Ask your patient to pull the scapulae together energizing the muscle, and see if it enhances the feel of the fiber direction. You should palpate horizontal fibers in the trapezius.

8. Palpate through the horizontal fibers of the trapezius to the next layer of muscle. Can you identify muscle fibers which course obliquely laterally from above downward? To assist you, offer resistance to the elbow on the ipsilateral side as the patient attempts to push the elbow caudad (Fig. 5.12). Another maneuver which will activate this muscle is placing the back of the patient's hand on the ipsilateral side against the back and resisting the palm of the hand as the patient attempts to

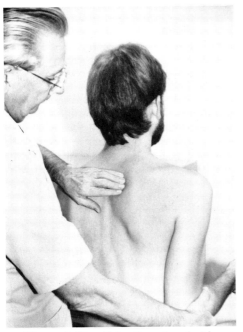

**Figure 5.12.** Palpation rhomboid.

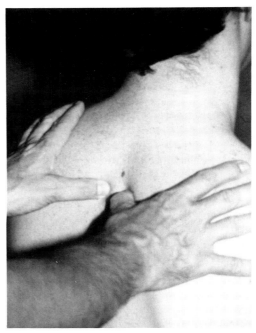

**Figure 5.13.** Palpation deep back muscles medial to longissimus.

push the hand away from the back. Each of these maneuvers will activate the rhomboid muscles and assist you in palpating their oblique fibers.

9. Palpate deeper by one muscle layer looking for the ropy structure called the erector spinae mass. At the deep fascia layer overlying the erector spinae mass it is possible to move your palpating thumbs or fingers from medial to lateral identifying a vertically oriented muscle group. The ropy structure you are palpating is primarily the longissimus muscle of the erector spinae mass, and on the medial and lateral side of it are deep fascial planes which allow you to go deeper into the structures of the back.

10. At the deep fascial plane on the medial side of the longissimus, palpate deeply (Fig. 5.13) until you encounter the fourth layer of muscle, the so-called single-segment

deep muscles of the back. Under your palpating digit are found the rotatores and the multifidi which are oriented in an oblique direction from medial to lateral from above downward (the same fiber direction as found in rhomboids). Palpate several levels of these deep fourth-layer muscles and see if it is possible to identify some that are more full and tense (and probably tender to the patient). This finding is usually due to hypertonicity of the fourth layer muscles, one of the cardinal diagnostic findings in vertebral segmental somatic dysfunction.

11. Palpate deeply along the lateral fascial plane of the longissimus muscle with the pads and tips of each thumb in a bilateral fashion. As you course deeper into the tissues go slightly medially from behind forward until you encounter resistance. At that level move your

thumbs cephalically and caudally looking for "bumps" and "hollows" similar to your grandmother's washboard. As you sense the bumps and hollows, you are palpating the posterior aspect of the transverse process at the bump and the intertransverse process space at the hollow. The ability to palpate paired transverse processes and follow them in their relationship to space is most valuable in motion testing of the vertebral segments (Fig. 5.14).

12. Bilaterally palpate the most posterior aspect of the thoracic cage from above downward. The contour should be smooth with a posterior convexity and somewhat divergent from above downward. You are palpating over the rib angles of the posterior aspect of each rib. At each rib angle palpate for tenderness and hypertonicity of the attached muscle. The ilio-

costalis muscles attached to the rib angles and tender hypertonicity at a given rib is a common finding in rib somatic dysfunction. Palpate to be sure that each rib angle is found within the convex contour of the posterior aspect of the thoracic cage. A rib angle more or less prominent than it should be in the normal posterior convexity is a very significant finding in a patient with rib somatic dysfunction of a specific type to be described later.

13. Palpate the posterior aspect of the shaft of each rib comparing it with the one above and the one below. Each rib shaft is convex posteriorly and has a sharp superior and inferior margin which is palpable. Normally the inferior margin is more easily palpable than the superior. While palpating the posterior contour of each rib, evaluate the intercostal space above and below looking for symmetry of the spaces. Ask yourself if one is narrower or wider than the one above or below, particularly in comparison with the opposite side. Palpate the intercostal muscle for hypertonicity in the same location. Alteration in the intercostal spare, hypertonicity of intercostal muscles, and increase or decrease in the palpable superior and inferior margin of a rib are all significant findings in certain rib somatic dysfunctions.

14. Return to the rib angle and palpate in a medial direction along the posterior shaft of the rib on each side (Fig. 5.15). Coursing from lateral to medial along the shaft you will eventually run into a "bump". This bump is the tip of the transverse process and you are palpating as close as possible to the costotransverse articulation of that rib with the transverse process on that side.

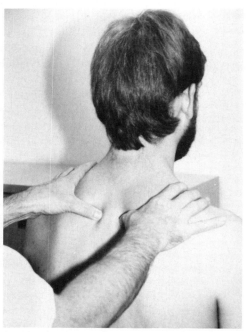

**Figure 5.14.** Palpating transverse processes lateral to longissimus.

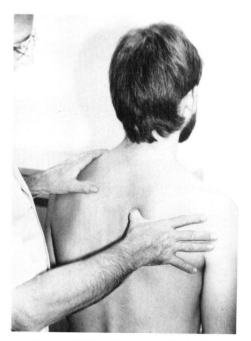

**Figure 5.15.** Palpation rib shaft.

This layer palpation exercise of the back will provide you with the ability to palpate the anatomical structures necessary for accurate diagnosis of the vertebral axis and the costal cage. Of particular importance are the ability to follow paired transverse processes through a range of movement and the ability to identify tender muscle hypertonicity of the fourth layer of deep muscles. Practice this exercise on a regular basis until it becomes habitual.

## VERTEBRAL MOTION

Certain conventions are used in describing all vertebral motion. The vertebral motion segment consists of the superior and inferior adjacent vertebra and the intervening disc and ligamentous structures. By convention, motion of the superior vertebra is described in relation to the inferior. Motion is further defined as the movement of the superior or anterior surface of the vertebral body. In describing rotation, the anterior surface is used rather than the elements of the posterior arch. For example, in rotation

of T3 to the right in relation to T4, the anterior surface of T3 turns to the right and the spinous process deviates to the left. Therefore, remember that descriptions relate to the anterior or superior surfaces of the vertebral body. In addition to describing characteristics of a vertebral motion segment, we also speak of movement of groups of vertebrae (three or more).

Vertebral motion is also described in relation to the anatomically oriented cardinal planes of the body using the right-handed orthogonal coordinate system. Most of the clinical literature relates to the anatomically described cardinal planes and axes, while the biomechanical research literature uses the coordinate system extensively. Motion can be described as rotation around an axis and translation along an axis with the body moving within one of the cardinal planes. By convention the horizontal axis is the x-axis; the vertical axis is the y-axis; and the anteroposterior axis is the z-axis. The coronal plane is the xy plane; the sagittal plane is the yz plane; and the horizontal plane is the xz plane. The ability to rotate around an axis and to translate along an axis results in six degrees of freedom for each vertebra. Vertebral motion can then be described as overturning moment (rotation around an axis) and translatory movement (translation along an axis).

## TERMINOLOGY

At the present time, convention in clinical practice describes vertebral motion in the following terms:

> Forward-bending
> Backward-bending
> Sidebending—right and left
> Rotation—right and left

***Forward-bending:*** A superior vertebra rotates anteriorly around the x-axis and translates somewhat forward along the z-axis. In forward-bending (Fig.5.16) the anterior longitudinal ligament becomes somewhat more lax, or posterior pressure is placed upon the intervertebral disc; the pos-

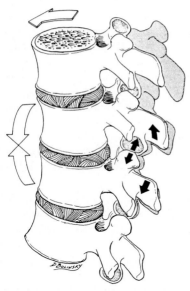

**Figure 5.16.**    Vertebral forward-bending.

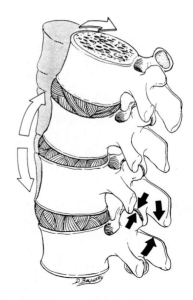

**Figure 5.17.**    Vertebral backward-bending.

terior longitudinal ligament becomes more tense as do the ligamentum flavum, and the interspinous and supraspinous ligaments. The inferior apophyseal facet of the superior vertebra moves superiorly in relation to the superior apophyseal facet of the inferior vertebra. This has been described as "opening" or "flexing" of the facet.

*Backward-Bending:*    In backward-bending the vertebra rotates backward around the x-axis and moves posteriorly along the z-axis (Fig. 5.17). The anterior longitudinal ligament becomes more tense. There is less tension on the posterior longitudinal ligament, the ligamentum flavum, and the interspinous and supraspinous ligaments. The inferior apophyseal facet of the superior segment slides inferiorly in relation to the superior apophyseal facet of the inferior vertebra. The facets are spoken of as having "closed" or "extended". Forward- and backward-bending result in an accordion-type movement of the opening and closing of the facet joints. If something interferes with the capacity of a facet joint to open or close, restriction of motion of either forward- or backward-bending will result.

*Sidebending:*    In sidebending there is rotation around the AP z-axis and transla-

tion along the horizontal x-axis. Sidebending is seldom a pure movement and is usually coupled with rotation. In sidebending to the right the right apophyseal joint "closes" and the left apophyseal joint "opens". Interference with a facet's capacity to open or close can interfere with sidebending and the coupled rotatory movement.

*Rotation:*    Rotation of a vertebra is described as rotation around the y-axis with the translatory movement being dependent upon the vertebral segment involved. Rotation is always coupled with sidebending with the exception of the atlantoaxial joint.

## COUPLED MOVEMENTS

As previously noted, sidebending and rotation are usually coupled movements and do not occur individually. In some instances rotation is coupled in the same direction as sidebending (e.g., sidebending right, rotation right) and at other times in opposite directions (e.g., sidebending right, rotation left). These coupled movements are by convention designated as type I, type II, and type III.

*Type I:*    Type I coupled movement results in sidebending and rotation occurring to opposite sides. This type of movement occurs most frequently when the patient is standing in the erect position with normal anteroposterior curves. For example, in the lumbar spine, with a normal lumbar lordosis present, sidebending of the trunk to the left results in rotation of lumbar vertebra to the right (Fig. 5.18). This can be clearly demonstrated by standing erect and placing the four fingers of your hand over the posterior aspect of the transverse processes of the lumbar spine. Now sidebend to the left and feel the tissues under your right hand become more full. This fullness is interpreted as posterior movement of the right transverse processes of lumbar vertebrae as they rotate right in response to sidebending left.

*Type II:* Type II coupled movement results in sidebending and rotation of a vertebra to the same side. This commonly occurs when there is alteration in the anteroposterior curve into forward or backward bending. For example, when standing and forward-bent at the waist, sidebending to the right results in rotation of lumbar vertebra to the right (Fig. 5.19). This can be felt on yourself by the following exercise. Place fingers of both hands overlying the posterior aspect of the transverse processes of your lumbar spine. While standing, forward-bend the trunk and then introduce sidebending to the right. You will feel fullness occur under the fingers of your right hand, interpreted as resulting from posterior orientation of the right transverse processes during a right rotational response to the right sidebending coupled movement. Return to the midline before returning to the erect position. The vertebral column is clearly at risk for dysfunction when type II vertebral mechanics are operative.

*Type III:* Type III movement refers to the fact that when motion is introduced within the vertebral column in one direction, motion in all other directions is reduced. To demonstrate this phenomenon have your patient sit erect on an examining couch and passively introduce rotation of the trunk to the right and to the left. Ascertain the range and quality of movement.

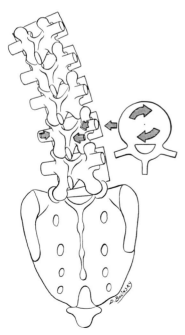

**Figure 5.18.** Type I (neutral) vertebral motion.

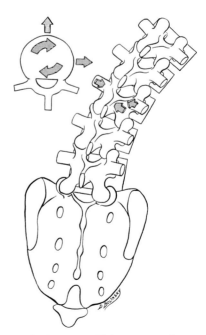

**Figure 5.19.** Type II (nonneutral) vertebral motion.

Now let your patient slump on the table with a posterior thoracolumbar convexity and again attempt to introduce trunk rotation to the right and left. Note the reduction in range, and the restricted quality of movement during the range, when the patient is in this slumped (forward-bent) position. Type III vertebral motion is employed therapeutically in localizing to dysfunctional segments and is a valuable concept to understand.

The type of coupled movement within the vertebral column varies from region to region and posture to posture. In those areas of the vertebral column which have the capacity for both type I and type II movement, the vertebra can become dysfunctional with either type of motion characteristic.

*Type of Motion Available*

### VERTEBRAL MOTION

| *SEGMENT(S)* | *TYPE(S)* |
|---|---|
| Co-C1 (occipitoatlantal) | I (always) |
| C1-C2 (atlantoaxial) | Rotation |
| C2-C7 (typical cervical) | II |
| C7-L5 (typical thoracic & lumbar) | I and II |

An understanding of the anatomy of the vertebral column, the ability to palpate the tissues found therein, and understanding of the concepts of vertebral motion are essential for understanding and diagnosing vertebral dysfunctions.

# 6

# CONCEPTS OF VERTEBRAL MOTION DYSFUNCTION

In the application of manual medicine procedures to the vertebral column, it is essential to make appropriate, accurate diagnosis of vertebral somatic dysfunction. Somatic dysfunction is altered function of the elements of the musculoskeletal system and their related vascular, lymphatic, and neural elements. This term is codable under current classifications systems and replaces old terminology such as osteopathic lesion, chiropractic subluxation, joint lock, loss of joint play, or minor vertebral derangement. Our concern with the function of the musculoskeletal system requires a method of evaluating motion within the vertebral complex to determine if it is normal, increased, or decreased. There is a spectrum of motion from the most advanced hypomobility (ankylosis) to normal motion, to hypermobility, to the most advanced states of hypermobility and instability. Manual medicine procedures are most appropriate for segments with hypomobility which retain the capacity to move.

There have been many theories proposed to explain the clinically observed phenomenon of hypomobility. One theory proposes that there is entrapment of synovial material or a synovial meniscoid between the two opposing joint surfaces. There is some anatomical evidence that meniscoids do occur but whether or not they actually cause joint restriction has not been demonstrated.

A second theory suggests that there is lack of congruence in the opposing surfaces of the articulation, particularly the point-to-point contact of the opposing joint surfaces. This theory postulates alteration in the normal tracking mechanism between the joint surfaces and that the role of manual medicine is to restore the joint to the "right track."

A third theory suggests an alteration in the physical and chemical properties of the synovial fluid and synovial surfaces. In essence, the smooth gliding capacity has been lost because the opposing surfaces have become "sticky." It has been demonstrated in both vertebral joints and extremity joints that following a high-velocity, low-amplitude thrusting procedure in which separation of the joint surfaces has occurred, there is an observable vacuum phenomena on x-ray. This suggests a change from the liquid to the gaseous state as a result of the thrusting procedure. This gaseous shadow is seen for a variable period of time and ultimately becomes no longer visible—ostensibly the gas has returned to a liquid state.

A fourth theory regards restriction of motion as due to altered tone and length of muscle. Muscle can become hypertonic, and bilateral muscle coordination is lost. Physiologically it appears that the antagonist of a hypertonic and shortened agonist muscle becomes lengthened and weaker. Alteration in muscle pathophysiology may extend to frank spasm and even into chronic contracture. Whether these changes in muscle are primary or secondary in the dysfunctional segment is still open to conjecture. However, clinically, it appears that alteration in muscle tone is a restrictor to normal movement and as such deserves attention during the treatment process.

A fifth theory considers changes in the biomechanical and biochemical properties of the myofascial elements of the musculoskeletal system, the capsule, the ligamentous structures, and fascia. When these structures are altered through traumatic, inflammatory, degenerative, or other changes, reduction of normal vertebral mobility can result.

Regardless of the theory to which one might subscribe, the clinical phenomenon of restricted vertebral motion can be viewed as the influence on the paired facets of the segment. We speak of the capacity of facets to open and close and refer primarily to the accordion-type movement, not separation-type movement. In forward-bending the facets should normally open and in backward-bending they should close. If something interferes with the capacity of both facets to open, forward-bending restriction will occur. Conversely, if something interferes with both facets' capacity to close, backward-bending restriction will occur. It is also possible for one facet to move normally and the other to become restricted. If, for example, the right facet does not open, but the left functions normally, right sidebending is possible but left sidebending is restricted. Since sidebending and rotation are coupled movements in the typical vertebral segments, rotation can also be affected by alteration in facet joint movement.

## DIAGNOSIS OF VERTEBRAL MOTION DYSFUNCTION

Dysfunctions in the vertebral column can be described as (*a*) single-segment dysfunctions involving one vertebral motion segment, and (*b*) group dysfunctions involving three or more vertebrae. After one completes a screening-and-scanning examination and fine-tunes the diagnostic process to segmental definition, one is particularly interested in the motion(s) lost by the vertebra(e) involved. There are many methods to accomplish the process. The most commonly employed is palpating the same bony prominence of two or more vertebrae (e.g., spinous processes or transverse processes) and actively and/or passively putting the segment(s) through successive ranges of movement into forward bending, backward bending, sidebending right, sidebending left, rotation right, and rotation left, comparing the motion of one segment with another. These procedures are most frequently done passively and the operator attempts to define restriction and quality of restriction of movement in one or more directions. While this method is frequently effective, it does have two serious drawbacks in this author's opinion. First, every time you introduce multiple-plane motion in a dysfunctional segment diagnostically, there is a therapeutic effect since you are accomplishing an articulatory (mobilization without impulse) procedure. This results in your finding being constantly under change. A second disadvantage is the difficulty in making an assessment following a treatment procedure, i.e., knowing whether or not you have modified the amount of range that were present prior to the procedure. It is difficult to remember accurately all of the nuances of motion restriction that were present prior to the therapeutic intervention.

A second method, preferred by this author, is to follow a pair of transverse processes through an arc of forward and backward bending and interpret the findings based upon the phenomena of facet opening and closing. Regardless of the method utilized, one can describe vertebral motion from the perspective of the motion available, the position in which the segment is restricted, or the motion of the segment that is restricted.

|  | Position | Motion Restriction |
|---|---|---|
| T3 on T4 | Flexed, left rotated | Extension, right rotation, |
|  | Left sidebent | Right sidebending |
|  | Extended | Flexion |
|  | Right rotated | Left rotation |
|  | Left sidebent | Right sidebending |

Notice the use of the suffix in each term. There will be either a static suffix representing the position of the segment or a motion suffix which describes the motion available or the motion lost. The current convention of describing vertebral dysfunction is either the position of the restricted segment or the motion that is lost in the restricted segment. Therefore, a segment that is backward bent (extended), right rotated, and right sidebent has forward bending (flexion), left sidebending, and left rotation restriction. A plea is made for the use of appropriate terminology either to describe position or motion restriction. One should learn to translate between the two systems of positional and motion restriction diagnosis but clearly a statement of terms is necessary for accurate communication between examiners.

## GROUP DYSFUNCTION

When three or more vertebral segments are involved in motion restriction, there will be alteration in the lateral curvature to one side. There is prominence on the side of the convexity of the group of segments due to the rotation of the vertebrae to the side of convexity. On palpation one finds a fullness overlying the transverse processes of three or more adjacent vertebrae. During a forward-bending—backward-bending movement arc, there may be change in the amount of fullness on the convex side, but there is no position in which the transverse processes on each side become symmetrical. The motion restriction found in this group of segments has minimal forward- or backward-bending restriction, but has restriction of sidebending to the side of convexity and rotation to the side of concavity (Fig. 6.1).

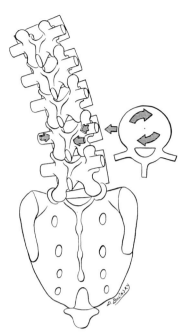

**Figure 6.1.** Vertebral group dysfunction.

The characteristics of a group dysfunction are

1. A group of segments (3 or more);
2. Minimal flexion or extension component of restriction;
3. Restriction of the group to sidebending in one direction and rotation in the opposite.

Group dysfunctions are also described as type I restrictions with the restricted coupled movement being sidebending to one side and rotation to the opposite. These group dysfunctions are present in compensatory scoliotic mechanisms and are frequently found above or below a single vertebral motion segment dysfunction with major restriction. They are frequently secondary to change elsewhere, but because they involve a large number of vertebral segments they receive a lot of diagnostic attention.

## DYSFUNCTIONS OF SINGLE VERTEBRAL MOTION SEGMENT

In examining for these dysfunctions the thumbs are placed on the posterior aspect of the transverse processes of a segment that is suspected of being dysfunctional, and the patient is put through a forward- or backward-bending movement arc either actively or passively. In the upper thoracic spine the active movement of the head on the trunk is frequently utilized while in the lower thoracic and lumbar spine the patient is examined in three different positions, fully forward bent, prone neutral on the table, and in full backward bending (Figs. 6.2, 6.3, 6.4). For the purpose of description, assume that something interferes with opening of the right facet joint. In the neutral position the right transverse process appears to be somewhat more posterior than the left. As the patient increases the amount of forward-bending, the right transverse process becomes more prominent compared to the left. The restricted right facet joint holds the right half of the posterior arch of that vertebra in a posterior position, while the free-moving facet joint on the left side allows the left half of the posterior arch to move forward and superior with the left transverse process seeming to become less prominent. In backward-bending both transverse processes appear to become more symmetric because the right transverse process is already held posterior by the restricted right facet joint, while the left facet closes in backward-bending allowing the left transverse process to move posteriorly and inferiorly becoming more symmetric in appearance (Fig. 6.5).

Now let us assume that something interferes with the left facet's ability to close. In this instance we usually find the right transverse process a little more prominent in the neutral position. In asking the patient to move into backward bending the right transverse process appears to become more prominent. This is the result of normal closure of the right facet allowing the transverse process to move posteriorly, while the left facet is restricted in its capacity to close and holds the left transverse process in a more anterior position. Upon forward-bending, both transverse processes become more symmetrical. The left transverse process is already held in an anterior position by the restricted left facet joint, and the motion of the right facet moving into an open position carries the right transverse process more anteriorly (Fig. 6.5).

These single vertebral motor unit dysfunctions are also described as type II dysfunctions because the restricted coupled movement is side-bending and rotation to the same side. They are also described as nonneutral dysfunctions for the same reason. The characteristics are as follows:

1. Single vertebral motion unit involved;
2. Includes either flexion or extension restriction component;
3. Motion restriction of sidebending and rotation to the same side.

We have described the phenomenon that occurs if one or the other facet loses the capacity to open or close. If there is a single vertebral motion segment involved in which both facets are restricted, the transverse processes remain in the same relative position throughout forward- and backward-bending movement. One can determine the case of bilateral facets being closed or bilateral facets being open by monitoring the interspace between the spinous process during forward and backward bending. If the facets are able to open, the interspinous distance will increase during forward bending. If the facets are able to close in a bilaterally symmetrical fashion, the interspinous distance becomes smaller during backward bending.

There are several reasons why this method of vertebral motion testing is recommended. First, this method remains consistent and reproducible over time. The challenge to the motion segment is in only one plane of movement. No multiaxial changes in movement characteristics are introduced, as in the procedure described earlier. This method does not put the segment through an articulatory procedure and thus is not changing the vertebral mechanics to any appreciable amount. This makes it possible for the examiner to be more confident

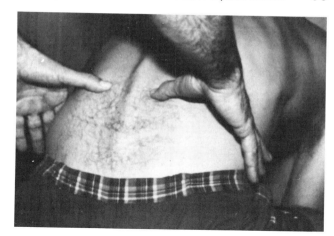

**Figure 6.2.** Vertebral motion
testing forward bent.

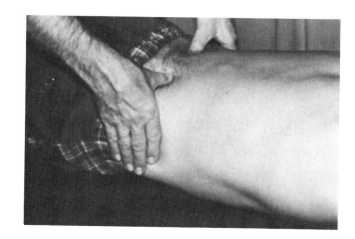

**Figure 6.3.** Vertebral motion
testing prone.

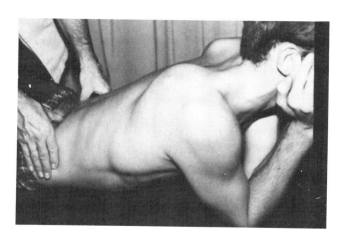

**Figure 6.4.** Vertebral motion
testing backward bent.

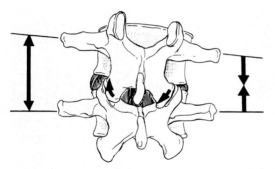

**Figure 6.5.** Dysfunction single vertebral segment.

in the posttreatment evaluation of a segment to be sure that, in fact, some change has occurred in the motion present before and after treatment.

Secondly, this procedure is easier for multiple examiners to apply because of the nontreatment aspect of the method. This allows more consistent student teaching and evaluation of vertebral diagnostic procedures. If five separate examiners tested a given segment by putting it through multiple ranges of movement, by the time the fifth examiner described the findings, the first examiner would think it was a different patient. Using this single-plane movement challenge, the findings remain much more consistent across examiners and across time.

A third reason to recommend this process is the examiner's capacity to differentiate between structural and functional asymmetry of a vertebral segment. Structural asymmetries do occur fairly frequently, and palpation of a posterior transverse process can not distinguish asymmetrical development from actual dysfunction of a rotational nature. If the prominent transverse process is due to type II, nonneutral, single vertebral motion segment dysfunction, the prominence of the transverse process will change during a forward- and backward-bending arc. In one position it will become worse, and in the other position it will become more symmetrical. If the transverse process is prominent because of asymmetrical development, and the segment is basically functional, the transverse process will retain the same amount of prominence throughout the forward-bending—backward-bending movement arc. There is a third possibility for the existence of a transverse process being more prominent on one side than the other. That can occur when one facet does not open and the other facet does not close. This bilateral restriction retains the same amount of prominence of the posterior transverse process throughout the movement arc. One can distinguish this bilateral restriction from a structural asymmetry by evaluating the forward-bending—backward-bending capacity while monitoring at the interspinous space.

## HYPERMOBILITY

Manual medicine procedures are appropriate for restriction of articular structures (hypomobility) but if used on hypermobile segments they could be detrimental, enhancing the hypermobility. In structural diagnosis we are concerned with three types of hypermobility: (*a*) hypermobility due to disease such as Ehlers-Danlos syndrome, Marfan's syndrome, the Marfanoid hypermobility syndrome, and others even more rare; (*b*) physiological hypermobility seen in certain body types (ectomorphic) and frequently observed in gymnasts, ballet dancers, and other athletic types; and (*c*) compensatory hypermobility due to hypomobility elsewhere in the musculoskeletal system.

The pathological hypermobilities are a group of conditions in which there is alteration in the histology and biochemistry of the connective tissues. In Ehlers-Danlos syndrome there is articular hypermobility, dermal extensibility, and frequent cutaneous scarring. This condition has been noted in circus performers who are classified as "elastic people." The classic Marfan syndrome demonstrates long slender (Lincolnesque) limbs; ectopic lentis, dilation of the ascending aorta, and mitral valve prolapse. While the severity of each of the components of the Marfan syndrome vary from patient to patient, all exhibit joint hypermobility. Following joint injury the hypermobility is increased and it is very difficult to manage patients with this condition who have somatic dysfunction superimposed upon their musculoskeletal anatomy. The Marfanoid hypermobility syndrome has the same musculoskeletal system findings but seems not to demonstrate either the eye or the vascular changes.

In the physiological hypermobility group there is hypermobility of fingers, thumbs, elbows, knees and trunk forward bending. A nine-point scale has been devised for the paired fingers, thumbs, elbows and knees with one point being assigned to trunk forward bending. Patients with this trait find it easy to become gymnasts and ballet dancers and increased mobility can result from training and exercise. In normal individuals joint mobility reduces rapidly during childhood and then more slowly during adulthood. Patients with increased physiological hypermobility are at risk for increased musculoskeletal system symptoms and diseases, particularly osteoarthritis.

It is in the secondary hypermobility states that the manual medicine practitioner becomes more involved. Compensatory hypermobility appears to develop in areas of the vertebral column as a secondary reaction to hypomobility within the complex. The segments of compensatory hypermobility can be either adjacent to, or some distance from, the area(s) of major joint hypomobility. Clinically, there also appears to be relative hypermobility on the opposite side of a segment that is restricted. The major difficulty encountered with these areas of secondary compensatory hypermobility is that they are frequently the ones that are symptomatic. Because they attempt to compensate for restricted motion elsewhere, they receive excess stimulation from increased mobility and frequently become painful and tender. As the painful areas, they receive a great deal of attention from the manual medicine practitioner, who can become trapped into treating the hypermobile segment because it is symptomatic,

and not realizing that the symptom is secondary to restricted mobility elsewhere. In most instances of compensatory hypermobility the condition requires little or no direct treatment but responds nicely to appropriate treatment of hypomobility elsewhere in the vertebral column. Many practitioners of musculoskeletal medicine use sclerosant-type injection into the tissues of a hypermobile segment as part of their treatment plan. Whether these solutions actually modify joint mobility or whether they result in chemical ablation of nociception is unknown. In this author's experience most areas of secondary, compensatory hypermobility are self-correcting once the hypomobility areas are adequately treated and the total musculoskeletal system is restored to functional balance.

One cannot discuss hypermobility without referring to instability. Instability occurs when the damage is sufficient and the opposing joint structures lose their anatomical integrity. The dividing line between extensive hypermobility and instability is very hard to define. In actual instability the appropriate treatment is either a stabilizing surgical procedure or a restraining orthopedic device.

## DIAGNOSING HYPERMOBILITY

The diagnosis of hypermobility in the Ehlers-Danlos and Marfan syndrome group is not difficult as long as the index of suspicion is present and the other physical findings are identified. The nine point scale mentioned above helps give an overall assessment of relative hypermobility. It is in the evaluation of local compensatory hypermobility that the difficulty exists. The diagnostic procedures are variations on regional segmental motion testing. In these procedures, one attempts to hold one segment and move the other in relation to it, comparing it with the perceived normals of the segments above and below the one suspected of hypermobility. Translatory motion challenges have been found to be the most effective (Fig. 6.6). With the lumbar

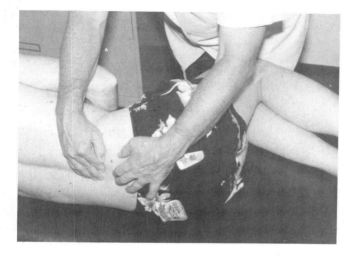

**Figure 6.6.** Hypermobility testing lateral recumbent.

spine, the patient can be in the lateral recumbent position while the operator monitors each vertebral segment. By grasping with the thumb and index finger two spinous processes, a to-and-fro lateral translatory movement can be introduced and compared above and below (Fig. 6.7). Using the same lateral recumbent position with the knees and hips flexed, the operator can monitor a given segment holding the superior one and then introducing an anteroposterior translatory movement by movement of the operator's thigh against the patient's knees (Fig. 6.8). Combined sidebending and rotation challenge can occur in the same position with the operator grasping the feet and ankles and lifting the extremities off the table (Fig. 6.9), and dropping them down below the table (Fig. 6.10), while monitoring the posterior elements of the lumbar vertebrae. Testing for hypermobility requires a great deal of practice and the judgment is highly individualistic. If one suspects significant segmental hypermobility, stress x-ray procedures in the flexion-extension and right and left sidebending modes should be used to assist in the diagnosis.

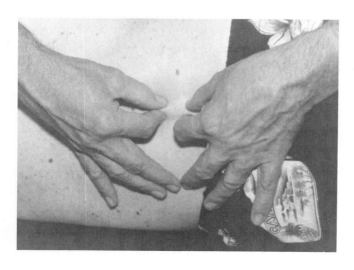

**Figure 6.7.** Hypermobility testing lateral translation.

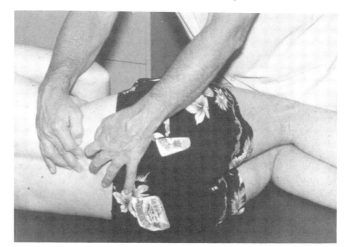

**Figure 6.8.** Hypermobility testing AP translation.

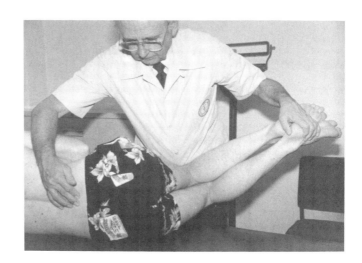

**Figure 6.9.** Hypermobility testing sidebending-rotation.

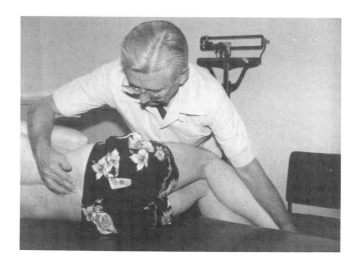

**Figure 6.10.** Hypermobility testing sidebending-rotation.

## CONCLUSION

While there is still a need for more research into the biomechanics of vertebral segmental motion and pathologies that might restrict vertebral motion, the concepts and methodologies described here will provide the practicing manual medicine clinician with sufficient accurate diagnostic information for treatment purposes, for accurate records, and for communicating with a colleague. The hallmark of structural diagnosis of restricted vertebral function is practice and experience.

# 7

# PRINCIPLES OF SOFT TISSUE AND ARTICULATORY (mobilization without impulse) TECHNIQUE

There are a great number of "hands-on" approaches to the body. They can all be classified as peripheral stimulation therapies. Chapter 4 mentioned soft tissue therapy procedures including Travell trigger points, Chapman's reflexes, acupuncture, and others. The soft tissue procedures to be described have had long acceptance and use in the field of manual medicine. Many of the procedures are the same as, or similar to, those found in traditional massage.

## DEFINITION

Soft tissue technique is defined as a "procedure directed towards tissues other than the skeleton while monitoring response and motion changes using diagnostic palpation. It usually involves lateral stretching, linear stretching, deep pressure, traction, and/or separation of muscle origin and insertion." (Glossary of Osteopathic Terminology, *J Am Osteopath Assoc. 80:552-567, 1981*)

## PURPOSE OF SOFT TISSUE TECHNIQUE

Soft tissue procedures are widely used in a combined diagnostic and therapeutic mode. They are frequently a prelude to other more definitive manual medicine procedures to the underlying articular structures. They prepare the soft tissues for other technique procedures. They are also employed as the only manual medicine intervention to achieve a specific therapeutic goal. These procedures have mechanical, circulatory, and neurological effects and are useful in both acute and chronic conditions. Soft tissue procedures can mechanically stretch the skin, fascia, and muscle tissues of the body to enhance their motion and pliability. These procedures are useful in encouraging circulation of fluid in and around the soft tissues of the musculoskeletal system, enhancing venous and lymphatic return, and decongesting parts of the body compromised by injury or a disease process. These same procedures can have a neurologic effect, particularly modifying muscle physiology to overcome hypertonicity and spasm. These neurological effects can be stimulatory or inhibitory depending upon how the procedure was applied. Another neurological effect is the relief of musculoskeletal pain following their use. This may result from the release of endogenous opioids and other neurohumoral substances. Another possible mechanism is the modulation of spinal reflex pathways by the stimulation of mechanoreceptors, proprioceptors, and nociceptors in the soft tissues.

Soft tissue procedures are also useful for their general "tonic" effect upon patients, particularly those who have been bedridden for any period of time due to illness or injury. They seem to enhance general physical tone and level of well-being. Since many of these procedures seem general in application, and result in various outcomes, the manual medicine practitioner must have a specific therapeutic goal in mind before instituting any soft tissue procedure. Once the objective is clear, the procedure can be adapted to fit the patient condition, patient location, and operator's strength and ability.

## TYPES OF SOFT TISSUE PROCEDURES

Soft tissue procedures are oriented toward the direction of a force being applied to the underlying muscle(s) (Fig. 7.1). A force at right angles to the long axis of the muscle is called *lateral stretch.* The force applied in the direction of the long axis of the muscle is called *linear or longitudinal stretch.* By apply-

ing a force in both directions along the long axis of a muscle we achieve *separation of origin and insertion.* If steady deep pressure is applied to a muscle close to its attachment to the bone, the procedure is called *deep pressure.* Although these procedures are described in relation to muscle and its fiber direction, remember that application of external force to the muscle area also involves skin, subcutaneous fascia, and the deep fascia surrounding muscle. All of these tissues are affected by soft tissue procedures.

## THERAPEUTIC PRINCIPLES OF SOFT TISSUE TECHNIQUE

As in all appropriate manual medicine procedures, the operator's body should be held in a posture that is comfortable and balanced to avoid undue strain or fatigue. The treatment table or bed should be at the appropriate height so that the operator need not bend forward unnecessarily (Fig. 7.2). The operator's stance should be relaxed with one foot slightly in front of the other so that the to-and-fro rocking of the operator's

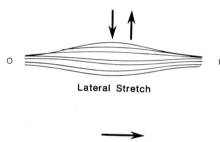

Lateral Stretch

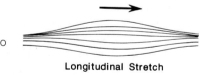

Longitudinal Stretch

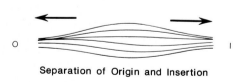

Separation of Origin and Insertion

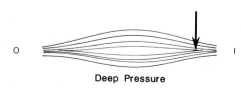

Deep Pressure

**Figure 7.1.    Soft tissue procedures.**

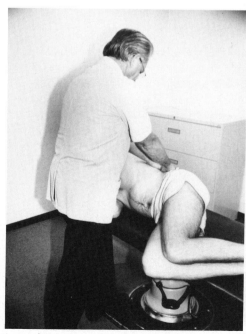

**Figure 7.2.    Operator's stance.**

body mass provides the force, not operator muscle activity.

The patient should be in a comfortable and relaxed position. If the prone position is used, the head should be turned toward the operator so that lateral force does not put undue strain on the cervicothoracic junction. If a lateral recumbent position is used, an appropriate pillow height should maintain the head and neck in the long axis of the trunk. It is useful to have the patient's feet and knees together with the knees and hips slightly flexed. This provides both comfort and stability to the patient. It is most important that the relationship of the patient and the operator be relaxed and synergistic.

The placement and use of the hands in soft tissue procedures becomes most important. These procedures use mainly the fingerpads, the thenar eminence of the hand, and the palmer aspect of the thumb. When the operator uses the fingerpads to engage the tissues, the distal interphalangeal joint flexion that occurs is a function of the flexor digitorum profundus (Fig. 7.3). Beginners in manual medicine have to practice

strengthening the profundus tendon flexor action in order to maintain appropriate application of force to soft tissues. The thenar eminence and palmer surface of the thumb can be laid along the long axis of muscle and used singly (Fig. 7.4), paired (Fig. 7.5), or with one hand reinforcing the other (Fig. 7.6). It is very important that the soft tissues be adequately and accurately engaged at the appropriate layer. In treating the erector spinae mass there are two common errors to be avoided. The first is pressure toward the spinous processes, instead of away from the spinous processes, on the side being treated. This causes compression of the erector spinae mass against the lateral side of the spinous process, is painful to the patient, and counterproductive. The second error is allowing the therapeutic hand to "snap over" an area of hypertonic muscle through failure of control at the muscle layer. Hand placement and control become most important.

The dosage of soft tissue procedures is modified by the rate, rhythm, and length of time of application, and, most importantly,

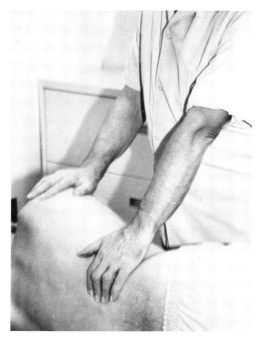

**Figure 7.3.    Soft tissue, finger pad contact.**

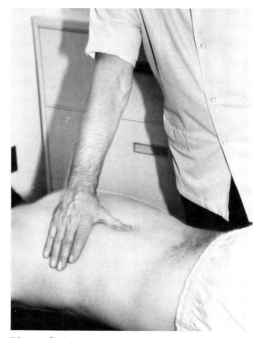

**Figure 7.4.    Single hand, soft tissue contact.**

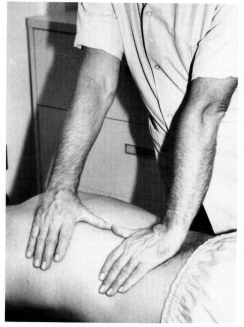

**Figure 7.5.   Paired hand, soft tissue contact.**

by the constant feedback from the tissues of the response obtained. Constant reassessment of the response is the hallmark of soft tissue procedures. The operator should continue until the desired response is obtained or stop as soon as it has been achieved. If the tissue response is not as anticipated, the procedure should be stopped and reassessment of the diagnosis and status of the patient should be made. Slow and steady soft tissue procedures appear to have inhibitory effects on the tissues. More rapid and vigorous applications of force appear to be stimulatory. The application of force is modified by the goal to be achieved and the response of the tissues. The operator must also be aware of other reactions within the patient in addition to those of the tissue being treated. Sometimes patients become quite agitated, other times they become very relaxed and almost euphoric. It must be remembered that although these procedures are passive, they are still fatiguing, and the length of treatment might well be modified by the response of the patient.

## SOFT TISSUE TECHNIQUES

### Cervical Spine

Procedure: Unilateral lateral stretch

1.  Patient is supine on table with operator on side of the table facing the patient (example left side) (Fig. 7.7).
2.  Operator's right hand stabilizes patient's forehead.
3.  Operator's left hand grasps the patient's right cervical paravertebral musculature with fingertips medial to the muscle mass and just lateral to the spinous processes.
4.  Lateral stretch is placed upon the cervical musculature by the operator's left hand pulling laterally and somewhat anteriorly with the operator's right hand maintaining the stability of the patient's head.
5.  Lateral stretch is applied and released rhythmically throughout the cervical musculature with particular

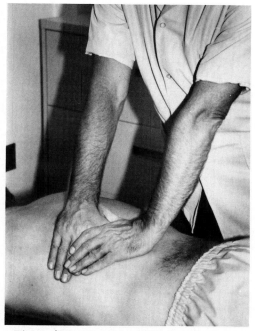

**Figure 7.6.   Combined hand, soft tissue contact.**

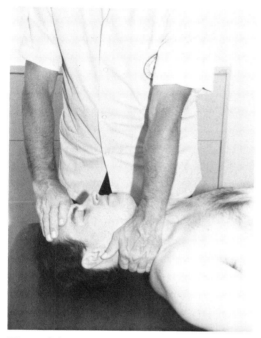

**Figure 7.7. Soft tissue, unilateral lateral stretch.**

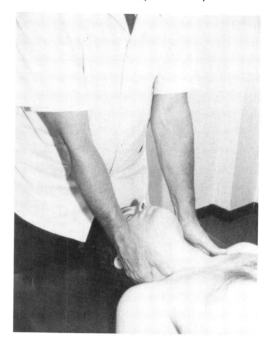

**Figure 7.8. Soft tissue, bilateral lateral stretch.**

reference to areas of increased muscle tone and soft tissue congestion.

6. The procedure can be varied to allow the patient's head to rotate toward the left during the application of force by the operator's left hand and a counter force can be applied by the operator's right hand in a "push-pull" manner.

7. The procedure can be repeated on the opposite side by having the operator now stand on the patient's right.

Procedure: Bilateral-lateral stretch

1. Patient is supine on table with operator standing at head of table (Fig. 7.8).

2. Operator's fingerpads contact the medial side of the cervical paravertebral musculature bilaterally.

3. The operator puts simultaneous lateral stretch on both sides of the cervical musculature, moving from above downward or below upward

and focusing upon side of greater tissue reaction and muscle hypertonicity.

Procedure: Long axis longitudinal stretch

1. Patient is supine with operator standing at head of table.

2. Operator's one hand cradles the skull with the index finger and thumb in contact with the insertion of the cervical musculature into the occiput and the chin held by the other hand (Fig. 7.9).

3. By the use of body weight, the operator puts long-axis extension (traction) in a cephalic direction and then releases.

4. Repeat as necessary.
   Caution: Too much traction is frequently counterproductive.

Procedure: Sub-occipital muscle deep pressure

1. Patient is supine with operator standing at head of table.

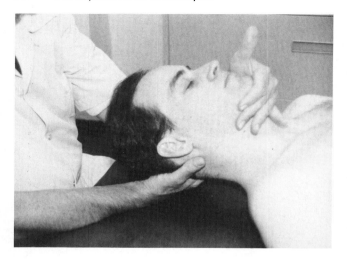

**Figure 7.9. Long-axis longitudinal stretch.**

2. Operator's fingertips of each hand contact the bony attachment of the deep cervical musculature at the suboccipital region.
3. By flexing the distal interphalangeal joints, the operator puts sustained deep pressure over the muscular attachment to the occipital bone (Fig. 7.10).
4. Pressure is applied on each side to achieve balance in tension and tone.
5. Pressure is released when bilateral relaxation occurs.

Procedure: Separation origin and insertion

1. Patient is supine with operator standing at head of table.
2. Operator's left hand is placed over the patient's occiput and controls head and neck position.
3. Operator's right hand is placed over the patient's right acromium process (Fig. 7.11).
4. Operator's left hand sidebends the head and neck to the left with some left rotation while right hand puts counterforce on the acromial proc-

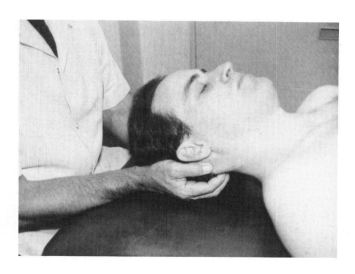

**Figure 7.10. Suboccipital muscle, deep pressure.**

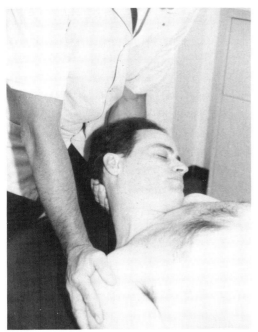

**Figure 7.11.  Separation of origin and insertion.**

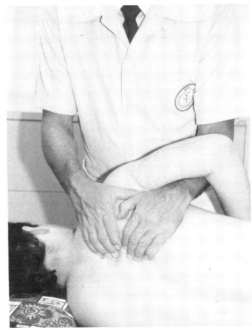

**Figure 7.12.  Lateral stretch, upper thoracic region.**

ess, separating the origin and insertion of the upper fibers of the trapezius.

5. By reversal of hand position the opposite side can be treated with the goal of symmetry of length and tone of each trapezius.

## Thoracic Spine

Procedure: Lateral stretch

1. Patient is in lateral recumbent position lying with involved side uppermost with operator standing and facing patient.

2. For upper thoracic region patient's right arm is draped over operator's left arm and fingerpads contact medial side of paravertebral musculature (Fig. 7.12).

3. Operator pulls thoracic paravertebral musculature laterally and releases in a rhythmical fashion.

4. A counterforce can be applied by the operator's right arm against the patient's right shoulder for additional leverage.

5. For midthoracic region the patient's right arm is held at the side of the body and the operator's right hand threads under the patient's arm. Again both fingerpads pull laterally in a rhythmical fashion on the thoracic paravertebral musculature (Fig. 7.13).

6. For rhomboid stretch the same body position as for upper thoracic spine but now fingerpads are in contact with vertebral border of scapula and the scapula is swept anterolaterally around the chest wall stretching in the direction of rhomboid fibers.

7. Repeat as necessary.

## Thoraco-lumbar Spine

Procedure: Lateral stretch

1. Patient lies in lateral recumbent position with involved side uppermost. Operator faces patient.

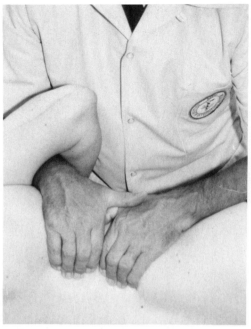

**Figure 7.13. Lateral stretch, midthoracic region.**

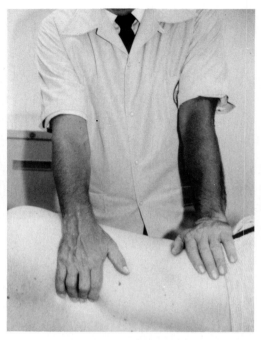

**Figure 7.14. Lateral stretch, midthoracic region.**

2. Operator's right hand grasps the thoracolumbar paravertebral muscle mass on the involved side (Fig. 7.14).
3. Operator's left hand is placed on patient's right ilium both to stabilize patient and as a counterforce.
4. Operator's right hand stretches paravertebral musculature laterally. Counterforce is applied by the left hand.
5. Repeat as necessary.
6. Variation sometimes allows patient's right arm to be flexed at the elbow and the operator's right hand to be threaded through before application to paravertebral musculature.

Procedure: Lateral and longitudinal stretch

1. Patient in lateral recumbent position with involved side uppermost. Operator faces patient.
2. Operator's right forearm is in patient's right axilla and right hand in

contact with paravertebral musculature.
3. Operator's left forearm is on superior aspect of the patient's right ilium with fingerpads in contact with paravertebral musculature.
4. Fingerpad contact of both hands stretches paravertebral musculature laterally while operator's forearms are separated, with right arm going cephalically and left going caudally, applying a longitudinal stretch.
5. Repeat as necessary.

Procedure: Prone lateral stretch

1. Patient lies prone on table with arms at side and face turned toward operator.
2. Operator stands at side of table.
3. Operator's thumbs and thenar eminences are placed on medial side of paravertebral musculature on involved side and lateral stretch is made rhythmically over involved areas (Fig. 7.15).

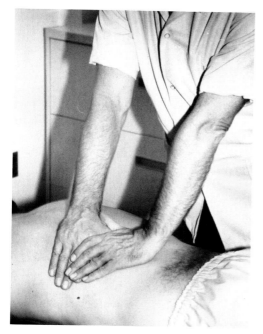

**Figure 7.15.    Prone, lateral stretch.**

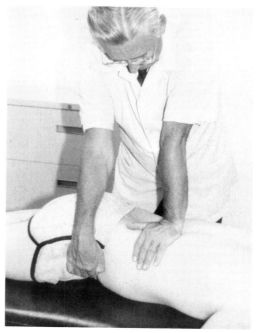

**Figure 7.16.    Prone, lateral stretch with counterforce.**

4.  A variation is using one hand on top of the other in a reinforced mode and applying lateral stretch.
5.  Another variation is to have the operator's right hand grasp the patient's right anterior superior iliac spine while the left thumb and thenar eminence puts lateral stretch on paravertebral musculature (Fig. 7.16). A counterforce can be applied by lifting the patient's right ilium.
6.  Repeat as necessary.

Procedure: Deep pressure

1.  Patient is prone on table.
2.  Operator places thumbs, or reinforced by hand, over area of hypertonic muscle attached to bone (Fig. 7.17).
3.  Steady pressure is applied in a ventral direction and sustained until muscle release is felt.
4.  Variation. The operator's olecronon process of the elbow can be

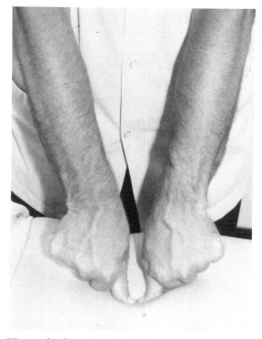

**Figure 7.17.    Deep inhibitory pressure with thumb.**

utilized as a contact point and body weight provides central direction pressure against hypertonic muscle (Fig. 7.18).

5.   Repeat as necessary.

### Gluteal Region

Procedure: Deep pressure

1.   Patient is in lateral recumbent position with involved side uppermost.
2.   Operator can stand in front or behind the patient.
3.   Reinforced thumbs are placed over hypertonic areas of gluteal musculature either near origin on the ilium, within the belly, or at insertion in greater trochanter (Fig. 7.19).
4.   Deep pressure is maintained until relaxation is felt.
5.   Variation can be the utilization of the olecronon process of the elbow as the contact point and body weight at the force (Fig. 7.20).
6.   Repeat as necessary.

### Lymphatic Pump

Procedure: Thoracic lymphatic pump

1.   Patient is supine on table with operator at head of table.
2.   Operator has both hands in contact with anterior aspect of the thoracic cage with heel of hand just below the clavicle (Fig. 7.21).
3.   Patient is instructed to inhale and then exhale.
4.   During exhalation phase the operator puts oscillatory compression on chest cage.
5.   At end of exhalation patient is instructed to breathe in while operator holds chest wall in exhalation position for a momentary period of time.
6.   Operator rapidly releases compression on chest during patient's inhalation effort.
7.   Repeat 2 through 6 several applications.

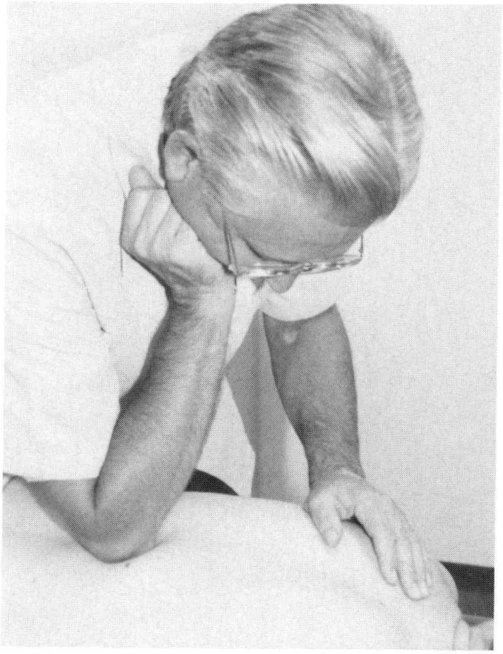

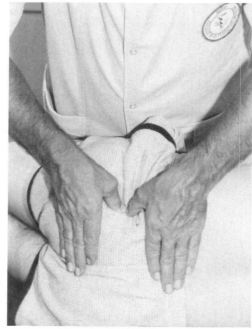

**Figure 7.18.   Deep inhibitory pressure with elbow.**

**Figure 7.19.   Deep inhibitory pressure with thumbs.**

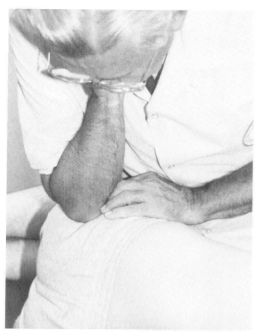

**Figure 7.20. Deep inhibitory pressure gluteal region.**

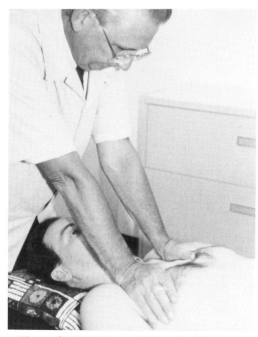

**Figure 7.21. Thoracic lymphatic pump.**

Procedure: Thoracic lymphatic pump (unilateral variation)

1. Patient is supine on table with operator at side of table.
2. Operator's left arm grasps the patient's right upper extremity.
3. Operator's right hand is in contact with right thoracic cage of patient (Fig. 7.22).
4. During inhalation operator puts traction on patient's right upper extremity.
5. During exhalation phase, traction on upper extremity is released, and operator puts oscillatory force against thoracic cage during exhalation effort.
6. Operator's right hand maintains compression on chest wall during initial phase of inhalation and gives rapid release, simultaneously cephalically lifting on patient's right upper extremity.
7. Repeat as necessary.
8. A variation can also be done in the lateral recumbent position with the treated side being uppermost. Steps 2-6 are repeated as necessary (Fig. 7.23).

Procedure: Lymphatic pump lower extremity

1. Patient is supine with operator at end of table.
2. Operator grasps dorsum of both feet with each hand.
3. Operator takes feet into plantar flexion (Fig. 7.24).
4. Operator applies oscillatory movement in a pedad direction and notes oscillatory wave of lower extremities to trunk.
5. Operator's hands now grasp ball of patient's foot and take foot into dorsi flexion (Fig. 7.25).
6. An oscillatory cephalic movement is placed on dorsiflexed feet.
7. Repeat each direction as necessary.

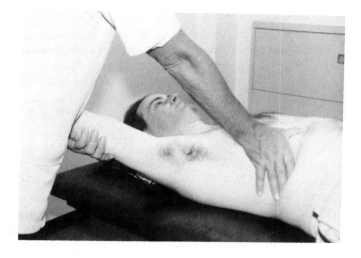

**Figure 7.22. Unilateral thoracic lymphatic pump.**

Procedure: Lymphatic pump upper extremity

1. Patient is supine and operator at head of table.
2. Patient raises both hands above head and operator grasps each wrist (Fig. 7.26).
3. Operator puts long-axis extension on patient's upper extremities.
4. Cephalic oscillatory movement is applied noting response in thoracic cage.

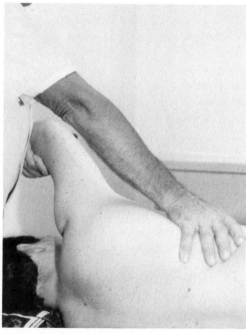

**Figure 7.23. Unilateral thoracic lymphatic pump, lateral recumbent.**

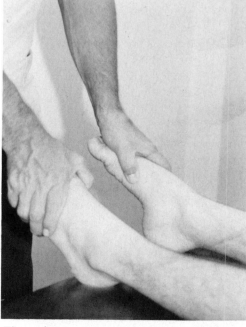

**Figure 7.24. Lower extremity, lymphatic pump, plantar flexion.**

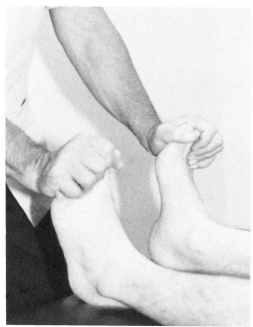

**Figure 7.25. Lower extremity, lymphatic pump, dorsiflexion.**

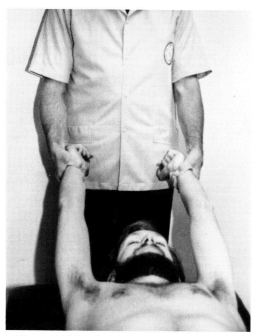

**Figure 7.26. Lymphatic pump, bilateral upper extremity.**

## Miscellaneous Soft Tissue Techniques

Procedure: Pectoral release

1. Patient is supine and operator at head of table.
2. Operator's two hands, particularly middle fingers, grasp inferior border of pectoral muscle of each side of patient (Fig. 7.27).
3. Cephalic traction is applied by the operator's hands on the inferior aspect of the pectoral muscles bilaterally.
4. Release of muscle tension is the response to be elicited.
5. Watch thorax and abdomen for change from thoracic to abdominal breathing.

Procedure: Diaphragmatic release supine technique

1. Patient is supine on table with operator standing on one side.
2. Operator's index finger and tips of other fingers are applied under the costal arch along the inferior surface of the diaphragm.
3. Operator's left hand contacts lower rib cage (Fig. 7.28).
4. As patient exhales, operator's right hand goes cephalically and deep, maintaining pressure on diaphragm and holds during next inhalation.
5. Operator's left hand folds thorax over the operator's right hand.
6. Several respiratory cycles are encouraged and release of diaphragmatic tension by palpating right hand is end point. Repeat on other side as necessary.

Procedure: Diaphragmatic release patient sitting

1. Patient sits on edge of table with operator behind.
2. Operator's fingerpads make contact along inferior surface of diaphragm just below costal arch on each side.

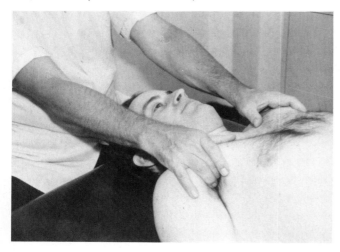

**Figure 7.27.  Pectoral release.**

3.  Patient slumps against operator with forward bending of the patient's trunk (Fig. 7.29).
4.  Operator maintains cephalic pressure on the inferior aspect of diaphragm. Exhalation effort is encouraged and maintained by fingertip compression until diaphragm is released.

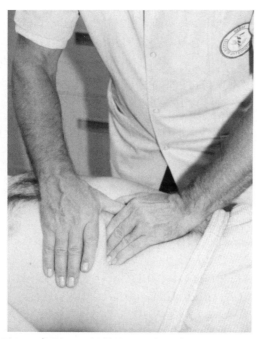

**Figure 7.28.  Diaphragmatic release, supine.**

5.  A variation can be used with the operator sitting in front of the patient. Thumbs are in contact with inferior surface of diaphragm below costal arch (Fig. 7.30). Patient slumps forward on operator's thumbs and exhalation effort is followed with upward pressure of operator's thumbs. Repeat until diaphragmatic release is obtained (Fig. 7.31).

Procedure: Pelvic diaphragm

1.  Patient is in lateral recumbent position, involved side uppermost, hips and knees flexed.
2.  Operator stands in front of patient and extended fingers of right hand are placed on medial side of ischial tuberosity (Fig. 7.32).
3.  Fingers are moved slowly along lateral side of ischiorectal fossa until tips of fingers in contact with pelvic diaphragm sensing tension.
4.  During exhalation, fingers flow more cephalically and hold as patient repeats inhalation cycle.
5.  When diaphragm has been released, it moves away from palpating fingers freely during exhalation and into fingers during inhalation.
6.  Repeat on opposite side as necessary.

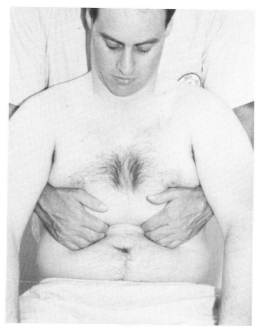

**Figure 7.29.** **Diaphragmatic release, sitting.**

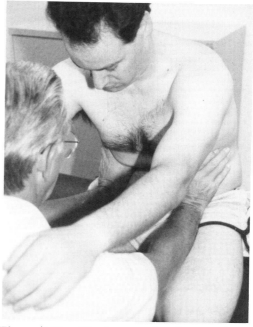

**Figure 7.31.** **Diaphragmatic release, exhalation effort.**

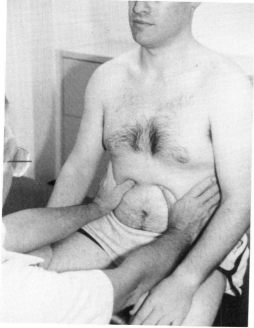

**Figure 7.30.** **Diaphragmatic release, thumb placement.**

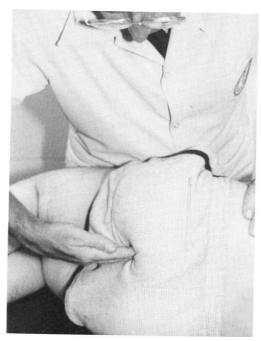

**Figure 7.32.** **Pelvic diaphragm, release.**

Procedure: Mesenteric release

1. Patient is supine on table with operator standing at side.
2. Operator places both hands on each
   side of the anterior abdomen.
3. Operator applies clockwise and
   counterclockwise rotation to the anterior abdominal wall with some abdominal compression (Fig. 7.33).
4. Sensation of release of underlying
   abdominal contents is end point.

Procedure: Mesenteric release prone
position

1. Patient is prone on table in knee-
   chest position.
2. Operator stands at side or head of
   table.
3. Operator places both hands over
   lower abdomen just above pubic
   bones (Fig. 7.34).
4. Operator's hands lift abdominal
   contents out of pelvis in slow oscillatory fashion until release is felt.

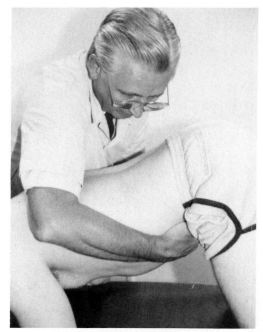

**Figure 7.34.   Mesenteric release, prone.**

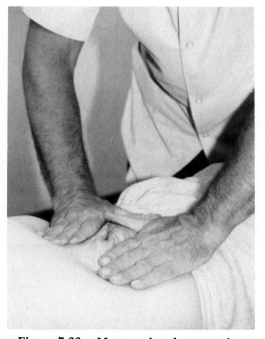

**Figure 7.33.   Mesenteric release, supine.**

## ARTICULATORY PROCEDURES

Articulatory procedures are nothing more
than an extension of motion testing procedures. Like soft tissue procedures, they are
repetitively applied and modified by the response of the tissues. In articulatory procedures one's goal is to increase the range of
motion in an articulation with some
hypomobility. Repetitive, oscillatory efforts
are applied by the operator against the resistant barrier in the arc or plane of restricted movement in the articulation.
These procedures require good visualiza-
tion of the articulation and the range and
arc of movement which is restricted. The
operator must constantly monitor the
endfeel of the motion introduced with the
goal of restoring the endfeel toward the
"normal". These procedures are also called
mobilization without impulse and have long
been part of manual medicine, particularly
as practiced by physiotherapists. A series of
gradations in mobilizing effort can be made
from one to four depending upon the
amount of motion introduced (one being

limited and four being maximum) and with increasing degrees of arc of movement. During articulatory procedures, one is interested in both the endfeel, and the quality of movement during the range. The goal is a smooth range of movement in the multiple planes possible within the treated joint. These procedures can be applied regionally to a group of segments or individually to a single articulation.

The purposes of articulatory technique are to restore range of motion and to stretch out the connective tissue surrounding the restricted articulation. One also anticipates modulation of neural activity both to relieve pain and to restore more normal reflex activity to the nerves and spinal cord segments related to the area. The admonitions given for soft tissue technique apply to articulatory technique, the relaxation of the patient, the relaxation and control by the operator, and the localization of the procedure to the appropriate area. These techniques are described as direct action (force applied against the restrictive barrier) and the activating force is extrinsic (by the operator in an oscillatory and rhythmic mode).

## CONCLUSION

Soft tissue and articulatory procedures are useful in a wide variety of acute to chronic patient conditions. They are applicable to all regions of the body. They are useful as independent procedures or can be combined with other manual medicine procedures. Experience in palpating the tissue response to both soft tissue and articulatory procedures is necessary to properly utilize them for the appropriate diagnosis.

# 8

# PRINCIPLES OF MUSCLE ENERGY TECHNIQUE

In the evolution of manual medicine a great deal of emphasis has been placed upon the osseous skeleton and its articulations. The heritage of the "bonesetters" gave all practitioners of manipulation the aura of "putting a bone back in place." The muscle component of the musculoskeletal system did not receive as much attention by manual medicine practitioners. Early techniques did speak of muscle relaxation with soft tissue procedures but specific manipulative approaches to muscle appear to be a 20th century phenomena. In osteopathic medicine, Dr. T. J. Ruddy developed techniques which he described as resistive duction. A series of muscle contractions against resistance were accomplished by the patient with a tempo approximating the pulse rate. He used these techniques in the cervical spine and around the orbit in his practice as an ophthalmologist-otorhinolaryngologist.

Dr. Fred L. Mitchell, Sr. is acknowledged as the father of the system which we now call muscle energy technique. He took many of Dr. Ruddy's principles and incorporated them in a system of manual medicine procedures which could be applicable to any region of the body or any particular articulation. Dr. Mitchell was a great student of anatomy and gifted osteopathic physician. He was a skilled practitioner and an excellent teacher who gave much time and effort to the educational programs of the

American Academy of Osteopathy. Early in his career, he lectured and demonstrated to large audiences, but it was later in small group tutorials that some of his most effective teaching occurred.

## WHAT IS MUSCLE ENERGY TECHNIQUE

Muscle energy technique is a manual medicine treatment procedure which involves the voluntary contraction of patient muscle in a precisely controlled direction, at varying levels of intensity, against a distinctly executed counterforce applied by the operator. Muscle energy procedures have wide application and are classified as active techniques in which the patient contributes the corrective force. The activating force is classified as intrinsic. The patient is responsible for the dosage applied.

Muscle energy technique has many clinical uses. It can be used to lengthen a shortened, contractured, or spastic muscle; to strengthen a physiologically weakened muscle or group of muscles; to reduce localized edema and relieve passive congestion (the muscles are the pump of the lymphatic and venous systems); and to mobilize an articulation with restricted mobility. The function of any articulation in the body which can be moved by voluntary muscle action, either directly or indirectly, can be influenced by muscle energy procedures. The amount of patient effort may vary from a minimal muscle twitch to a maximal muscle contraction. The duration of the effort may vary from a fraction of a second to a sustained effort lasting several seconds.

## TYPES OF MUSCULAR CONTRACTION

There are four different types of muscle contraction in muscle energy technique. They are

1. Isometric
2. Concentric isotonic
3. Eccentric isotonic
4. "Isolytic"

With an isometric contraction the distance between the origin and the insertion of the muscle is maintained at a constant length. A fixed tension develops in the muscle as the patient contracts the muscle against an equal counterforce applied by the operator preventing shortening of the muscle from the origin to the insertion.

A concentric isotonic contraction occurs when the muscle tension causes the origin and insertion to approximate.

An eccentric isotonic contraction is one in which there is muscle tension which allows the origin and insertion to separate. In fact the muscle actually lengthens.

An "isolytic" contraction is a nonphysiological event in which the contraction of the patient attempts to be concentric with approximation of the origin and insertion but an external force applied by the operator occurs in the opposite direction.

With the elbow as an example, let us see how each of these contractions operates. With the patient's elbow flexed, the operator holds the distal forearm and shoulder. The patient is instructed to bring the wrist to the shoulder while the operator holds the wrist and shoulder in the same relative position. The force inserted by the patient's contracting biceps has an equal counterforce applied by the operator. This results in isometric contraction of the biceps

brachii muscle. Muscle tone increases but the origin and insertion do not approximate.

A concentric isotonic contraction occurs during the process of holding a weight in the hand and bringing it to the shoulder by increasing the flexion at the elbow. The concentric isotonic contraction of the biceps brachii increases muscle tone, and the origin and insertion are approximated.

An eccentric isotonic contraction occurs when the weight which had been brought to the shoulder is now returned to the starting position by increasing the amount of elbow extension. There is tone within the biceps brachii allowing the origin and insertion to separate in a smooth and easy fashion as the elbow extends and the weight is taken away from the shoulder.

An "isolytic" contraction occurs when the elbow is flexed at 90° and the patient attempts to increase the flexion of the elbow by bringing the hand to the shoulder while the operator holds the shoulder and wrist, forcefully extending the elbow against the effort of the patient to concentrically contract the biceps brachii. An isolytic procedure must be used cautiously to lengthen a severely contracted or hypertonic muscle because rupture of musculotendinous junction, insertion of tendon into bone, or muscle fibers themselves can occur.

## MUSCLE PHYSIOLOGY AND PRINCIPLES

It is beyond the scope of this volume to describe all of the elements of muscle physiology that underlie muscle energy technique. The reader is referred to a physiology text for those details. Knowledge of a few principles of muscle physiology are necessary for the manual medicine practitioner to use these techniques appropriately.

Isometric muscle energy techniques primarily reduce the tone in a hypertonic muscle and reestablish its normal resting length. Shortened and hypertonic muscles are frequently identified as the major component of restricted motion of an articulation or group of articulations. The length and tone of a muscle are in large measure controlled by the fusiform motor system to the intrafusal fibers. The gamma system provides the neural control for this fusimotor mechanism and some people have explained muscle hypertonicity as the result of gamma gain. The reflexes are somewhat complex (Fig. 8.1). Afferents from both Golgi tendon receptors and gamma afferents from spindle receptors feed back to the cord; gamma efferents return to the intrafusal fibers resetting their resting length; and this changes the resting length of the extrafusal fibers of the muscle. There is a slight delay after the muscle isometric contraction before it can be taken to a new resting length. Simply put, after an isometric contraction, a hypertonic muscle can be passively lengthened to a new resting length.

When using isotonic procedures, two other muscle physiological principles are considered. The first is the classic law of reciprocal innervation and inhibition (Fig. 8.2). When an agonist muscle contracts and shortens, its antagonist must relax and lengthen so that motion can occur under the influence of the agonist muscle. The contraction of the agonist reciprocally inhibits its antagonist allowing smooth motion. The harder the agonist contracts, the more inhibition occurs in the antagonist, in effect relaxing the antagonist. The second principle of isotonic muscle energy technique is increasing the tonus and improving the performance of a muscle that is too weak for its

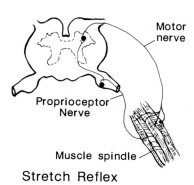

**Stretch Reflex**

**Figure 8.1.   Muscle spindle reflexes.**

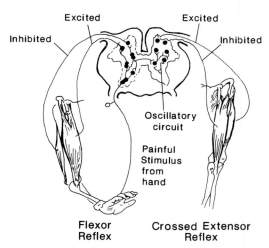

**Figure 8.2.   Reciprocal inhibitation reflex arc.**

musculoskeletal function. As a series of repetitions of isotonic concentric contraction occur in the muscle, against progressively increasing resistance, extrafusal muscle fiber participation in the contraction increases. Isotonic muscle energy procedures reduce hypertonicity in a shortened antagonist and increase the strength of the agonist.

All of these muscle contractions influence the surrounding fascia, connective tissue ground substance, and interstitial fluids, and alter muscle physiology by reflex mechanisms. Fascial length and tone is altered by muscle contraction. Alteration in fascia influences not only its biomechanical function, but also the biochemical and immunological functions. The patient's muscle effort requires energy and the metabolic process of muscle contraction results in carbon dioxide, lactic acid, and other metabolic waste products which must be transported and metabolized. It is for this reason that the patient will frequently experience some increase in muscle soreness within the first 12 to 36 hours following a muscle energy technique treatment. Muscle energy procedures provide safety for the patient since the activating force is intrinsic and the dosage can be easily controlled by the patient, but it must be remembered that this effort comes at a price. It is easy for the inexperienced practitioner to overdo these procedures, and, in essence, overdose the patient.

## ELEMENTS OF MUSCLE ENERGY PROCEDURES

1. Patient-active muscle contraction
2. Controlled joint position
3. Muscle contraction in a specific direction
4. Operator-applied distinct counter-force
5. Controlled contraction intensity

These five elements are essential for any successful muscle energy procedure. The patient is told to contract a muscle while the operator holds an articulation or portion of the musculoskeletal system in a specific position. The patient is instructed to contract in a certain direction with a specified amount of force, either in ounces or pounds. The operator applies a counterforce; one that prevents any approximation of the origin insertion (making the procedure isometric), one to allow yielding (for a concentric isotonic contraction), or one that overpowers the muscle effort (resulting in a "isolytic" procedure).

The common errors patients make during muscle energy procedures are that they contract too hard; contract in the wrong direction; sustain the contraction for too short a time; or do not relax appropriately following the muscle contraction. The most common operator errors are not accurately controlling the joint position in relation to the barrier to movement; not providing the counterforce in the correct direction; not giving the patient accurate instructions; and moving to a new joint position too soon after the patient stops contracting. The operator must wait for the refractory period following an isometric contraction before the muscle can be stretched to a new resting length.

Clinical experience has shown that three to five repetitions of muscle effort for 3 to 7 seconds each are effective in accomplishing the therapeutic goal. Experience will tell the operator when longer contraction or more repetitions are needed.

### Comparison

| Compare | |
| --- | --- |
| ISOMETRIC | ISOTONIC |
| 1. Careful positioning | 1. Careful positioning |
| 2. Light to moderate contraction | 2. Hard to maximal contraction |
| 3. Unyielding counterforce | 3. Counterforce permits controlled |
| 4. Relaxation after contraction | 4. Relaxation after contraction |
| 5. Repositioning | 5. Repositioning |

The isometric contraction need not be too hard. It is important that it be sustained and that the muscle length be maintained as nearly isometric as possible. Following the sustained but light contraction, a momentary pause should occur before the operator stretches the shortened and contracted muscle to a new resting length. Isotonic procedures require forceful contraction by the patient since the operator wants to recruit the firing of muscle fibers and make them work as hard as possible, resulting in relaxation of the antagonist. The muscle should contract over its total range. After any muscle energy procedure the patient should relax before repositioning against a new resistant barrier.

## MUSCLE ENERGY TECHNIQUES

In succeeding chapters muscle energy techniques will be described for specific regions. Here we shall use the elbow as an example. Assume that there is restriction of elbow movement into full extension, i.e., the elbow is flexed. One etiology for restricted elbow extension is hypertonicity and shortening of the biceps brachii muscle. The operator might choose an isometric muscle energy technique to treat this condition as follows:

1. Patient sits comfortably on the treatment table with the operator standing in front.
2. Operator grasps patient's shoulder with one hand and distal forearm with the other hand (Fig. 8.3).
3. Operator extends the elbow until the first barrier to extension movement is felt.
4. Operator instructs the patient to attempt to bring the forearm to the shoulder utilizing a few ounces of force in a sustained manner.
5. Operator provides equal counterforce to the patient's effort.
6. Following 3-7 seconds of contraction the patient is instructed to stop contracting and relax.
7. Operator waits until the patient is completely relaxed after the contracting effort and extends the elbow until a new resistant barrier is felt.
8. Steps 2-7 are repeated three to five times until full elbow extension is restored.

The restriction of elbow extension might also be the result of length and strength imbalance between the biceps muscle as the elbow flexor and the triceps muscle as the elbow extender. A weak triceps could prevent full elbow extension. The operator might choose an isotonic muscle energy technique to treat this condition as follows:

1. Patient sitting on table with operator in front.
2. Operator grasps shoulder and distal forearm and takes elbow into full flexion.
3. Patient is instructed to extend the elbow with as much effort as possible, perhaps several pounds (Fig. 8.4).
4. The operator provides a yielding counterforce which allows the elbow to slowly but steadily extend throughout its maximal range (Fig. 8.5).
5. Operator returns elbow to full flexion and the patient repeats the con-

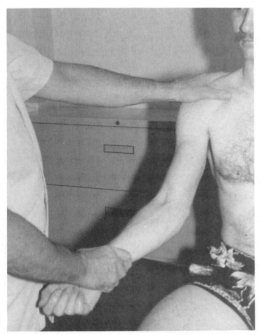

**Figure 8.3. Isometric muscle contraction, biceps.**

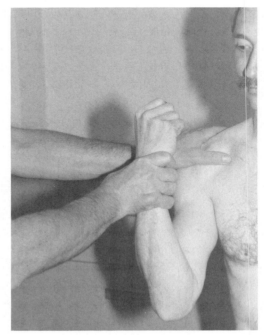

**Figure 8.4. Isotonic muscle energy technique, triceps.**

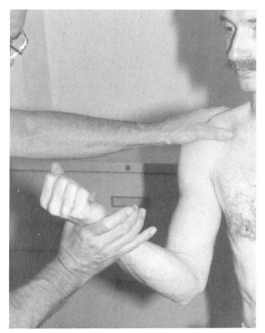

**Figure 8.5.   Elbow extension.**

traction of the triceps to extend the elbow, but this time the operator provides increasing resistance to elbow extension.

6. Several repetitive efforts are accomplished with the operator providing increasing resistance each time and with the patient endeavoring to take the elbow through full extension with each effort.

7. Approximately three to five repetitions are usually necessary to achieve full elbow extension.

In any of these muscle energy procedures, it is important to accurately assess the resistant barrier. With an isometric technique the first barrier sensed must be the point where the careful joint position is held by the operator. If the operator "crashes into" the muscle resistant barrier in positioning the joint, an increase in the muscle hypertonicity will result, just the opposite of the desired therapeutic effort. Secondly, when using these procedures in a joint with multiple planes of movement available, each motion barrier must be engaged in the same fashion. In the vertebral column with motion restriction around and along three different axes, precision in the engagement of the restrictive barrier is essential for therapeutic effectiveness.

Successful muscle energy technique can be assured if the operator will constantly keep in mind the following three words:

Control
Balance
Localization

Both the operator and patient must be balanced and the operator must be in control of the localization against the resistant barrier. There must be continued control of the muscle effort by the patient and the yielding or unyielding counterforce by the operator. Each element is essential with each effort during the procedure.

In this author's opinion, muscle energy is one of the most valuable forms of manual medicine therapy because many therapeutic effects result from a single procedure and the procedures are physiologically and anatomically quite safe. It is possible to achieve increased joint movement, normalization of muscle strength and length, stretch of shortened fascia, and removal of passive congestion, all during a single procedure. Not only have you used muscle effort to move a joint, but you have restored more normal physiology to the muscle.

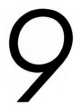

# 9

# PRINCIPLES OF HIGH-VELOCITY, LOW-AMPLITUDE THRUST TECHNIQUE (Mobilization with Impulse)

High-velocity, low-amplitude thrust technique is one of the oldest and most widely used forms of manual medicine. The scientific advisory committee of the International Federation of Manual Medicine, during its work in the 1980s, recommended the term *mobilization with impulse* to designate this form of manual therapy. Previously, the term *manipulation* was used to designate mobilization procedures with an operator-applied extrinsic thrusting force. It was felt that the term manipulation would be better applied to the "therapeutic use of the hands" rather than designating a specific therapeutic method. These procedures have long been deemed the treatment of choice for the "manipulable lesion". Terms such as "joint lock", "joint blockage", and "chiropractic subluxation", all emphasize alteration in articular function.

The use of an extrinsic applied force was found to be useful in overcoming restricted articular movement. Despite recent developments in manual medicine procedures (e.g., muscle energy technique, functional and indirect technique, myofascial release, craniosacral technique, etc.), high-velocity, low-amplitude thrust remains one of the most frequently used forms of manual medicine. Because it is commonly used, there is the danger of inappropriate usage yielding poor or no therapeutic result and

the risk of complications. As with all therapeutic interventions, these procedures should be applied after an appropriate diagnosis and in a proper manner.

## JOINT PLAY

Mennell is credited with contributing the concept of joint play to manual medicine. He defines joint play as movement within a synovial joint that is independent of, and cannot be introduced by, voluntary muscle contraction. The movements are small (less than 1/8 inch in any plane), with a precise range that depends upon the contour of the opposing joint surfaces. These joint-play movements are deemed essential for the normal, pain-free, non-restricted, movement of the particular articulation. If these movements are absent, normal voluntary movements are restricted and frequently painful. Mennell defines joint dysfunction as loss of joint-play movement that cannot be recovered by the action of voluntary muscle, i.e., joint dysfunction is loss of joint play. These principles apply to all synovial joints and are applicable in both the spine and the extremities. Mennell's diagnostic system tests for normal joint play movements in each articulation, and introduces therapeutic joint manipulation to restore movement and function. Mennell's ten rules of therapeutic manipulation are

1. Patient must be relaxed.
2. Therapist must be relaxed. Therapeutic grasp must be painless, firm, and protective.
3. One joint is mobilized at a time.
4. One movement in a joint is restored at a time.
5. In performance of movement, one aspect of joint is moved upon the other which is stabilized.
6. Extent of movement is not greater than that assessed in the same joint on opposite unaffected limb.
7. No forceful or abnormal movement must ever be used.
8. The manipulative movement is a sharp thrust, with *velocity*; to result in approximately 1/8" gapping at the joint.
9. Therapeutic movement occurs when all of the *"slack"* in the joint has been taken up.
10. No therapeutic maneuver is done in the presence of joint or bone inflammation or disease (heat, redness, swelling, etc.).

These ten rules are applicable to all procedures described as high-velocity, low-amplitude thrust techniques or mobilization with impulse.

## THEORIES OF JOINT DYSFUNCTION

There have been many theories proposed for the cause of joint dysfunction, and the therapeutic effect of mobilization with impulse. These theories have focused on alteration in the relationship of the opposing joint surfaces, the articular capsules and associated meniscoids, and, more recently, upon neural mechanisms from the mechanoreceptors and nociceptors of the articulation, and their associated neural effects on segmentally related muscle function. At this time, all of these are considered working hypotheses. The joint surface theories are "lack of tracking" of opposing joint surfaces and "hitching within the joint". Some have suggested a change in the thixotropic prop-

erty of the synovial fluid which makes it more "sticky". An articular capsular theory postulates that a fringe of synovium might be caught between two opposing surfaces. Many authors have found meniscoids in the apophyseal joints of the spine. It seems reasonable that they might become entrapped between the two opposing joint surfaces, but to date this has not been demonstrated and it remains controversial. More recently it has been postulated that stress on the capsule of the involved joint alters the afferent nerve traffic from the type one mechanoreceptors so that central control of motion cannot determine the joint's spatial relationship. This alteration in neural control is postulated to affect the length and tone of the segmentally related muscles, further restricting normal joint movement.

There is some research evidence on the effect of a high-velocity, low-amplitude thrusting procedure. It has been demonstrated that a "cavitation" phenomena occurs at the time of the "audible joint." Radiographically, a negative shadow which appears to have the density of nitrogen is seen within the joint. This gas shadow is present for a variable period of time, usually less than 20 minutes. The cavitation phenomena suggests that the synovial fluid changes from a liquid to a gaseous state. Whether or not this influences the "stickiness" of the synovial fluid is unknown. A second phenomena has been observed in the segmentally related musculature of a spinal apophyseal joint undergoing a thrusting procedure. Following the procedure there is temporary electrical silence of the segmental muscles, with a refractory period before electrical activity returns. The hypothesis is that the segmentally related muscles have more normal function after the thrusting procedure, and thus contribute to the positive therapeutic response. Despite the fact that more research is needed, clinical experience shows an area of joint dysfunction (somatic dysfunction) for which mobilization with impulse technique appears to be effective.

### Indications for the Use of Mobilization with Impulse

These procedures appear to be most effective in somatic dysfunction when the restriction is in and closely around the joint itself, the so-called "short restrictors". They are usually applied as precisely as possible to a single joint level and for specific joint motion loss. Although Mennell states that a therapeutic procedure should occur in only one plane, it is possible to influence all three planes of vertebral movement simultaneously by specific localization and leverage application. These procedures appear to be much more effective in subacute and chronic conditions than in acute somatic dysfunction. While most are designed for a single joint and its motion loss, some of the procedures can be applied in a regional fashion. The procedures advocated by Zink, for use with his respiratory-circulatory model, are designed to mobilize regions of the body to enhance fluid circulation, not to overcome a specific joint restriction. The difference between specific and nonspecific mobilization with impulse lies with the principle of localization and locking described below.

High-velocity, low-amplitude thrusting procedures are used in direct and exaggeration methods. The most common usage is direct, with engagement of the restrictive barrier and thrusting through the barrier to achieve more normal joint motion. Some authors advocate the exaggeration method (also called "rebound thrust") in which the thrust is against the normal physiological barrier in the direction opposite the motion loss. This author uses only the direct method, and would use something other than an exaggeration thrust, if a direct action thrust was not possible. The activating force is extrinsic, a thrusting procedure by the operator. Other assisting forces are gravity (patient seated or standing versus recumbency) and patient respiratory efforts, both for relaxation and for influence upon joint position desired.

### PRINCIPLES OF TECHNIQUE APPLICATION

The first principle is *joint gapping*. All thrusting procedures result in gapping of the joint, which requires that the operator know the anatomical joint contour and the type of movement possible at that articulation. The gapping can be in the plane of the joint, at right angles to the plane, or with joint distraction. With any successful thrusting procedure there is some element of joint distraction and gapping. It is this joint gapping that appears to result in the audible joint pop or click, but it must be remembered that the production of joint noise is not the therapeutic goal. In fact, Kimberly states that the goal of a successful thrusting procedure is "painless and noiseless restoration of maximum joint function."

*Localization* is the second principle of successful thrusting procedures. Localization limits the thrusting procedure to the joint needing treatment; other joints do receive the mobilizing impulse. This relates to Mennell's principle of holding one bone of the articulation and moving the other bone in relation to it. Localization involves the application of the principle of levers and locking. Levers are classified as short or long. The short lever is one in which a portion of one vertebra (spinous process) is held firmly while force is applied to a bony prominence of the adjacent vertebra (spinous process, transverse process, mamillary process); the force is applied with sufficient velocity to move one segment on the other. Long levers involve the use of either one of the extremities or multiple segments within the vertebral column in a "locking" maneuver. Long levers have the advantages of reducing the required force and increasing the distance through which the force travels. Long lever technique requires precise localization and limitation of force.

Establishing a long lever in the vertebral column involves the principles of "locking". A ligamentous lock occurs when the spine is sufficiently forward-bent to put maximum tension on the posterior ligamentous structures surrounding the articulation. A joint lock occurs when the spine is backward-bent with engagement of the posterior apophyseal joints. Both of these maneuvers reduce vertebral mobility. A third principle involves the introduction of concept three of normal vertebral motion in which introduction of movement in one direction reduces vertebral motion in all other directions. The introduction of type I vertebral movement (sidebending and rotation to opposite sides) will restrict movement of the vertebrae as far up or down the vertebral column as the motion is introduced. In locking maneuvers, the goal is to reduce all movement above and below the joint level to be treated. One does not wish to "lock" the segmental level to be treated, but rather to localize to that level and its restrictive barrier. For example, if L3 is dysfunctional in relation to L4, a locking procedure will be introduced from above downward to L3, and from below upward to L4 leaving the L3, 4 joint(s) "free". The L3, 4 level must have sufficient slack remaining so that the restrictive barrier to movement can be appropriately engaged, and the extrinsic thrust applied through the elastic barrier to accomplish mobilization. If the L3, 4 level is "locked" the articulation will not move. Frequently excessive force is applied to a "locked" localized joint in an attempt to overcome poor localization.

There is another principle of localization that is most useful—the introduction of convexities in two different planes localized to the segment to be treated. The first convexity to be introduced is either forward-bending or backward-bending of the body, to introduce localization to the forward-bending or backward-bending restrictor of the vertebra to be treated. The goal is to place the segment under treatment at the apex of the convexity introduced. For example, if L1 has forward-bending restriction in relation to L2, forward-bending of the trunk is introduced from above downward through the thoracic spine down to

L1. Flexion of the lower extremities, pelvis, and lumbar spine from below upward is introduced up to L2. The L1, L2 interspace becomes the apex of the forward-bending curve introduced. If the segment to be treated is in the upper to midthoracic region less forward-bending is introduced from above downward and more from below upward, and vice versa for segments below L1, 2. The second convexity to be introduced is that of sidebending to introduce a convexity right or left. If in our example of L1, 2, the sidebending and rotation restrictions coupled to the right side, sidebending to the right is introduced in order to establish a convexity of the thoracolumbar spine to the left with the apex of the convexity introduced to occur at the L1-L2 interspace. It is usually helpful to introduce both of these convexities not only by forward-bending—backward-bending, or sidebending right or left, but also by the use of translatory movement from front-to-back and from side-to-side. The introduction of a front-to-back convexity, and a sidebending convexity, with the apex of both convexities at the segment to be treated, is the principle used when treating type II, or nonneutral, vertebral dysfunctions in which there is either forward- or backward-bending restriction, and with sidebending and rotation restriction to the same side.

In the treatment of type I, or neutral, vertebral dysfunctions, the locking principle utilized is the introduction of sidebending and rotation to opposite sides from above downward and from below upward to the segment requiring treatment. In this instance no forward-bending or backward-bending locking maneuver is introduced; the amount of forward-bending or backward-bending that is introduced is sufficient only to put the joint under treatment at its point of maximum ease in the forward-bending or backward-bending arc of movement at that vertebral level. This principle is best demonstrated in the use of the lateral recumbent "lumbar roll" technique. With the patient in the left lateral recumbent position with the L1, 2 area in the "neutral" position in the forward-bending and backward-bending arc, as the operator pulls the patient's left upper extremity anteriorly and caudad, there is introduction of sidebending left and rotation right of the thoracolumbar spine. When movement is first felt at the L1 level, motion stops. As the operator rolls the pelvis forward, there is introduction of rotation to the left from below upward until L2 is reached. This results in neutral locking of L1-L2 and any thrusting force will summate at that level. The lower in the lumbar spine that localization is desired, the more movement is introduced from above downward and less from below upward. The higher in the lumbar spine or into the lower thoracic spine, the less is introduced from above downward and the more from below upward. Again the goal is to achieve localization so that the segment under treatment is maintained in the coronal (XY) plane.

*Velocity* is the third principle. Velocity means speed not force. In mobilization with impulse technique the velocity is high. The maneuver should have quickness. The common mistake made is that the maneuver is a "push" rather than a "quick thrust". The thrust should be high in velocity and short in time. A second mistake made when applying the thrusting maneuver is that the "slack" within the joint is removed before the thrust is given. Remember that added force does not make up for poor velocity or poor localization.

*Amplitude* is the fourth principle. In high-velocity, low-amplitude thrusting procedures, the goal is to achieve movement of 1/8th inch at the joint under treatment. The thrusting force should be applied quickly and for a short distance. With short lever technique the amplitude of the thrust to achieve 1/8th inch at the joint is considerable less than that with long lever technique to achieve the same movement at the joint being treated. It is frequently observed, when two long levers are utilized, that a great deal of movement is introduced by the operator to the patient. What must be

remembered is that the summation of all of that movement should result in amplitude of thrust at the joint under treatment of 1/8th inch.

*Balance and control* is the fifth principle. As in any successful manual medicine procedure both the operator and the patient must be in body positions that are comfortable, easily controlled, and balanced. Then the patient can be completely relaxed, while the operator can apply the thrust with maximum efficiency. Lack of control and balance is frequently seen in the application of the lateral recumbent lumbar roll technique. Often using a table that is too high will compromise the operator's ability to control a patient in the lateral recumbent position. Frequently the patient is either too far away or too close to the operator while lying on the table. If too far away, the operator cannot control the localization, and if too close, the patient may fear falling and not be relaxed. Some operators attempt to introduce the thrust by an adduction movement of the arm placed upon the pelvis, rather than with a total body movement. It is most difficult to provide appropriate velocity, amplitude, and direction with an adductor muscular movement of the operator's upper extremity. It is much easier to apply the proper thrust by the weight transfer of the operator's body (with the arm contacting the patient being incorporated as part of the operator's body) or with the arm fully extended, and the thrust applied by a balanced movement of the operator's body in the right direction.

### Therapeutic Goals of High-Velocity, Low-Amplitude Thrust Technique

These procedures are useful in increasing range of movement of an articulation that has dysfunction (loss of joint play). Although the motion loss seemed to be only in one direction, a successful thrust procedure will increase range of movement in all possible directions. While moving the joint, one might attempt to realign the skeletal parts in their normal anatomical relationship, intending to restore normal joint receptor activity at that level. An additional outcome is reduction of muscle hypertonicity and/or spasm in an attempt to restore balance to the segmentally related musculature. Another therapeutic outcome might be the stretching of shortened connective tissues surrounding the articulation. The fascial connective tissues may be shortened and tightened as the result of the altered position of the articulation, the healing of the inflammatory process following injury. As suggested earlier, the therapeutic goal might be the movement of fluid, both intra- and extravascular, by "wringing out" the tissues. One or more of these therapeutic goals might be the objective of a procedure, but many of the others would be operative simultaneously. These procedures seem most effective for sub-acute and chronic dysfunctions which appear to be due to short restrictors.

## Contraindications

As in all forms of manual medicine, accurate diagnosis is essential and precision and accuracy of therapeutic intervention is required. When these criteria are met for mobilization with impulse, the contraindications become fewer. However, these procedures have more contraindications, both absolute and relative, than others. Absolute contraindications for mobilization with impulse are hypermobility and instability of an articulation and the presence of inflammatory joint disease.

There are many relative contraindications and authors classify them differently. For example, in the cervical spine there is a major concern about these procedures and the vertebral artery. The vertebral artery is anatomically at risk at the craniocervical junction, and movements of extension and rotation will narrow normal arteries. In the presence of disease of the vertebral arteries, these movements become even more potentially dangerous. The need for precision of diagnosis and application of technique be-

comes crucial in the presence of disease of the vertebral arteries. In the cervical spine there are also developmental and congenital situations which might contraindicate a thrusting procedure. Conditions such as agenesis of the odontoid process and Down's syndrome are but two. Throughout the vertebral column there is concern for metabolic and systemic bone disease. Particularly with metastatic disease and osteoporosis, there is the potential risk of osseous damage from a thrusting procedure. However, with very careful and precise localization and with appropriate amounts of force, these procedures can restore the lost joint play despite the alteration in osseous architecture. Another relative contraindication is the presence of degenerative joint disease, particularly of the apophyseal and uncovertebral joints of Luschka. Degenerative joint disease does alter the capacity of the apophyseal joints to function and a thrusting procedure inappropriately applied could damage these joints. However, degenerative joint disease can also be complicated by joint dysfunction, and joint dysfunction can be successfully treated with a thrusting procedure if the principles are applied properly. The thrust should be operative between the elastic barrier of the joint dysfunction and the altered anatomical barrier due to the degenerative joint disease. An interesting question regarding relative contraindications is that of acute disk disease. Some authors feel that manipulation of this type is the treatment of choice for disk derangement. Others feel that thrusting procedures, particularly long lever techniques using rotation torque, should not be utilized in the lumbar spine because of the possibility of exacerbating an acute disk into increased herniation and sequestration. The potential danger of an acute cauda equinus syndrome should always be considered. This author has utilized high-velocity, low-amplitude thrusting procedures in the known presence of disk herniation (as demonstrated by lumbar myelography) with a successful therapeutic result, but with no objective evidence of myelographic change of the disk herniation. It would appear that accuracy of diagnosis and precision of the therapeutic intervention remain essential.

## CONCLUSION

High-velocity low-amplitude thrusting procedures (mobilization with impulse) are most valuable in the armamentarium of the manual medicine practitioner. They require accuracy of diagnosis and precision of therapeutic intervention. The appropriate use of velocity rather than force is a competence to be mastered when utilizing these techniques.

# 10
# *PRINCIPLES OF FUNCTIONAL (Indirect) TECHNIQUE*

The procedures found within this category are not as well known as many others in the field of manual medicine. Interest in these procedures increased in the 1950s in the United States through the efforts of members of the New England Academy of Osteopathy on the East Coast and a group of physicians working with the Drs. Hoover on the West Coast. It is somewhat paradoxical that these procedures are viewed by many as being highly complex while the principles are relatively simple and straightforward.

These procedures focus on the interrelationship of structure and function in the body and the tendency to self-regulation. However, they look at this interrelationship of structure and function from the functional and not from the structural perspective. In viewing a vertebral segment that is dysfunctional, the thought is not that the bone is out of place but that it behaves as though it were. The classic structural approach would be to put the bone back in place, while the functional approach would be to restore its coordination and cooperation with other segments within the vertebral column. The same analogy can be applied to a dysfunctional vertebral segment as Korr does in describing the facilitated segment of the spinal cord. Imagine that one soldier, marching in a rank of soldiers, is out of step. Because he is out of step,

he is easily visible. The functional view of a dysfunctional vertebral segment is the same. The soldier is in line in the rank (i.e., he is not out of place), but he behaves as though he is, because he is "out of step." He does not function in a coordinated manner with his fellow soldiers on either side. To take the analogy further, the sergeant would not take the soldier out of the rank and put him elsewhere but he would change his stride so that it matched the remaining soldiers in the rank. The physician using functional technique does not change the vertebral position but changes its interaction with its fellow segments.

These procedures focus more upon motion than on position. Chapter 3 described the difference in normal and restrictive barriers and, in the presence of dysfunction, defined the "pathological" neutral point as being the point of maximum ease or freedom between the restrictive barrier on one side and the physiological barrier on the other. Functional technique is more interested in the behavior of the motion present than in its specific relationship to the barrier. One becomes more interested in the quality of motion, rather than the quantity, and particularly how a dysfunctional segment behaves when motion is introduced. Functional diagnosis looks for a range of motion that would normally and reasonably be expected—coordinated and synchronized—and a quality and ease of movement sufficient for its participation.

Functional technique is based upon the premise that the dysfunction has altered neural function. Hypothetically, abnormal behavior stimulates abnormal afferent impulses from the mechanoreceptors and nociceptors which are transmitted to the spinal cord for processing, either locally or centrally, and result in abnormal efferent signals to the body, particularly the musculoskeletal system. The working hypothesis is that restoration of proper afferent signals to the central nervous system will return the neural traffic in the spinal cord segment to a more normal level and elicit a more normal neural response. Searching for alteration in the behavior of each segment within the musculoskeletal system, and attempting to restore it to normal, requires that each potentially dysfunctional segment receive appropriate attention.

### EASE-BIND CONCEPT

In functional technique one looks for the quality of movement rather than the range. Does movement appear to be easy and free (ease), or is the movement restricted and difficult (bind)? The spectrum runs from maximum ease to maximum bind with many gradations between. Functional diagnosis searches for the ease-bind interface. The gradations between ease and bind determine the manner and process in which functional technique is applied.

In seeking ease and bind the procedure is as follows. A palpating hand is placed over the segment suspected of being dysfunctional; this is called the "listening hand". Contact is maintained in a quiet and noninvasive fashion, focusing upon changes which occur in the adnexal tissues surrounding the dysfunctional segment. The listening hand introduces no movement or energy, it is a "receiver" of information. The operator's other hand makes contact with some area of the musculoskeletal system distant from the dysfunctional segment and is used either to introduce motion or to monitor the motion the patient introduces under verbal commands. This hand is called the "motor hand", and it introduces the movement that the listening hand monitors as a response of either ease or bind. The process requires a motion demand and a response. The motion hand initiates the demand and the listening hand monitors the response.

In functional technique there is a constant diagnostic and treatment interface. The motion hand can introduce both diagnostic and therapeutic motions and the listening hand monitors the response throughout the movement process. The diagnosis-treatment procedure is a constant assessment process like a cybernetic loop of continuous input and feedback. Because of this dynamic process, practitioners of functional technique may look as though they are doing different things with little standardization of these procedures. In fact, the converse is true. Irrespective of how the motion is introduced, the effect is constantly monitored by the listening hand.

### THERAPEUTIC USES

Functional technique can be valuable in both acute and chronic conditions. It is particularly useful in acute conditions because it is nontraumatic and can be performed often. Results depend on tissue response, not a structural change. Acute conditions respond quickly to these procedures which can be done in any location. They do not require extensive study of a technique manual, and they can be done by a relative neophyte. They are also very effective in chronic conditions because they attempt to overcome the programmed abnormal neural response, and not just alter position. It does little good to restore the position of a dysfunctional vertebral segment without restoring the neuromuscular mechanisms which control its function. Functional technique is also useful in chronic conditions because it monitors tissue response and behavior irrespective of the therapeutic intervention.

Functional diagnosis also has prognostic value. It can assess the therapeutic response at a dysfunctional level, even though the therapy might not be a functional technique procedure. For example, lift therapy for an apparent short lower extremity and pelvic tilt mechanism (a structural intervention) will change the function of the entire musculoskeletal system. Functional diagnosis can help determine whether or not the structural intervention of the lift has accomplished improvement in musculoskeletal function, both locally and distantly.

## TYPES OF FUNCTIONAL TECHNIQUE

Functional techniques can be placed within one of three categories

> Balance and hold
> Dynamic functional procedures
> Release by positioning

## BALANCE AND HOLD

These procedures can be accomplished in any body position, standing, sitting, supine, prone, or lateral recumbent. A listening hand monitors the dysfunctional segment and the patient's response to motion introduced either by a physician, passively, or by the patient actively assuming a body position under the physician's verbal commands. Motion is introduced sequentially in seven different directions and the balance point of maximum ease within each range is held in a stacking fashion. The ranges introduced are as follows:

> Forward bending-backward bending
> Sidebending right-sidebending left
> Rotation right-rotation left
> Translation anterior-posterior
> Translation laterally-both right and
>   left
> Translation cephalic-caudad
> Respiration-inhalation-exhalation

The stacking sequence of the first six makes little difference. The last movement introduced is respiratory. Once the dysfunctional segment has been "stacked" at the point of maximum ease in the first six movements, the respiratory effort is introduced. The phase of respiration found to be the most free is then held by the patient as long as comfortably possible. This is usually for 5 to 30 seconds. When the patient can no longer hold the breath comfortably in that phase of respiration, instruction is given to breathe normally and naturally. A new balance point is sought in each motion direction and the respiratory effort is repeated. The entire process is repeated until release of restriction is felt and increased mobility is obtained. In these procedures the operator senses that the neutral point is returning more and more toward normal and that its range is increasing.

The second category of functional technique is described as "dynamic functional" and focuses upon the restoration of normalcy to the apparently abnormal tracking mechanism. In dynamic functional technique the listening hand again monitors a series of motions introduced by the motive hand and attempts to direct the motion demand along a new track of increased ease. The goal is to restore a more normal movement pattern and the operator attempts to "ride out" the dysfunction. Because of the dynamic motion patterns introduced, these techniques look quite varied. They can be standardized by the formula C-C-T-E-T. C stands for contact over the adnexal tissue of the dysfunctional segment. The second C stands for the control of the introduced movement by the motor hand. T stands for testing of the adnexal tissue response. E stands for evaluation of the compliance of the segment as normal or abnormal, looking for significant lesion(s). T stands for treatment by constantly monitoring the bind-ease point of the dysfunctional segment through the contact (listening) hand, based on the demands placed by the motor hand.

The third category of functional technique is released by positioning. This system, described as *counterstrain*, was originated and popularized by Lawrence Jones, D.O., F.A.A.O. The system identifies the body position in which the patient has the least pain.

Any number of different body positions can be employed, frequently including combined sitting and recumbent positions. The second feature is the identification and monitoring of palpable tender points in specific locations throughout the musculoskeletal system. Many of these points coincide with locations reported by other authors (Travell, myofascial trigger points; Chapman's reflexes; and acupuncture points), but in these procedures the tender points are used both diagnostically and to monitor the therapeutic intervention. When a tender point is identified, a body position is assumed which reduces both the patient's pain and the tenderness and tissue feel by the operator. This position is held for 90 seconds. At the end of this time the patient is slowly returned to a more normal body posture and reevaluated. A specific exercise program supports these procedures. A study of *Strain and Counterstrain*, (Jones, LH, Colorado Springs, CO, American Academy of Osteopathy, 1981) is recommended before using this technique.

## FUNCTIONAL PALPATION EXERCISE

The following exercise is useful in learning the principles of functional diagnosis and treatment.

1. Have the patient sit on an examining table in an erect position with both arms folded across the chest, each hand holding the opposite shoulder.
2. The operator stands behind and to the side of the patient and places the fingertips in the upper thoracic region and waits. The listening hand should be as quiet as possible and the operator waits until the listening hand feels nothing.
3. The operator's other hand becomes the motor hand by being placed on top of the head and is used to lead the patient through certain movements much in the fashion of the use of the reins on the bridle of a horse. The motor hand monitors the response of the patient to verbal commands and also introduces passive movement.

4. Introduce forward-bending slowly and smoothly and attempt to identify (with the listening hand) changes from maximum to decreasing ease to increasing bind to maximum bind. Then reverse the procedure into backward-bending. Repeat several times and constantly concentrate on the range of ease to bind.
5. With the patient returned to the starting position introduce (with the motor hand) sidebending to the right and rotation to the left of the head and neck on the trunk. This introduces type I vertebral movement. Again monitor the range of this coupled movement through the ease and bind phenomena. Reverse to sidebending left and rotation right. Is there symmetry to the ease and bind phenomena? As you modulate sidebending and rotation, is there a difference in the ease and bind of each component part?
6. Return to the starting position and introduce a small amount of forward-bending, right sidebending, and right rotation of the head and neck on the trunk. This introduces a type II coupled movement and again the listening hand monitors ease and bind of this motion. Repeat to the left side. Are they symmetrical in quality?

This exercise can be repeated throughout the vertebral axis in a number of positions. Diagnostically one is attempting to classify a segment as normal, marginally dysfunctional, or significantly dysfunctional. The normal segment has a wide range of minimal signaling throughout the procedure and a significantly dysfunctional segment has a narrow range of rapid signaling in the ease-bind range. It is not uncommon to find a segment that is marginally dysfunctional and it is important to make a decision about its significance within the total musculoskeletal complex. Fortunately this can be achieved by experience, but experience is the only teacher.

## CONCLUSION

Functional-indirect techniques are based on a common neurological model in which reducing the flow of abnormal afferent impulses into the central nervous system reprograms the "central computer" to more normal function. These procedures focus on the quality of movement, particularly the quality on the initiation of motion, rather than the amount of range or the feel of its endpoint. They are primarily nontraumatic and easily used in a variety of patient conditions and health care settings. They require considerable practice to educate the senses to the ease and bind phenomena and to the point of maximum pain-free position for the tissues of the musculoskeletal system. The value of these procedures in patient care warrants the expenditure of time and effort needed for the student to acquire proficiency.

# 11
## *PRINCIPLES OF MYOFASCIAL RELEASE TECHNIQUE*

Myofascial release technique is a relatively recent addition to the field of manual medicine. It can be classified as a combined technique using some principles from soft tissue technique, muscle energy technique, and inherent force craniosacral technique. There are many combinations, and different authors and teachers of myofascial release technique show similarities and differences. Myofascial release technique has been described by Ward as a "bridging" technique spanning the spectrum of manual medicine procedures. It combines soft tissue changes, faulty body mechanics, and altered reflex mechanisms in both diagnosis and treatment. Fascia had received attention from such individuals as the osteopathic physician Neidner, who used twisting forces on the extremities to restore fascial balance and symmetry. The famous Ida Rolf used deep pressure and stretching of the fascia, from the top of the head to the tips of the toes. Rolfing requires extensive investment in time and energy, by both patient and operator, and the process is not always comfortable.

Myofascial release technique as described here can be classified as either direct or indirect, and frequently is used in a combined fashion. The resistant barrier may be engaged directly; the tissue may be stretched in the direction away from the barrier in an indirect fashion; or the barriers can be addressed in each direction. The activating forces are both intrinsic and extrinsic. Of the intrinsic forces, the inherent force of body rhythm and the capacity to restore homeostatic balance, are utilized throughout the procedure. The extrinsic activating forces are applied by the operator, and force is applied in both a traction and twisting manner to achieve the appropriate tension on the soft tissues to effect both biomechanical and reflex changes. This technique is useful in both regional and local dysfunctions. It shares the common goal of all manual medicine procedures of attempting to achieve symmetrical function of the entire musculoskeletal system in postural balance.

## FASCIA

To use myofascial release technique adequately, the operator must have a working knowledge of the continuity and integrative nature of fascia. While variously named, in actual fact, the fascia of the body is continuous from region to region and totally invests all other elements of the body.

The fascia can be simply described as consisting of three layers. The superficial fascia is attached to the undersurface of the skin and is loosely knit, fibroelastic, areolar tissue. Within the superficial fascia are found fat, vascular structures (including capillary networks and lymphatic channels), and nervous tissues, particularly the pacinian corpuscles referred to as skin receptors. Because of the loosely knit nature of superficial fascia, the skin can be moved in many directions over the deeper structures, and there is potential space for the accumulation of fluid and other metabolites.

The deep fascia is tougher, tighter, and more compact. It can be described as compartmentalizing the body. It envelops and separates muscles; surrounds and separates internal visceral organs; and contributes greatly to the contour and function of the body. Specialized elements of the deep fascia include the peritoneum, the pericardium, and the pleura. The deep fascia is quite tough and resilient and as such can be quite confining. One need only recall the problems created by "compartment syndromes". Acute trauma with hemorrhage in the anterior compartment of the lower leg and swelling and hemorrhage inside the investing fascia can be highly detrimental to the sensitive nerve structures within the compartment. It is for this and similar conditions that surgical fasciectomy is performed.

The subserous fascia is the loose aerolar tissue which covers all of the internal visceral organs. It provides the small amount of fluid which lubricates the surfaces of the internal viscera and contains many small circulatory channels.

Fascia has many functions. It provides support for vessels and nerves as they course throughout the body. It enables adjacent tissues to move upon each other and gives stability and contour to many structures. It provides fluid for lubrication between structures for both movement and nutrition. It participates in reflex mechanisms by reporting afferent impulse from the pacinian corpuscles in the superficial fascia. Fascia, as we have described it, is continuous with specialized elements of fascia such as ligaments and tendons. While these tissues have unique characteristics, they share with the general fascia collagen fibers, elastic fibers, cellular elements, and ground substance. Within these specialized elements of fascia are found specialized mechanoreceptors and proprioceptors, which constantly report information to the spinal cord and brain on body position and movement, both normal and abnormal. Fascia also functions within the immune system of the body. Fascia can contract and relax, and has an elasticity which helps it to retain its shape and respond to deformation. Fascia behaves, while mechanically under load, with both elastic and plastic deformation. Usually under load, it will recover its original shape when the load is removed (elastic deformation), but depending upon the load, its type, amount, and duration, fascia may not recover its original size and shape after plastic deformation. Fascia has the capacity to "creep", that is, when subjected to an extension load and held constant, the tissue relaxes and "creeps" so that it has less resistance to a second application of load. This has significance when we look at the effects of injury and long-term stress on these connective tissues. Fascia also has the capacity to change and lose energy when it is subjected to stress. This phenomena, called hysteresis, is utilized therapeutically in myofascial release technique.

When fascia is subjected to stress, from acute injury or long-standing microtrauma (such as postural imbalance due to anatomical short leg), certain responses occur. The first is the inflammatory process of injury which can span the spectrum from acute to chronic changes. The inflammatory fluid can be absorbed easily in the superficial fascia, but within the tight compartments of deep fascia it can become quite detrimental. These changes in fascia are palpable by the trained hand and contribute greatly to the tissue texture abnormalities so characteristic and diagnostic of somatic dysfunction.

Fascia under stress also responds biomechanically. Depending upon the amount and type of load, deformation may be temporary or permanent. In large measure, the number and type of collagen and elastic fibers within the connective tissue and the type of load applied determine the result of the biomechanical stress. The stress of injury causes the receptors within the connective tissue to report information to the central nervous system for processing. The ability of the receptors to adapt and the facility of the central nervous system to adjust, determines the short- or long-term effect on neural integration that results from the connective tissue injury.

Biochemical and immunological changes can occur within the ground substance of the fascia and have general systemic effects which seem quite far removed from the injury to the soft tissues themselves. Scarring during the healing process frequently interferes with the functions of support, movement, and lubrication. The resultant functional alteration can be quite detrimental to the patient and can produce symptoms which cannot be measured "objectively". These soft tissue changes frequently lead to persistent symptoms long after the acute injury should have healed. The controversies surrounding patients with flexion-extension-type cervical spine injuries (whiplash injury) in automobile accidents is a classic example.

## MUSCLE

Muscle is the second main focus of myofascial release. Muscles have both the function of maintenance of posture (so-called static muscles), and the function of movement (so-called phasic muscles). Most muscles have both functions, but one will predominate. For each muscle action there is usually an equal and opposite muscle action (the agonist-antagonist principle). There are sophisticated neuromuscular reflexes which constantly maintain body posture and prepare for, initiate, and continue, movement. Sherrington's law of reciprocal innervation and inhibition constantly works on muscles to balance the tone and function of agonist and antagonist. Groups of muscles are classified as strong or weak. In the lower extremity, the hamstrings are a strong group and the gluteals are weak; in the upper extremities the pectorals are strong

and the rhomboids are weak. This is a relative classification based on clinical observations.

The function of muscles in the musculoskeletal system is totally integrated and involves all muscles from the attachment at the skull to the distal attachment of both upper and lower extremities. This muscle integration is highly complex. Fortunately homeostasis maintains high levels of integration. Alteration in this integrative function of muscle is frequently observed in patients with chronic musculoskeletal symptoms. The control of muscle function is both voluntary and involuntary and is mediated by the central nervous system. When this control mechanism is working at normal efficiency, movement patterns are symmetrical, coordinated, and free. One need only contrast the performance of an olympic-level runner and a patient with far advanced Parkinson's disease. Gradations between these two extremes span the spectrum from hypertonicity to hypotonicity and integrative coordination problems, as seen in patients with minimal brain dysfunction.

Injury to muscle can interfere with its anatomy and basic function. During acute injury there can be muscle tears and disturbances at the myotendinous junction and at the insertion of tendon into bone. These undergo the same fibrotic healing process as other injuries to soft tissues and a certain amount of functional loss may result. Even if injury is not so severe as to cause permanent anatomical damage to muscle, it frequently alters neuroreflexive control of muscle function and can contribute to the persistence of long term symtomotolgy. Muscle, like the fascia with which it is intimately connected, can undergo both biomechanical and neurophsiologic change.

### Concepts in Myofascial Release Technique

The first concept in this system is that of *tight-loose*. This concept is that tightness creates and weakness permits asymmetry.

There are both biomechanical and neural reflexive elements to this tight-loose concept. Increased stimulation causes an agonist muscle to become tight, and the tighter it becomes, the looser its antagonist becomes by reciprocal inhibition. Shortening of the fascia surrounding the hypertonic, contracted muscle requires loosening of the fascia in the opposite direction in accommodation. One cannot step a mast on a boat by pulling up on the forestay if the backstay is not loose enough to permit movement. In acute conditions the cycle can be described as continuing spasm—pain—spasm. This results in tightness and can progress from the acute condition of muscle contraction to actual contracture of muscle leading to chronicity. In the chronic condition the cycle is described as pain—looseness—pain. All manual medicine practitioners are familiar with the painful symptoms of hypermobility. The application of this tight-loose concept is fundamental to the therapeutic use of myofascial procedures.

The second concept is that of the role of palpation in myofascial pain syndromes. There are many diagnostic and therapeutic systems built upon peripheral stimulation (acupuncture, acupressure, Chapman's reflexes, Travell's trigger points, Jones' pain points). Palpation of the myofascial elements can frequently identify a site of initiation for myofascial pain which can be therapeutically addressed by the hands. A significant proportion of myofascial sensitivity appears to be mediated by the autonomic nervous system; some of the symptoms found with myofascial pain are probably mediated by sympathetic nervous system reflexes. It is interesting to note the frequent occurrence of myofascial pain in the areas of soft tissue looseness.

The third concept deals with the neuroreflexive change that occurs with the application of manual force on the musculoskeletal system. The hands-on approach offers afferent stimulation through receptors, which require central processing at the spinal cord and cortical levels for a response. Afferent stimulation frequently results in efferent inhibition. This principle is used in myofascial release technique when the afferent stimulation of a stretch is applied and the operator waits for efferent inhibition to occur so that relaxation results in tight tissues. Neuroreflexive response is individualistic and appears to be modified by the amount of patient pain, the patient's pain behavior, the level of wellness (particularly the nutritional status), stress response, and the basic life-style of the individual, particularly the use/abuse of alcohol, tobacco, and drugs, including medications.

The fourth concept is that of the "release" phenomenon. This concept is shared with other forms of manual medicine, particularly the craniosacral technique and the ease-bind principle of functional-indirect technique. Release, in the myofascial release concept, is the tissue relaxation (including muscle relaxation), which follows the appropriate application of stress on the tissue. The tightness "gives way" or "melts" under the application of load. Release becomes an enabling and terminal objective of the application of myofascial release. Release of tightness is sought to achieve improvement in symmetry of form and function. The student of these procedures must search for and feel the release phenomena as a guide through the treatment process.

## PRINCIPLES OF MYOFASCIAL RELEASE EVALUATION

Ward has coined the mnemonic M A I (N)4 for the evaluative process. *M* stands for analysis of the mechanics of the musculoskeletal system, symmetry- asymmetry, looseness-tightness, etc. *A* stands for anatomy, particularly the analysis of functional anatomy of the body. One is interested in both symmetry of form and symmetry of function. One needs a sense of three-dimensional anatomical relationships, the integration of neural control and muscle function, and joint mechanics. *I* stands for immunology and focuses upon the response mechanisms of the patient to stress. How does the patient's complex immune system respond and influence the level of general wellness? Are there systemic factors which influence musculoskeletal system response? Does the patient have rheumatic tendencies? The first *N* stands for neurologic findings. Are the demonstrable central or peripheral (upper or lower motor neuron) neurologic abnormalities? Are the reflexes hyper- or hyporeactive? Are they symmetrical? Is the pain pattern radicular or just referred? The second *N* stands for neurogenic considerations. Are there alterations in autonomic nervous system balance and tone? Is there evidence of neuroendocrine imbalance? Is the patient anxious or depressed? How does the patient's life-style effect the neurogenic response? The third *N* stands for nociceptive considerations. How does the patient respond to pain? Is there aberrant pain behavior? Has sensitization or habituation occurred? How does the patient's lifestyle influence the nociceptive response? The fourth *N* stands for nutritional status. It has long been known that altered nutrition, particularly inadequacy of B- complex vitamins results in abnormal nervous system function. How does the patient's nutrition affect the response? Is there excessive weight gain or loss? Is there use or abuse of alcohol and tobacco? What medications or other drugs are used?

The myofascial release concept attempts to integrate the biologic, psychologic, and social aspects of the patient.

## MYOFASCIAL RELEASE TREATMENT CONCEPTS

Myofascial release technique is directed toward a biomechanical effect and a neurophysiological effect. Ward has coined the mnemonic $P O E (T)^2$. $P O E$ stands for point of entry into the musculoskeletal system. Entry may be from the lower extremity, the upper extremity, through the thoracic cage, through the abdomen, or from the cranial cervical junction. The two *T*s stand for traction and twist. In most of the techniques traction produces stretch along the long axis of the myofascial elements that are shortened and tightened. The stretch should always be applied in the long axis rather than transversely across myofascial elements. Introduction of a twisting force provides the opportunity to localize the traction, not only at the point of contact with the patient, but also at points some distance away. The beginner should develop the ability to feel change (tightness, looseness, release) at some distance from the point of contact. For example, when grasping the lower extremity near the ankle the operator attempts to feel through the extremity to the knee, thigh, hip, sacroiliac joint, and into the vertebral column, and sense changes occurring at each of these levels as perceived at the contact point at the ankle. This is a skill which requires concentration, practice, and an appreciation for the three-dimensional aspects of the musculoskeletal system.

Patients treated with these techniques are given exercise programs specifically designed for them. Specific stretching exercises are given to maintain the added length of the tight tissues, and strengthening exercises are given to strengthen the weaker muscles. In treatment of muscle imbalance, first stretch the short, tight muscle groups and follow with strengthening exercise for the weaker, loose muscle groups. Exercise programs to enhance integrative muscle balance are frequently useful. Such exercises as a cross-pattern pep walk, swimming, square dancing, rebounding, etc., can be used. The goal is not only to increase mobility and strength, but also to enhance muscular coordination.

Because the concept is more than just biomechanical, attention should be given to general health issues such as life-style, coping mechanisms, appropriate use of alcohol and other medications, discontinuance of tobacco, and adequate and appropriate nutrition with resultant appropriate weight control.

## EXERCISES IN PALPATION

Myofascial release procedures require skill at palpating the musculoskeletal system for something other than one bone moving on the other. One must learn to "read the tissues" for their tightness-looseness and their inherent mobility, in addition to the usual soft tissue texture abnormalities of hard-soft, cool-warm, smooth-rough, etc., referred to in Chapter 2. One needs to develop increased sensitivity to the patient's tissues both at point of contact and at some distance. There are many exercises in palpation that can be useful and the following are but a few.

Place the fingertips of all five fingers together without contact with the rest of the hand. Introduce force from one hand to the other and then reverse. Sense what goes on with the hand generating the force and the one receiving the force. Are they different from side-to-side? Now take one hand and stroke with the fingerpads down the volar surface of the fingers and palms, first with light stroking and then with increased pressure. Repeat using the other hand as the motor hand. Sense the difference in the sensitivity of the hand being stroked, as well as the sensation of touch by the fingerpads of the motor hand. In order to properly sense what goes on in the patient, you must have an awareness of your own palpable skills and sensations and your own self-body awareness.

Fold your hands together interlacing all your fingers. You will find that either the right or the left second metacarpophalangeal joint is on top. Now reverse the position so that the other metacarpophalangeal joint is on top. Sense the difference, with one appearing to be more comfortable than the other, and with the less comfortable one feeling tighter.

Stretch your arms out ahead of you crossing them at the wrist and pronating both hands until the palmer surfaces meet. Interlace your fingers and raise the extended arms over your head. As you reach toward the ceiling feel the difference in tension between the right and left sides of your body. Return to the starting position, reverse the way in which your wrists are crossed, and repeat the procedure. Again, note the difference in tension from side to side and the difference introduced by altered crossing of the wrists.

Working with a patient partner, return to the forearm described in Chapter 2. This time start with your palpating hand some distance from the forearm and slowly move toward the forearm until you begin to feel radiant energy from the patient. This is usually sensed as heat. Repeat the procedure several times with your eyes closed to see if you can repeatedly stop at the point where you first feel the sensation and if the distance from your palpating hand to the forearm is consistent. Continue to approach the forearm until you are palpating just the superficial hair and course up and down over the forearm, attempting to sense what is going on under your hand. See if you can identify differences in the proximal forearm, distal forearm, wrist, and hand. Place your hand in contact with the skin and concentrate, applying no motion of your own, but attempting to sense the inherent movement of the patient's tissues under your hand. It takes several seconds to several minutes to begin to sense an inherent oscillating-type movement within the forearm.

When you have mastered the ability to apply pressure but not movement, and the ability to sense inherent movement within your patient, place the palm of your hand in contact with the bony sacrum. This should be done both in the supine and prone position. The contour of the sacrum fits nicely in the palm of your hand. In the prone position it is sometimes necessary to use a slight compressive force to begin to feel the inherent motion of the sacrum. In a supine position the patient's body weight on your hand is sufficient to initiate inherent sacral movement. Try to follow the sacrum in the directions in which it wishes to move. Do not attempt to direct it. What is the rhythm, amplitude, and direction of the sacrum moving in space? When you have been able to identify inherent soft tissue and bony movement, you are well on your way to being able to use myofascial release technique.

## CONCLUSION

Myofascial release techniques utilize both direct and indirect action with activating forces that are both extrinsic and intrinsic. They influence the biomechanics of the musculoskeletal system and the reflexes which direct, integrate, and modify movement. The goal is restoring functional balance to all of the integrative tissues in the musculoskeletal system, and the techniques are useful in acute, sub-acute, and chronic conditions, with simple and complex problems. The techniques can be used in multiple patient positions. They usually consist of symmetrical placement of the operator's hands introducing some twisting force to engage the tissues and then following directly or indirectly along fascial planes to sense areas of tightness and looseness. Traction is placed upon the tight area awaiting the sensation of release. Release is hypothesized as following reflex neural efferent inhibition and biomechanical hysteresis within the tissues. The techniques are highly individualized to the patient's need and the operator's training and experience.

# 12

# PRINCIPLES OF CRANIOSACRAL (Inherent Force) TECHNIQUE

Craniosacral technique was added to the armamentarium of manual medicine around 1940 through the work of William G. Sutherland, D.O. The principles were developed following many years of study of the anatomy of the skull, meninges, brain, spinal cord, and sacrum, together with clinical experimentation upon both himself and patients. Although these procedures, like many others in manual medicine, were not readily received, craniosacral technique has become increasingly popular through Sutherland's work and the contributions of many generations of students. Craniosacral technique was developed by Sutherland as an extension of Andrew Taylor Still's principles on the articulations of the skull. Sutherland reasoned that the sutures forming the joints between bones of the skull were intricately fashioned for the maintenance of motion. The sutures are present throughout life, have consistent areas of bevel change, and consistently separate when the skull is "exploded" (filled with beans through the foramen magnum, then immersed in water). The bones of the skull don't fracture, the sutures separate. Sutherland further hypothesized that the skull would have normal mobility during health and would show restrictions in response to trauma or systemic disease. His clinical observations were consistent with this hypothesis. The use of craniosacral technique requires that the practitioner make an intense study of the osseous cranium, sutures, and meninges, and finely tune a palpatory sense to perceive inherent mobility within the craniosacral mechanism and apply manual technique with precision, depth, and dexterity.

## Anatomy

The skull can be divided into three elements: *(a)* the vault, consisting of portions of the frontal bone, the two parietal bones, the occipital squama, and the temporal squama which develop from membrane; *(b)* the base, consisting of the body of the sphenoid, the petrous and mastoid portions of the temporals, the basilar and condylar portions of the occiput which form in cartilage; and *(c)* the facial bones. The bones of the skull can be divided into those that are paired and those that are unpaired. The unpaired midline bones are the occiput, sphenoid, ethmoid, and vomer. The motion of these midline bones is primarily flexion and extension with an overturning moment around a transverse (x-axis). The flexion-extension movement occurs at the sphenobasilar junction, a synchondrosis. During this movement the sphenoid and occiput rotate in opposite directions. During sphenobasilar flexion, the sphenoid rotates anteriorly with the basisphenoid being elevated and the pterygoid process moving inferiorly (tθ + X), and the occiput rotating posteriorly (tθ − X) with the basiocciput being elevated, and the squama and condylar parts being depressed (caudad). During sphenobasilar flexion, the ethmoid rotates in the opposite direction to the sphenoid and in the same direction as the occiput. During sphenobasilar flexion, the vomer is carried caudad as the anterior portion of the sphenoid moves in that direction. During sphenobasilar extension all of the motions are reversed. The paired bones consist of the parietal, temporal, frontal, zygoma, maxilla, palatine and nasal bones. Their motion is described as paired internal and external rotation and is normally synchronous with sphenobasilar flexion and extension. During sphenobasilar flexion, there is external rotation of the paired bones.

The combined flexion and extension of the midline unpaired bones coupled with the internal-external rotational movement of the paired bones, causes observable change in cranial contour during sphenobasilar flexion and extension. With flexion, the transverse diameter of the skull increases, the AP diameter decreases, and the vertex flattens. With sphenobasilar extension, the transverse diameter decreases, the AP diameter increases, and the vertex becomes more prominent. The facial bones and the sphenoid can be viewed as being suspended from the frontal bone. The sphenoid determines the motion characteristics of the paired facial bones. The meninges are strongly attached at the foramen magnum, continue down the spinal canal with attachment to the upper two or three cervical segments, and then remain free until they attach to the sacrum at approximately the second sacral segment. It is through this membranous attachment that the sacral component of the craniosacral mechanism is controlled. As one of its many movements, the sacrum has an involuntary nutation-counternutation movement that is synchronous with flexion-extension at the sphenobasilar junction. During sphenobasilar flexion the foramen magnum is elevated, and the tension on the dura causes the base of the sacrum to move posteriorly and the apex to move anteriorly. This is described as sacral flexion. During sphenobasilar extension, the foramen magnum moves inferiorly, releasing tension on the dura, the sacral base moves anteriorly, and the apex posteriorly. This is called sacral extension. Note that the use of the terms flexion and extension here is the reverse of the usage in a postural- structural model of sacral mechanics. Despite the confusion in terminology, the concept that must be understood is the interrelationship of movement of the occiput and sacrum, normally in synchronous directions.

The sutures are the joints which join the bones of the skull. The sutures have many variations and appear to be intricately designed to permit and direct certain types of movement between opposing cranial bones. Found within the sutures are extensions of the dura and other connective tissue, primarily Sharpey's fibers. Study of the sutures will show that fiber direction is not haphazard and random, but rather specific at each sutural level. Within the sutures are blood vessels with accompanying nerves for vasomotor control. Other neural elements found within the sutures include free nerve endings with unmyelinated fibers, suggesting the possibility of pain perception and transmission. A detailed description of the cranial sutures is beyond the scope of this text. The reader is urged to study not only the classical anatomical descriptions, but also, in detail, the sutures found on each bone of a disarticulated skull. The following palpation exercise is useful in identifying palpable sutures in a living subject:

Palpate the extreme vertex of the skull slightly more than halfway posteriorly to feel the sagittal suture through the scalp. Use the fingerpads and move from side to side feeling the serrated sutural contour.

Follow that sagittal suture in an anterior direction until you arrive at a small depression which may feel somewhat triangular. This is the bregma, the junction of the sagittal and coronal suture.

Starting from the bregma, palpate bilaterally along the coronal suture, feeling the articulation of the frontal with the parietal bone on each side.

At the inferior extremity of the coronal suture the palpating finger moves over a bony prominence, goes somewhat deeper, and ends at the suture for the sphenoid.

The palpating finger now lies at the pterion which is the junction of the sphenoid, frontal, parietal, and temporal squama. Just inferior to this junction is the palpable tip of the great wing of the sphenoid which is the point of palpatory contact both for diagnosis and treatment.

From the pterion follow a suture line posteriorly following the junction of the parietal and the temporal squama. This suture courses in a circular fashion over the top of the ear and arrives posteriorly at a depression which is called the asterion and is the junction of the temporal, parietal, and occiput.

Just anterior to the asterion one can palpate a short amount of suture between the parietal bone and the mastoid portion of the temporal.

From the asterion course medially and superiorly along the lambdoidal suture until arriving at the midline where it joins with the sagittal suture at the lambda.

Returning to the asterion palpate in a caudad direction posterior to the mastoid process and follow the occipital mastoid suture until it is lost under the soft tissues of the attachment of the neck to the head.

Starting at the upper outer margin of the orbit, follow the orbit around laterally and inferiorly until you feel the frontozygomatic suture.

Continue to follow the lateral aspect of the orbit until you feel the zygomaticomaxillary suture.

Continue medially along the inferior aspect of the orbit and up its medial wall palpating the suture at the maxillae-nasal junction and the maxillae-frontal junction.

This exercise should be repeated on multiple patients until one becomes confident of the ability to palpate and control the bones within the skull.

The meninges are divided into three layers, the pia, arachnoid, and dura. Within the cranium the external layer of the dura is continuous with the periostium and the internal layer has several duplications which separate segments of the brain and encircle the venous sinuses. The three dural duplications have intricate fiber directions throughout. The falx cerebri attaches anteriorly to the crista galli of the ethmoid, the frontal bone, both parietal bones, and the occipital squama. At its osseous attachment it encloses the superior sagittal sinous. The falx cerebri separates the two cerebral hemispheres and at its free margin encloses the inferior sagittal sinus. The tentorium cerebelli separates the cerebrum and cerebellum and attaches to the occipital, parietal, and temporal bones. It is attached to the anterior and posterior clinoid processes of the sphenoid and where it attaches to the falx cerebri, it encloses the straight sinus. There are two other dural duplications and folds, the falx cerebelli which separates the two hemispheres of the cerebellum, and the diaphragma sellae which covers the sella turcica of the sphenoid. The falx cerebri and the tentorium cerebelli meet at the reciprocal tension membrane, or "Sutherland fulcrum". These dura membranes are under constant and dynamic tension so that tension of one requires relaxation of another and vice versa. During sphenobasilar flexion there is flattening of the tent and shortening of the falx from before backward. During sphenobasilar extension, the reverse occurs. Craniosacral motion then becomes a combination of articular mobility and change in the tensions within the membranes. It is through this membranous attachment that the synchronous movement of the cranium and the sacrum occurs. The dura is intimately attached at the foramen magnum of the occiput, to the upper two or three cervical segments, and then is free until it attaches to the sacrum at approximately S2. The continuity of the dural attachment allows for the influence of the cranium upon the sacrum, and the sacrum upon the cranium.

Sphenobasilar flexion and extension are also related to and influenced by respiratory activity. Inhalation enhances sphenobasilar flexion, and exhalation enhances sphenobasilar extension. The tentorium cerebelli can be viewed as the diaphragm of the craniosacral mechanism. It descends and flattens during inhalation as does the thoracoabdominal diaphragm. The pelvic diaphragm is also observed to descend during inhalation. The pelvic diaphragm is intimately related to the sacrum within the osseous pelvis. One can then view the body from the perspective of three diaphragms: the tentorium cerebelli, the thoracoabdominal diaphragm, and the pelvic diaphragm. In health these diaphragms should function in a synchronous fashion. If dysfunction interferes with the capacity of any of the three, it is reasonable to assume that the other two will be altered as well. That is what is observed in clinical practice.

## PRIMARY RESPIRATORY MECHANISM

If one places both hands upon the lateral aspects of the skull and waits a sufficient period of time the palpatory sensation of widening and narrowing of the skull is perceived. This sensation normally occurs at a rate of 10 to 14 times per minute and is of a relatively low amplitude. This sensation, called the cranial rhythmic impulse, is interpreted as the result of the function of the time component primary respiratory mechanism.

*Inherent mobility of brain and spinal cord.* The brain is living tissue which appears to have an inherent mobility readily observable during a craniotomy procedure. The motion appears to be that of coiling and uncoiling of the cerebral hemispheres. During the uncoiling process the cerebral hemispheres appear to swing upward, and the paired and unpaired bones of the cranium respond with their normal flexion mobility. During the coiling process, the cerebral hemispheres descend and the cranial bones move into the extension mode. This inherent brain mobility is one of the biological rhythms that currently cannot be artificially restored if lost.

*Fluctuation of the cerebral spinal fluid.* The cerebral spinal fluid (CSF) is found within the lateral ventricles, the third ventricle, the fourth ventricle, the cisterns within the skull, and the spinal dura. Obstruction to the flow of cerebral spinal fluid in certain locations lead to pathological conditions such as hydrocephalus. The CSF is formed in the choroid plexuses of the lateral ventricles. Where the CSF exits the system is less well known, but it appears to follow along the dural attachment to the spinal nerves to the spinal nerves themselves. The coiling maneuver of the brain seems to increase the volume of the cerebral ventricles while uncoiling appears to compress them. Perhaps this mechanism produces the circulatory CSF flow.

*Motility of intracranial and intraspinal membranes.* As noted previously, the falx cerebri, falx cerebelli, and tentorium cerebelli are all duplications of the intracranial dura and the membranes within these structures have an intimate and intricate pattern. The intracranial membranes are continuously under dynamic tension so that a change in one requires adaptive change in another. During flexion movement the tent descends and flattens and the falx cerebri shortens from before backward. In extension movement just the reverse occurs. The intracranial membranes are connected with the intraspinal membranes through a continuation from the firm attachment at the foramen magnum down the spinal canal to the upper two or three cervical vertebra, and then they traverse freely down the spinal canal until attachment to the sacrum at approximately S2. With movement of the foramen magnum there is alteration in tension on the anterior and posterior aspects of the spinal dura, and this movement influences the motion and position of the sacrum between the two innominates.

*Articular mobility of cranial bones.* As stated previously, the sutures appear to be organized to permit and guide certain types of movement between the cranial bones. The cranial bones and sutures are intimately attached to the dura, and the sutures contain vascular and nervous system elements. The fibers within the sutures appear to be present in directions which permit and yield to certain motions.

*The involuntary mobility of the sacrum between the ilia.* The sacrum is suspended between the two ilia by the ligaments at the sacroiliac joints. The posterior sacroiliac ligaments are both thick and strong with multiple fiber directions, analogous to the strong ropes of a child's swing. The anterior sacroiliac ligaments are not only anterior but inferior as well, and appear to support the sacrum from below like the seat of a child's swing. With the patient in either the prone or supine position, the sacrum can be cupped in the examiner's hand, and with a light palpatory compression one can feel, in the normal patient, the to-and-fro oscillating movement of the base and apex of the sacrum which is synchronous with that which was palpated at the cranium.

The primary respiratory mechanism and its related cranial rhythmical impulse (CRI) is influenced by trauma, disease processes, psychological stress, exercise, respiration, and the skilled application of craniosacral manual medicine procedures.

The rate of the CRI is quite close to the patient's respiratory rate. Patients can voluntary control diaphragmatic respiration but cannot directly influence the primary respiratory mechanism. Voluntary respiratory effort of inhalation and exhalation can influence the CRI and the inherent mobility of the osseous and membraneous cranium.

## Craniosacral Diagnosis

As in all other areas of manual medicine the diagnostic process begins with the screening examination, observation and palpation. The operator looks at the skull for symmetry from the anterior, posterior, superior, and both lateral views. One looks at the frontal bosses to see if they are symmetrical, the orbits, nose, zygoma, maxillae, mandible, the level of the ears, and the overall cranial contour. The second stage of the screening examination is palpation of the contours in all dimensions, specifically the palpable sutures as described earlier. One looks for sutural widening, narrowing, tenderness, and any other changes present. Palpation proceeds to the overall resiliency of the skull answering the question, is it more hard and less resilient than normal? Bilateral palpation is performed over the parietotemporal region to ascertain the rate, rhythm, and amplitude of the CRI.

The screening procedure also includes the osseous sacrum to ascertain its movement characteristics between the two ilii with the patient at rest either prone or supine. Is there a normal anterior-posterior nodding movement that is palpable and synchronous with the cranially palpated CRI? Is the movement exaggerated, depressed, or irregular, and is the movement something other than the normally anticipated anterior and posterior nodding range?

If the screening examination provides sufficient evidence for dysfunction of the craniosacral mechanism, additional scanning and segmental-definition examinations proceed. Attention to sphenobasilar mechanics is accomplished by placing the palms of the hands over each side of the skull with the index fingers on the great wings of the sphenoid just behind the midportion of the orbit, with the middle and ring fingers in front of, and behind, the ear, and with the little fingers on the occiput just posterior to the occipitomastoid suture. The two index and two little fingers give four-point contact to the sphenoid and occiput to evaluate sphenobasilar mechanics. With sphenobasilar flexion the index and little fingers separate as they move in a caudad direction, and with extension the fingers on each side come closer together as the hands move cephalically. With sphenobasilar sidebending-rotation to the right, the skull on the right side becomes more convex and the right hand finger contact has the separation in the caudad direction while the fingertip contact on the left side narrows and moves in a cephalic direction. Sphenobasilar left sidebending-rotation provides just the opposite findings. Testing for torsional movement at the sphenobasilar junction is accomplished by maintaining the four point contact and alternately turning one hand forward while the other turns backward. The hand that moves anteriorly carries the sphenoid caudad on that side and elevates the occiput on the same side. The hand that rotates posteriorly carries the sphenoid high on that side and the occiput low on the same side. This torsional movement should be symmetrical bilaterally but if restricted, the dysfunction is named for the side with the sphenoid held in a cephalic (high) position.

The tests to this point are evaluating the pattern of movement at the sphenobasilar junction and the flexion-extension, sidebending-rotation, and torsional movements are all present physiologically. Other disturbances at the sphenobasilar junction are usually the result of traumatic episodes and include lateral strain, vertical strain, and sphenobasilar compression. Injury to the skull from before backward can easily result in sphenobasilar compression which, if present, restricts the midline sphenobasilar movement patterns. The skull usually compensates for this restriction by increased internal and external rotation of the paired lateral bones. Lateral strain occurs when some traumatic episode comes from the side and alters the sphenoidal-occipital relationship in the horizontal plane. Trauma from above can alter the relationship of the sphenobasilar junction in the sagittal plane. Both of these strain mechanisms alter the central axis through the sphenobasilar junction. Traumatic lateral and vertical strains and compressions significantly alter the relationships of the rest of the mechanism. Traumatic sphenobasilar mechanics are more easily tested by a frontooccipital hold in which one hand grasps the occiput posterior to the occipital mastoid junction, and the other hand spans the whole frontal bone with the thumb on one great wing of the sphenoid and the long middle finger on the opposite sphenoid. The two hands can now introduce side to side translatory movement, cephalic to caudad translatory movement, and impaction and distraction. Lateral strain at the sphenobasilar junction will be identified by altered translatory movement from side to side, vertical strain by translatory movements cephalic to caudad, and sphenobasilar compression by distraction through separation of the two hands.

Once the evaluation of sphenobasilar mechanics is made, specific motion tests of each suture of each bone within the mechanism can be evaluated. Specific sutural motion testing is beyond the scope of this volume and the reader is referred to standard texts in the field. Following analysis of the sphenobasilar mechanics and the paired lateral bones of the vault, evaluation of facial mechanics can be made.

## PRINCIPLES OF CRANIOSACRAL TREATMENT

The goals of craniosacral technique are to improve motion in articular restrictions, reduce membranous tension restrictions, improve circulation (particularly of the venous system), reduce the potential for neural entrapment from exit foraman at the base of the skull, and increase the vitality of the cranial rhythmical impulse. All of the specific goals are directed toward improvement in the level of wellness of the patient, and techniques can have local effects within the head and neck region, as well as distal effects throughout the body. Simply, the goal of craniosacral treatment is to restore balanced membranous tension. The normal dynamic reciprocal tension of the falx and tent cannot occur in the presence of restriction or alteration in relationship of cranial bones. Because of the relationship of the membranes to the venous sinuses within the skull, venous drainage cannot be enhanced if abnormal membranous tension persists. The membranes are intimately attached to the periosteum on the internal surface of the skull bones and each of the exit foramen of the skull. Tension in these regions could contribute to neural entrapment and negative neural function. Therefore, restoring maximum mobility to the osseous cranium allows the homeostatic mechanisms to restore balanced membranous tension, enhance venous flow, reduce neural entrapment, and permit normal CRI rate, rhythm, and amplitude.

The most effective treatment sequence is first the sphenobasilar mechanism, then the paired bones of the vault, and finally the facial bones. Treatment of the mechanism from the sacral end can follow, precede, or be done concurrently with treatment at the cranium. This is largely an individual decision, but all successful practitioners of craniosacral technique strive to balance the function of both the cranial and sacral limbs of the mechanism.

## METHODS OF CRANIOSACRAL TECHNIQUE

As in other forms of manual medicine, the methods can be direct, indirect, or exaggeration. In addition, there are two others, disengagement, and molding. The direct action method is the application of effort directly into the barrier to motion. The direction of motion loss is engaged and the activating force(s) are directed against the barrier. Exaggeration method moves the parts in the direction opposite to restriction and into the physiological barrier in the opposite direction. The indirect method attempts to find the neutral point between the area of normal motion in one direction and restricted motion in the opposite, and hold in that position while the activating forces are working. The disengagement method is the application of an activating force to separate sutures; it is particularly used at pivot areas within a suture. Molding technique attempts to modify the resiliency and contour of bone(s) by the application of external force while waiting for intrinsic activating forces to alter the contour and resiliency of the bone.

## ACTIVATING FORCES

The primary activating force in craniosacral technique is the inherent force of the primary respiratory mechanism. The fluctuation of the cerebral spinal fluid can be a powerful, inherent and intrinsic activating force, easily directed from the exterior of the skull. The fluid fluctuation force can be directed by finger contact exactly opposite the area of restriction within the skull. This is used frequently in V-spread technique. If a suture is found to be restricted (e.g., the left occipitomastoid), the index finger of the left hand is put on the posterior aspect of the mastoid process and the middle finger is placed on the occiput posterior to the occipitomastoid suture. The left index and ring fingers are then separated and the index finger of the right hand is placed over the right frontal bone opposite to the left occipitomastoid region. One frequently has the sensation of surf-like pounding until the restricted joint appears to release. This fluid fluctuation activating force is also used in some of the molding method techniques.

The second activating force is respiratory assistance. Voluntary inhalation enhances flexion movement of the mechanism, and voluntary exhalation enhances extension movement of the mechanism. Forced inhalation or exhalation and holding in that extreme of respiration, can be most useful as an activating force to enhance motion in any direction.

The third activating force is enhancement of dural tension by application of effort at the sacrum and from the feet. Flexion and extension movement enhancement can be made directly from the sacrum by the operator's hand enhancing either motion direction at the sacral level. It has been noted that dorsiflexion of the foot, either voluntarily by the patient, or passively by an operator, enhances the intrinsic activating force. One again uses the longest diagonal and, if working on the left side of the skull, dorsiflexion of the right foot; if working on the right side, dorsiflexion of the left foot is used.

The fourth activating force is the procedure "CV 4". This is accomplished by the application of force by the thenar eminences of both hands against the occiput to resist flexion, and maintaining that resistance. This induces a phenomenon called the "still point" during which, for a temporary period of time, no motion is felt. One holds this for approximately five cycles and waits for the fluctuation to return and push the hands away. This maneuver seems to enhance the movement of fluid, changes the rhythm of the diaphragms, and increases temperature in the suboccipital region. A still point can be instituted by compression in places other than the occiput.

Although the aforementioned are all methods of enhancing activating forces in craniosacral technique, the main activating force continues to be the inherent mobility of the brain, meninges, and cerebrospinal fluid. It can be termed inherent force technique and is intrinsic. Enhancement by fluctuation of the CSF, by respiratory insistence, by sacral or extremity force application, or by the CV 4 maneuver, all depend ultimately upon the intrinsic inherent force to reestablish normal mobility.

## Craniosacral Techniques

*Venous sinus technique.*  This procedure is directed toward enhancing the flow of venous blood through the venous sinuses and out from the skull through the jugular foramen. It is particularly useful when the initial palpatory screening examination revealed a hard, rigid skull with loss of resiliency. Venous congestion is believed to contribute greatly to this hard, rigid sensation, and one attempts to enhance venous return to the central venous circulation.

This procedure is initiated at the external occipital protuberance of the occipital bone. Fingertip contact is made with both middle fingers over the protuberance and the weight of the head is carried on these fingerpads. The operator waits for a softening sensation and the beginning of freer mobility. The fingers are then moved sequentially along the midline of the occiput in the direction of the foramen magnum, awaiting the same softening sensation. When this is accomplished, one returns to the external occipital protuberance and, with the pads of all four fingers applied to the occiput along the superior nuchal line, firm pressure is maintained until softening is felt. This reduces congestion within the transverse sinuses. You then return to the external occipital protuberance and address the superior sagittal sinus from behind forward. A thumb is placed on each side of the sagittal suture, palmar surfaces of the hand against the head, and a separation force is applied with each thumb until softening occurs. One works anteriorly from the posterior aspect of the sagittal suture until arriving at the bregma. The last phase is the application of four fingers on either side of the midline of the frontal bone from the bregma to the nasion. Compression and lateral distraction on the frontal bone are made simultaneously by both hands, again waiting for the sensation of softening and release. Frequently, this venous sinus technique is used before approaching specific articular restrictions.

*Condylar Decompression.*  In this procedure the patient lies supine with the operator at the head of the table, the skull in the palms of the hands. The pads of the middle fingers are placed along the inferior aspect of the occiput and slid forward as far as possible and as close to the midline as possible. With some individuals you can reach the posterior margin of the foramen magnum. Pressure is placed upon the occiput by flexing the distal interphalangeal joints of your middle fingers, putting cephalic and posterior traction on the occiput. The operator's elbows are then brought together resulting in supination of both hands and separation of the middle fingers. The resultant force vector is cephalic and posterolateral on each side of the occiput just posterior to the foramen magnum. This is held until release of tension is felt, particularly the sensation of equal softening on each side of the occipital bone.

*CV 4: (Bulb Compression).* This technique has been described above under activating forces. It can be used independently or in combination with other approaches to the craniosacral mechanism.

*Sphenobasilar Junction.* Dysfunctions at the sphenobasilar junction, both physiological and traumatic, can be addressed by an occipitofrontal hold. One hand holds the posterior aspect of the skull (the occiput) in the palm with the thumb and middle finger controlling the occiput posterior to the occipitomastoid region. The other hand grasps the front of the skull with the frontal bone in the palm and with the thumb and middle finger grasping the greater wing of the sphenoid on each side. One hand controls the occiput while the other controls the sphenoid. Sphenobasilar dysfunction can be addressed in either a direct method, an exaggeration method, or an indirect procedure. Respiratory assistance is frequently used concurrently.

*Temporal Rocking.* In this technique the patient is supine on the table with the operator at the head of the table; the occiput is held in the palms of both hands. A thumb is placed behind each ear in front of the mastoid process. The thumbs can now control the temporal bone on each side. Pressure by the distal phalanx of the thumb on the inferior aspect of the mastoid process introduces external rotation. Compression with

the heel of the hand on the base of the mastoid process can enhance internal rotation. Therefore, by movement of the thumbs, the temporals can be rocked into internal and external rotation, either synchronously (both into internal rotation or both into external rotation), or nonsynchronously (one turning into internal rotation and the other into external rotation). Asynchronous rocking through several cycles changes the fluid fluctuation from a to-and- fro movement from front to back to a to-and-fro movement from side to side. Once that becomes symmetrical from side to side, synchronous rocking is then performed to restore the more normal anteroposterior to-and-fro fluid fluctuation. Synchronous movement of the two temporal bones is most important for the maintenance of function at the temporomandibular joint (TMJ). Many patients with TMJ problems have asymmetrical relationship and movement of the two temporal bones.

*V Spread.* This procedure is used to separate restricted and impacted sutures wherever present. It is frequently used at the occipitomastoid suture and is accomplished by placing the index finger and the ring finger on opposite sides of the suture and applying a separation stress. Fluid fluctuation is used as an activating force by applying pressure with the opposite hand at a point most distant and opposite to the suture, in this instance, over the opposite frontal bone.

*Lift Techniques.* There are a number of lift techniques which vary depending upon which bone is engaged and "lifted". A frontal lift involves the application of force by one or two hands on the lateral aspects of each frontal bone with the patient in a supine position on the table. A lifting force toward the ceiling is applied and held for a sense of release. This procedure can be useful in putting longitudinal tension on the falx cerebri and in lifting the frontal from the sphenoid. A parietal lift applies cephalic traction by hands on each parital bone just above the squamoparietal suture and below the attachment of the temporalis muscle.

The principle of all lift techniques is to distract one bone from the other.

### Sequence of Treatment

The sequence of treatment procedures will vary from practitioner to practitioner, from patient to patient, and from one treatment to the next. However, there are some useful general principles which can be individually adapted. First and foremost, the craniosacral mechanism must be viewed within the context of the total musculoskeletal system. Dysfunctions within the craniosacral mechanism may be primary, secondary, or of little import. Cranial dysfunction may be the result of alteration elsewhere, and, if that is not addressed, treatment of the cranial dysfunction will be less than satisfactory. Conversely, continued attention to dysfunction in the musculoskeletal system elsewhere, without addressing the craniosacral dysfunction, will give less than satisfactory results.

When the decision is made to treat the craniosacral mechanism some of the following are useful. If the flexion-extension capability of the sphenobasilar junction is markedly restricted and rigid, and if the head feels as though it is "hard", then venous sinus technique, condylar decompression, and CV 4 technique can be used to begin to obtain some mobility. Once rigidity is addressed, then the sphenobasilar junction should be treated for its nonphysiologic and traumatic dysfunctions of sphenobasilar compression, vertical strain, and lateral strain. Subsequently, the physiological sphenobasilar dysfunctions of sidebending, rotation, torsion, and flexion and extension can be addressed. Attention is then given to the temporal bones to achieve bilateral synchronous temporal rocking. If it is asynchronous, treatment of specific sutural restrictions at all sutural levels of the temporal bone may be necessary. Once temporal synchronous movement is restored, then one can address individual facial bone restrictions, and individual restrictions of other bones in the vault. At the conclusion of treatment, one should assess the mechanism again for overall mobility and for the rate, rhythm, and amplitude of the cranial rhythmic impulse.

These techniques, like any others in manual medicine, need to be prescribed in the dosage appropriate to the individual patient need. Although these procedures do not appear to be active and forceful, they are still powerful and, if inappropriately applied, can be quite detrimental to the patient. As in all other aspects of medicine, the admonition of "primum non nocere" (first do not harm) applies when using craniosacral technique.

# Section II  TECHNIQUE PROCEDURES

# 13

## *CERVICAL SPINE TECHNIQUE*

The cervical spine is of great importance in the field of manual medicine and is one area which receives a great deal of attention by manual therapists. The region is subjected to acute injuries, such as the flexion-extension "whiplash" injury, as well as chronic, repetitive injury from improper posture and abnormal positions of the head and neck. The region is where most of the reported complications of manual medicine procedures have occurred. Traumatic insult to the vertebral-basilar artery system is a rare but catastrophic event. Congenital, inflammatory, and traumatic alterations in the upper cervical region can place the cervical spinal cord at risk from improper diagnostic and manual medicine therapeutic methods. A few such conditions are Down's syndrome, rheumatoid arthritis, agenesis of the odontoid process, and fracture of the odontoid base.

The function of the cervical spine is important, and a myriad of head, neck, and upper extremity symptoms have been clinically observed when this function is altered. Symptomatic conditions in the area can be categorized as cervical-cephalic syndromes, cervical syndromes, and cervical-brachial syndromes. The cervical-cephalic syndromes include those in which pain and restriction of motion of the upper cervical spine is related to pain in the head, both superficial or deep, functional alteration in

vision, vertigo, dizziness, and nystagmus. Cervical syndromes include painful and stiff necks of severity varying from quite mild to an acute spastic torticollis. The cervical-brachial syndromes include all conditions of the shoulder girdle and upper extremity which are related to dysfunctions in the cervical spine, from either altered nervous system functions to the brachial plexus, or altered vascularity (arterial, venous, or lymphatic) resulting from dysfunction at the thoracic inlet. The student and practitioner must know the anatomy and physiology of the region to understand the therapeutic role of manual medicine in this area and avoid its potential complications.

### *FUNCTIONAL ANATOMY*

The cervical spine can be divided into the atypical segments of the upper cervical complex: occipitoatlantal (CO-C1), atlantoaxial (C1-C2), and C2, an atypical vertebra on its superior aspect, and a typical cervical vertebra on its inferior aspect. C3 to C7 are the typical cervical segments.

The C0-C3 complex functions as an integrated unit, whose biomechanics are under intense research and study. For practical purposes it is useful to look at each level individually, recognizing that each contributes appropriately to the function of the overall complex.

**125**

The occipitoatlantal junction (C0-C1) consists of the two articulations formed by the occipital condyles and the superior articular facets of the atlas. The occipital condyles are convex from front to back and from side to side, and the superior articular facets of the atlas are concave from front to back and from side to side. The two articulations are divergent from before backward. The primary movement is that of forward-bending and backward-bending. There is coupled sidebending and rotation movement to opposite sides which is quite small, but becomes highly significant clinically when lost. The sidebending movement occurs with the occipital condyles sliding upward on one side of the atlas and downward on the other. This sidebending arc is probably less than 5° from side to side. The coupled rotation is to the opposite side from sidebending and appears to be a function of the ligamentous attachments of the occiput to the atlas and axis, and the relationship of the slope of the sides of the superior facets of the atlas and their divergence posteriorly. The amount of rotation is quite small.

The atlantoaxial articulations (C1-C2) consist of the right and left apophyseal joints in which the inferior facet of the atlas, which becomes slightly convex when the articular cartilage is present, articulates with the convex superior facets of the axis, resulting in a unique convex-to-convex apposition. The superior articular facets of the axis face superiorly and laterally and give the appearance of a pair of shoulders. Other articulations at the atlantoaxial junction are *(a)* the small facet on the posterior aspect of the anterior arch of the atlas which articulates with the anterior surface of the odontoid of the axis, and *(b)* the articulation of the posterior aspect of the odontoid of the axis and the transaxial ligament. The integrated function of all of these articulations, modified by the ligamentous and muscular attachments, result in a small amount of forward-bending, and backward-bending, and sidebending; but the primary motion is rotation to the right and left. Because of the unique convex-to-convex articular apposi-

tion of the apophyseal joints, there is a range of cephalic-to-caudad translatory movement during rotation. As the atlas turns to the right on the axis, the right facet of the atlas slides downward on a posterior aspect of the right facet of the axis, and the left inferior facet of the atlas slides downward on the anterior aspect of the left facet of the axis resulting in some caudad translation. Upon returning to neutral, the inferior facets of the atlas "crawl back up" the articular shoulders of the axis resulting in a cephalic translatory movement.

The C2-C3 articulation has typical cervical spine characteristics. However, because of the relationship of the superior aspect of C2 to the atlas as well as to the occiput through ligamentous and muscular attachment, C2 functions as a transitional segment and has some unique functional characteristics.

The typical cervical segments from C3 to C7 articulate at the vertebral bodies with an intevertebral disk. The superior surface of the vertebral body is convex from before backward and concave from side to side while the inferior surface of the vertebral body is convex from side to side and concave from before backward. This configuration results in a "universal-type" joint at the intervertebral disc level. At the posterolateral corner of the vertebral body is found the uncovertebral joint of Luschka which appears to have some function in guiding movement during forward-bending and backward-bending. These joints also seem to protect the posterolateral aspect of the intervertebral disk from herniation in that direction. These synovial joints are subject to degenerative change with productive lipping, which occasionally encroaches upon the anterior aspect of the lateral intervertebral canal. The apophyseal joints of the typical cervical vertebra face backward and upward at an angle of approximately 45° and provide for forward-bending, backward-bending, and a coupled sidebending-and-rotation movement. Because of the facing of the apophyseal joints, the universal characteristic of the vertebral bodies, and the intervening intervertebral disk, the coupled sidebending-rotation movement is *always* to the same side.

There are several other anatomical relationships in the cervical spine of importance to manual medicine. The first is the course of the vertebral artery. Its intimate relationship to the cervical spine begins at the level of C6 and 7 where it enters between the transverse processes and immediately turns cephalic. It runs through the intertransverse foramen of the cervical vertebrae and exits from the superior side of the transverse process of C1. At this level it travels acutely posteriorly over the posterior arch of the atlas and penetrates the posterior occipitoatlantal membrane, entering the foramen magnum. Here it joins the vertebral artery of the opposite side to form the basilar artery. It can be seen that the vertebral artery is at risk at the acute angulation at C6-7; by productive change in and around the intertransverse foramen from C7 to C1; and at the occipitoatlantal junction. Another phenomenon affecting the vertebral artery is its narrowing on the side contralateral to cervical rotation. This normal phenomenon is exacerbated when accomplished in backward-bending of the head on the neck and is complicated by the presence of congenital or degenerative vessel disease. There are provocative diagnostic tests, such as the hanging (De Kleyn) test, in which the examiner backward-bends the neck over the head of the table and introduces rotation to the right and to the left, testing for the development of nystagmus. This author does not advocate such testing as it appears to put the vertebral artery at unnecessary risk. A comprehensive history and physical examination should alert the examiner to the potential presence of vascular disease in the vertebrobasilar system. One of the earliest symptoms of cerebral anoxia is acute anxiety and panic, and if occurring during a structural diagnostic or manual medicine procedure in the cervical spine, should alert the examiner to stop and institute immediate evaluation and treatment for potential vascular complications.

A second anatomical feature of the cervical spine is the wealth of mechano- and nociceptors present in the articulations and particular structures. Dysfunction in the cervical spine can result in increased afferent stimulation from these mechanoreceptors and nocireceptors and influence the integrative function of the musculoskeletal system as well as contribute to the production of local and regional symptoms.

The relationship of the superior cervical ganglion to the cervical spine also appears to be clinically significant. The sympathetic autonomic nervous system control of cerebral blood flow emanates from the superior cervical ganglia. This structure is intimately related to the longus colli muscle and the anterior surface of C2. It is intimately bound down by deep connective fascia and appears to respond to dysfunction at the upper cervical spine, particularly at C2. It has been observed that C2 dysfunction is frequent in cervicocephalic syndromes and internal visceral disease. It has been reported that there is a small branch of the second cervical nerve which connects with the vagus as it descends through the neck. It is hypothesized that this neural connection may be responsible for the clinical observation of dysfunction at C2 with visceral disease.

## STRUCTURAL DIAGNOSIS

In the typical cervical segments the coupled sidebending-and-rotation movement is to the same side (type II). This coupled movement is most easily evaluated by employing a right-to-left translatory movement to introduce the sidebending component. While restriction of this translatory movement does occur when the cervical lordosis is in neutral, in most dysfunctions of the typical cervical segment there will be either a forward-bending or backward-bending motion restriction component.

The anatomical structure available for structural diagnosis of the typical cervical segments is the posterolateral aspect of the articular pillar. The articular pillar can be palpated by following the deep fascial band between the semispinalis medially and the longissimus laterally. With paired fingers the examiner can palpate and localize to the right and left articular pillars of a given cervical segment; fixing that segment and translating it right to left introduces motion testing for sidebending and rotation. The articular pillars in the typical cervical spine are about the size of the examiner's fingerpad, and localization to a given segment can be accomplished in the following fashion. The spinous process of C2 is easily palpable in the midline posteriorly and the articular pillars are lateral at the same level. The transverse processes of C7 are easily palpable on the lateral aspect of the neck just anterior to the trapezius muscle. C7 articular pillars are at the same level. The examiner places the four fingers of each hand, overlying the articular pillars, with the index finger just superior to the transverse process of C7 and the little fingers just below the spinous process of C2. The index fingers will be on C6, the middle fingers on C5, the ring fingers on C4, and the little fingers on C3. This gives one the ability to localize to a specific cervical segment.

Palpating in this region allows the examiner to detect tissue texture abnormality, particularly muscle hypertonicity. These areas are quite tender in the cervical area and in some systems are called zones of irritation. Once identifying an area of tissue texture abnormality, with a screening procedure indicating cervical dysfunction, the examiner proceeds to specifically identify motion restriction at the dysfunctional segment. The procedure is as follows:

—The examiner palpates and stabilizes the superior segment at the dysfunctional level with paired fingers overlying the articular pillar.

—The operator's heel of the hands controls the patient's head so that all movement above the segment being tested is controlled.

—The operator introduces translatory movement to the right and to the left to test the coupled sidebending-and-rotation movement to the same side.

—Translation from right to left of C5 on C6, tests the capacity of C5 to right side bend and right rotate on C6.

—Translation from right to left without abnormal resistance requires the right facet to close and the left facet to open.

—If resistance of translation from right to left is encountered, there is restriction of right sidebending and right rotation of C5 on C6.

The examiner now proceeds to evaluate for the presence of forward-bending and backward-bending restriction together with the coupled sidebending-and-rotation restriction to the same side.

—The examiner's fingertips contact the articular pillars of the superior vertebra of the vertebral motion segment being tested (e.g., C5 on C6).

—With the patient supine on the examining table, the examiner, sitting or standing at the head of the table, lifts the fingers toward the ceiling introducing backward bending at the C5, 6 level (Fig.13.1).

—The head is translated to the left and then to the right sensing for resistance to the translatory movement with the head and neck in the backward-bent position.

—The eyes should remain in the horizontal (x) plane so that the sidebending is introduced by the translatory effort. Sidebending is not introduced by cocking the head to one side or to the other.

—If resistance is encountered with the translatory movement from the right to the left while the head is backward bent, a diagnosis of restriction of backward bending, right sidebending, and

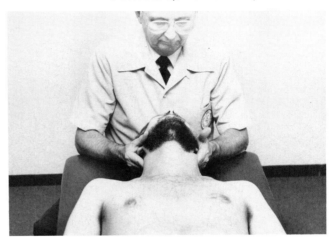

**Figure 13.1.** Motion tests C5, 6 backward-bending.

right rotation is made. Positionally the segment will be flexed, rotated left, sidebent left (FRS left) (Fig. 13.2).

—If the resistance is noted in translation from left to right while the head is backward bent, the motion restriction is backward-bending, left sidebending, left rotation. The segment is flexed, rotated right, sidebent right (FRS right) (Fig. 13.3).

—If resistance was encountered in translation from right to left, the right facet did not close. If resistance was met in translation from left to right, the left facet did not close.

To test the presence of forward bending restriction the examiner now proceeds as follows:

—The patient is supine on the table with the operator standing or sitting at the head.

—The examiner grasps the head in the heels of the hand with the palpating finger over the posterior aspect of the articular pillar of the superior vertebra of the vertebral motion segment (e.g., C5 on C6).

—The examiner rotates the head forward and forward-bends the neck

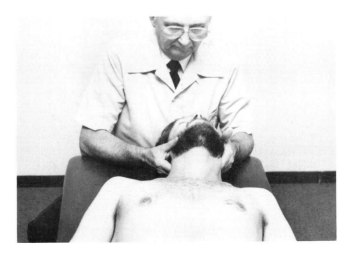

**Figure 13.2.** Motion tests C5, 6 backward-bending, translation right to left.

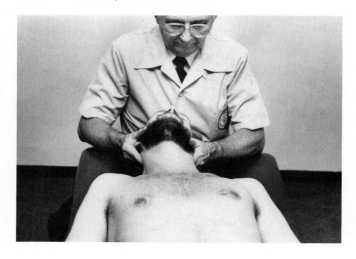

**Figure 13.3.** Motion tests C5, 6 backward-bending, translation left to right.

down to the segment being tested (Fig. 13.4).

—The examiner introduces translatory movement from right to left. If resistance is encountered, a diagnosis is made of forward-bending, right sidebending, and right rotation restriction. Positionally the segment is extended, rotated left, sidebent left (ERS left) (Fig.13.5).

—If resistance is encountered in translation from left to right, a diagnosis is made of restriction of forward-bending, left sidebending, left rotation. Positionally, the segment is extended,

tated right, sidebent right (ERS right) (Fig.13.6).

—If resistance was encountered in translation from right to left the left facet did not open. If a resistance is encountered in translation from left to right, the right facet did not open.

Occasionally there is resistance to the same translatory movement in both forward-bending and backward-bending. This is interpreted as a restriction of both facets, i.e., one does not open and the other does not close. There is undoubtedly a component of this in most typical cervical vertebra dysfunctions, but usually there is a major re-

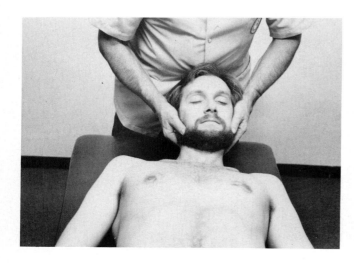

**Figure 13.4.** Motion tests C5, 6 forward-bending.

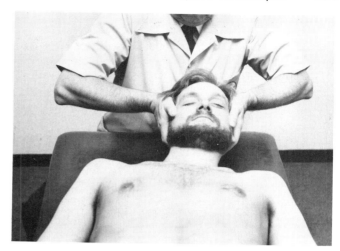

**Figure 13.5.** Motion tests C5, 6 forward-bending, translation right to left.

strictor in one direction, which when appropriately treated restores maximal function to that segment. The typical cervical vertebra should be evaluated and treated segment by segment. While it is possible for several consecutive vertebral motion segments to become dysfunctional, this does not result in a group (type I) dysfunction. They are a series of single vertebral motion segment dysfunctions, which must be treated individually. Group dysfunctions do not occur in the cervical spine.

After restoration of function to the typical cervical segments, the examiner proceeds cephalically and evaluates the atlanto-axial articulation. Since rotation makes up approximately 90° of the mobility of this articulation, it is tested. If there is restriction of rotation there is undoubtedly some restriction of the minor movements as well, however restoration of the rotational function appears to restore normal motion to the minor movements. The test is accomplished as follows:

— The patient is supine on the table with the operator standing at the head.

— The operator grasps the head in the two hands and flexes the head on the neck to approximately 45° (Fig. 13.7).

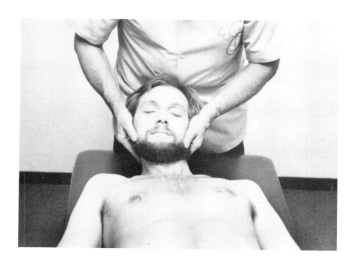

**Figure 13.6.** Motion tests C5, 6 forward-bending, translation left to right.

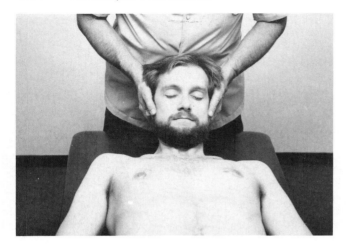

**Figure 13.7.**   Motion tests C1, 2 flexed starting position.

—While retaining the 45° forward-bending, the operator introduces rotation to the right and then to the left testing for resistance to the rotational movement.

—Resistance to rotation to the right makes a diagnosis of right atlas restriction. Positionally the atlas is left rotated (Fig. 13.8).

—Resistance of rotation to the left results in a diagnosis of restriction of atlas rotation to the left. Positionally the atlas is rotated right (Fig. 13.9).

Once the atlantoaxial component of the upper cervical complex has been diagnosed as dysfunctional, it should be appropriately treated before evaluation of the occipitoatlantal junction.

The examiner is now prepared to evaluate the occipitoatlantal articulation for its motion contribution to the upper cervical complex at the craniocervical junction. Translatory movement is again utilized to introduce the sidebending-motion test. Rotation is not actively tested but restriction of rotation is detected by restriction of sidebending. At the occipitoatlantal articulation sidebending and rotation are always coupled to opposite sides. The procedure is as follows:

—The patient is supine on the table with the operator sitting or standing at the head.

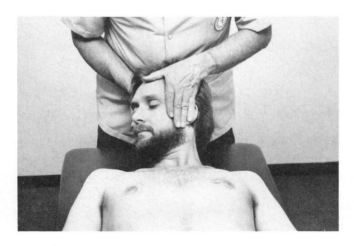

**Figure 13.8.**   Motion tests C1, 2 right rotation.

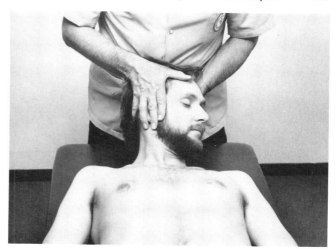

**Figure 13.9.** Motion tests C1, 2 left rotation.

—The operator grasps the patient's head in the two hands overlying the temporoparietal regions.

—The operator introduces backward-bending by rotating the head around an approximate axis through the external auditory meatus (Fig. 13.10).

—With the head backward-bent (but not off the table) the operator introduces translatory movement from right to left, keeping the eyes in the horizontal plane. If resistance is encountered a diagnosis is made of restriction of occipitoatlantal backward-bending, right sidebending, and left

rotation. Positionally the occiput is flexed, sidebent left, rotated right ($FS_L R_R$) (Fig. 13.11).

—With the head remaining in a backward-bent position, translation is introduced from left to right. If resistance is encountered, it is interpreted as a diagnosis of restriction of the occiput to backward-bending, left sidebending, right rotation. Positionally the occiput is flexed, sidebent right, rotated left ($FS_R R_L$) (Fig. 13.12).

—The operator introduces forward-bending of the head around an ap-

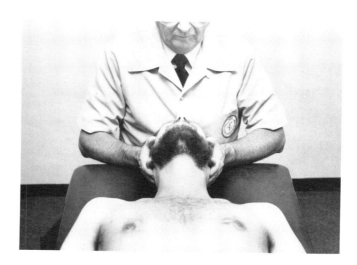

**Figure 13.10.** Motion tests C0-C1 backward-bending.

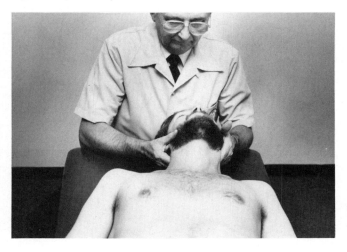

**Figure 13.11.** Motion tests C0-C1 backward-bending, translation right to left.

proximate axis through the external auditory meatus (Fig. 13.13).

—With the head forward-bent, translatory movement from left to right. If resistance is encountered, a diagnosis is made of restriction of occipitoatlantal forward-bending, left sidebending and right rotation. Positionally the occiput is extended, right sidebent, and left rotated ($ES_RR_L$) (Fig. 13.14).

—With the head still forward-bent, translatory movement is introduced from right to left. If resistance is encountered, a diagnosis is made of restriction of occipitoatlantal forward-bending, right sidebending, and left rotation. Positionally the occiput is extended, left sidebent and right rotated ($FS_LR_R$).

This diagnostic process allows the examiner to evaluate all the motion characteristics of the occipitoatlantal, atlantoaxial, and typical cervical articulations.

### Manual Medicine Therapeutic Procedures

A direct action, muscle energy procedure for a segment that has backward-bending restriction is as follows:

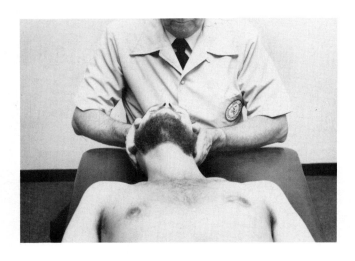

**Figure 13.12.** Motion tests C0-C1 backward-bending, translation left to right.

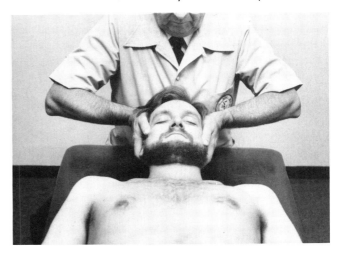

**Figure 13.13.** Motion tests C0-C1 forward-bending.

*Typical cervical vertebra*
Diagnosis
Position: Flexed, rotated right, sidebent right (FRS$_{Rt}$)
Motion restriction: Extension, left rotation, left sidebending

1. Patient supine on table with operator sitting at head of table.
2. Operator's fingertips palpate the pillar of the inferior vertebra of the dysfunctional vertebral motion segment to hold that segment so that the superior can be moved upon it (Fig. 13.15).

3. The operator's other hand controls the patient's head to introduce side-bending and rotation (Fig. 13.16).
4. The operator lifts the fingerpads in contact with the articular pillar toward the ceiling introducing backward-bending while simultaneously the other hand introduces rotation and sidebending toward the restriction of the barrier.
5. The patient is asked to exert a small isometric effort against the operator's resistant hand into either side-bending or rotation, or to lift the head off the table for forward-bending.

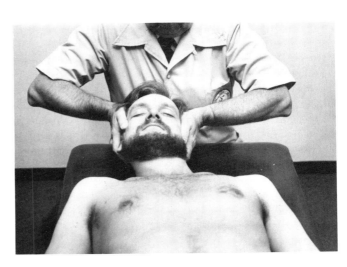

**Figure 13.14.** Motion tests C0-C1 forward-bending, translation left to right.

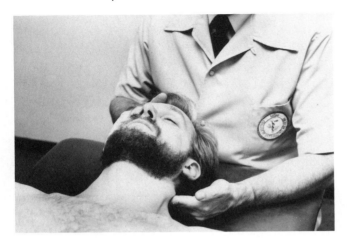

**Figure 13.15.** Muscle energy technique, typical cervical vertebra, pillar contact.

6. Following a 3- to 5-second muscle effort, the patient relaxes and the operator increases the backward-bending, sidebending and rotation against the next barrier. The process is repeated approximately 3 to 5 times.

7. Retest.
   Note: An alternative activating force could be eye movement. In the example of restriction of backward-bending, left sidebending, left rotation, the patient's activating force could be to look to the right against resistance and the new barrier is engaged during relaxation when the patient looks to the left.

The high-velocity, low-amplitude procedure for the same diagnosis is as follows:

*Cervical spine*

Typical cervical vertebra

Diagnosis
Position: Flexed, rotated left, sidebent left ($FRS_{Lt}$)
Motion restriction: Extension, right rotation, right sidebending
Facet-closing thrust

1. Patient supine on table with operator sitting at head of table.

2. Operator's left hand controls left side of the patient's head.

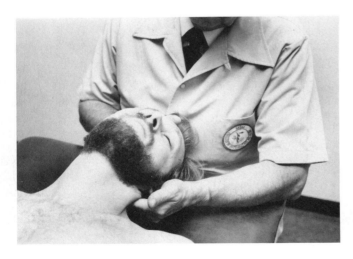

**Figure 13.16.** Muscle energy technique, typical cervical vertebra, engagement of sidebending rotation barrier.

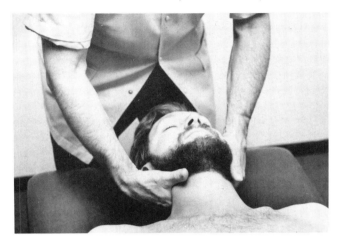

**Figure 13.17.** Typical cervical vertebra, facet-closing thrust, superior pillar contact.

3. Operator's second metacarpophalangeal joint is in contact with the articular pillar of the *superior* segment of the vertebral motion unit (Fig. 13.17).
4. Extension, right sidebending is introduced and localized at the involved segments (Fig.13.18).
5. When extension and right-sidebending barrier is engaged, a high-velocity, low-amplitude, low-force thrust is applied caudad in the direction of the spinous process of T1.
6. Retest.
   Note: Regardless of which cervical segment is dysfunctional, the thrust is always in the direction of T1.

A direct action muscle energy procedure for a typical cervical vertebra that has forward-bending restriction with side bending and rotation restriction of the same side is as follows:

*Cervical spine*
Typical cervical vertebra
    Diagnosis
        Position: Extended, rotated right, sidebent right ($ERS_{Rt}$)
        Motion restriction: Forward-bending, rotation left, sidebending left

1. Patient supine on table with operator standing at head of table.

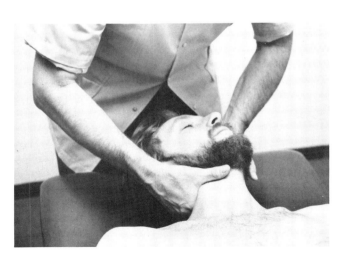

**Figure 13.18.** Typical cervical facet-closing thrust engaging backward-bending right sidebending barrier.

2. Operator's heel and palm of the left hand supports the patient's occiput and the operator's thumb and index finger contact the two facet joints at the dysfunctional level.

3. The operator's right hand controls the patient's head.

4. The head and neck are forward-bent down to the first forward-bending barrier palpated by the operator's index and ring fingers (Fig. 13.19).

5. Sidebending and rotation left are introduced by the operator's right hand (note: a right translatory movement of the operator's left hand localizes this maneuver to the dysfunctional segment) (Fig. 13.20).

6. Patient is instructed to isometrically put the head backward into the palm of the operator's hand or to sidebend the head to the right against resistance.

7. Three to five efforts follow with the engagement of new barrier between each effort.

8. Retest.
   Note: Again, eye movement can be utilized with looking to the right as the activating force against resistance with new slack being taken up to left sidebending and left rotation when the patient looks to the left.

There are two variations of high-velocity low-amplitude thrusting procedures for diagnosis of forward-bending restriction of the typical cervical segments. They are as follows:

*Cervical spine*
Typical cervical vertebra (variation #1)
"Opening facet thrust"
  Diagnosis
      Position: Extended, rotated right, sidebent right (ERS$_{Rt}$)
      Motion restriction: Flexion, rotation left, sidebending left

1. Patient supine on table, operator standing at head of table.

2. Operator's left second metacarpophalangeal joint is in contact with the left facet joint of the involved segment (Fig. 13.21).

3. The head is flexed and sidebent to the left with localization of sidebending at the involved segment (Fig. 13.22).

4. When resistance is engaged with flexion, left sidebending and left rotation, a high-velocity, low-amplitude, low-force thrust is applied horizontally in the plane of the involved joint. (Facet on right side "gaps" open.)

5. Retest.

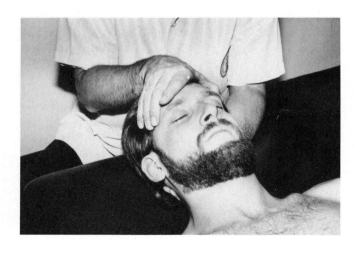

**Figure 13.19.** Typical cervical vertebra, muscle energy starting position.

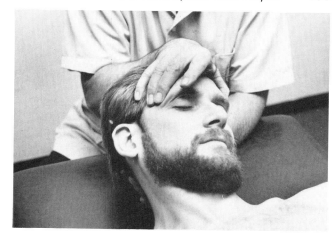

**Figure 13.20.** Typical cervical vertebra, muscle energy engaging barrier of forward-bending, left sidebending, and left rotation barrier.

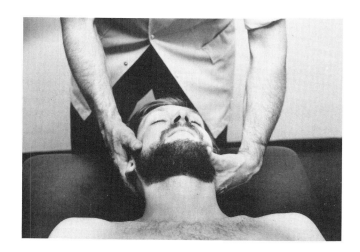

**Figure 13.21.** Typical cervical vertebra, opening facet thrust, contact on left facet joint.

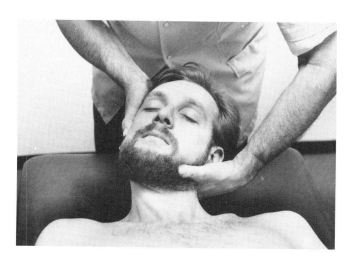

**Figure 13.22.** Typical cervical vertebra, opening facet thrust, localization of forward-bending, left sidebending, left rotation barrier.

*Cervical spine*
Typical cervical vertebra (variation #2)
"Opening facet thrust"
> Diagnosis
>> Position: Extended, rotated right, sidebent right ($ERS_{Rt}$)
>> Motion restriction: Flexion, rotation left, sidebending left

1. Patient supine on table, operator sitting at head of table.
2. Operator's two hands control patient's head with thenar eminences on both temporal regions (Fig. 13.23).
3. With left index and middle fingers blocking the facet joint on the left side; flexion, sidebending, and rotation left are introduced.
4. The operator's right second metacarpophalangeal joint contacts the right articular pillar of the superior segment of the vertebral motion unit.
5. When the flexion, left sidebending, left rotational barrier is engaged, a rotary thrust of high-velocity, low-amplitude, low-force is introduced in a left rotary fashion pivoting around the blocking fingers of the operator's left hand (Fig. 13.24)
6. Retest.

A direct action muscle energy procedure for the atlantoaxial joint is as follows:

*Cervical spine*
Atlantoaxial junction
> Diagnosis
>> Position: Atlas rotated right
>> Motion restriction: Atlas resistant to left rotation on axis

1. Patient supine on table with operator sitting or standing at head of table.
2. Operator grasps the head in the palms of the hands and flexes the head to 45° (Fig. 13.25).
3. The operator introduces rotation left until the restricted barrier is engaged (Fig. 13.26).
4. The patient is instructed to turn the head to the right against resistance with a light isometric muscle energy procedure.
5. Following 3- to 5-second contraction and subsequent relaxation, the operator increases rotation to the left.
6. Patient repeats right rotational effort against resistance approximately three to five times.
7. Retest.
   Note: An eye movement activating force can be utilized as well, with in-

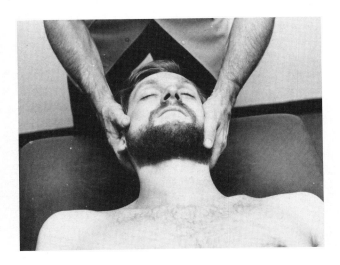

**Figure 13.23.** Typical cervical vertebra, opening facet thrust, hand contact.

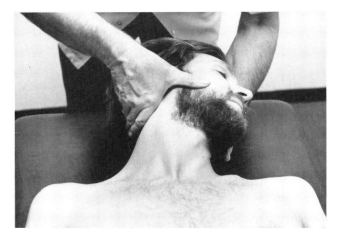

**Figure 13.24.** Typical cervical vertebra, opening facet thrust, into forward-bending, left sidebending, and left rotation.

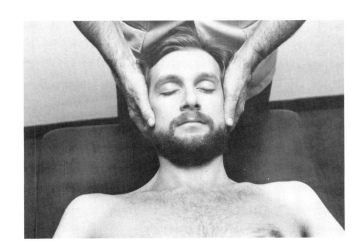

**Figure 13.25.** Muscle energy C1-2, head flexed 45°

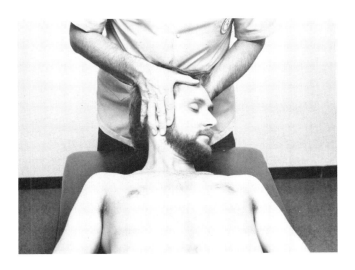

**Figure 13.26.** Muscle energy C1-2, engaging left rotation restriction barrier.

struction to the patient to look to the right. During the relaxation phase, left rotational barrier can be engaged with the patient looking to the left.

High-velocity, low-amplitude, direct action thrust procedures for the atlantoaxial junction are as follows:

*Cervical spine*
Atlantoaxial junction (variation #1)
> Diagnosis
>> Position: Atlas rotated right
>> Motion restriction: Atlas resistant to left rotation on axis

1. Patient supine on table, operator standing at head of table.
2. Operator's left hand cradles left side of patient's head by overlying parietotemporal area.
3. Operator's right hand is on the right posterior arch of the atlas (Fig. 13.27).
4. Patient's head is rotated left to the left rotation restriction barrier (Fig. 13.28).
5. A rotary high-velocity, low-amplitude, low-thrust force is applied simultaneously by both hands, but localized by the operator's right metacarpophalangeal joint in contact with the right posterior arch of the atlas.
6. Retest.

*Cervical spine*
Atlantoaxial junction (variation #2)
> Diagnosis
>> Position: Atlas rotated left
>> Motion restriction: Atlas restricted right rotation at axis

1. Patient supine on table, operator standing at head of table.
2. Operator's two hands cradle the patient's head overlying the temporal regions, with fingers monitoring at posterior arch of atlas bilaterally.
3. Patient's head is flexed to approximately 45° (Fig. 13.29).
4. Rotation is introduced to the right rotational barrier (Fig. 13.30).
5. A rotary-type, high-velocity, low-amplitude, low-force thrust is applied in a right rotary direction.
6. Retest.

A direct action muscle energy procedure for the occipitoatlantal joint which resist backward-bending is as follows:

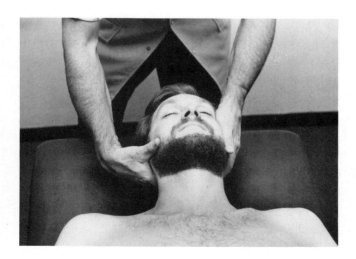

**Figure 13.27.** C1-2 direct action thrust, contact on right atlas.

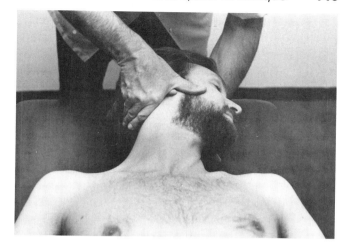

**Figure 13.28.** C1-C2 thrust against left rotation barrier.

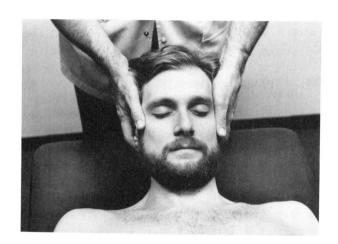

**Figure 13.29.** C1-C2 thrust, starting position.

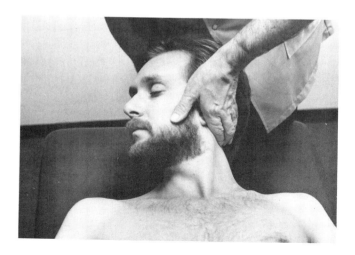

**Figure 13.30.** C1-C2 thrust into right rotational barrier.

*Cervical spine*
Occipitoatlantal junction
    Diagnosis
        Position: Flexed, sidebent
        right, rotated left ($FS_R R_L$)
        Motion restriction: Back-
        ward-bending, left side-
        bending, right rotation

1. Patient supine on table with operator standing or sitting at head.
2. Operator's left hand grasps the patient's occiput with the web of the
   thumb on the nuchal line.
3. Operator's right hand grasps the patient's chin with the right forearm in
   contact with the right temporoparietal area of the patient (Fig.
   13.31).
4. The backward-bending barrier is
   first engaged by the operator's two
   hands rotating the head
   posteriorly.
5. Left sidebending is introduced by
   the operator's right forearm while
   maintaining the chin in the midline.
   (Note: rotation is not actively introduced.) (Fig. 13.32).
6. The patient is instructed to pull the
   chin toward the chest against resistance offered by the operator's right
   hand for 3–5 seconds of a light isometric muscle energy contraction.

7. Following relaxation the slack is
   again taken up in backward-bending
   and left sidebending.
8. Patient's muscle energy effort is repeated 3–5 times.
9. Retest.
   Note: An eye movement activating
   force can be utilized with the instruction to the patient to look forcibly down toward the feet with engagement of a new barrier taken
   when the patient looks up toward
   the operator.

A high-velocity, low-amplitude, thrust
procedure for an occiput with backward-
bending restriction is as follows:

*Cervical spine*
Occipitoatlantal junction
    Diagnosis
        Position: Flexed, sidebent
        left, rotated right ($FS_L R_R$)
        Motion restriction: Exten-
        sion, sidebending right, ro-
        tation left

1. Patient supine on table, operator sitting at head of table.
2. Operator's right hand cradles
   occiput with web of thumb and index
   finger on bone at insertion of spinal
   extensor muscles (not over posterior
   occipitoatlantal membrane.)

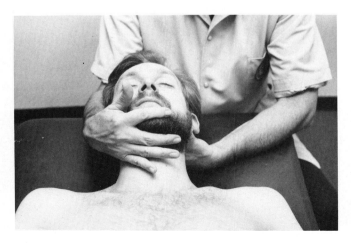

**Figure 13.31.** C0-C1 muscle energy, starting position.

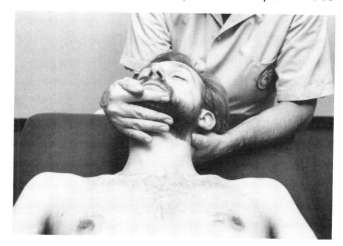

**Figure 13.32.** C0-C1 muscle energy, engaging backward-bending, left sidebending, right rotation barrier.

3. Operator's left hand cradles patient's chin with left forearm along left side of patient's mandible and temporal region (Fig. 13.33).
4. Extension is introduced to barrier sensed by operator's left hand.
5. Right sidebending of patient's head is introduced by the operator's left forearm, (note that patient's chin remains in the midline, resulting in left rotation) (Fig. 13.34).
6. When barrier engaged in extension, right sidebending and left rotation, a high-velocity, low-amplitude, low-force thrust is applied in a cephalic direction with simultaneous action of operator's two hands.
7. Retest.

A direct action muscle energy procedure for the occipitoatlantal junction in which the occiput resists forward-bending is as follows:

*Cervical spine*
Occipitoatlantal junction
    Diagnosis
        Position: Extended, sidebent right, rotated left ($ES_RR_L$)
        Motion restriction: Forward-bending, left sidebending, right rotation

1. Patient supine on the table with operator sitting at the head.
2. Operator's left hand grasps the occiput with the web of the thumb

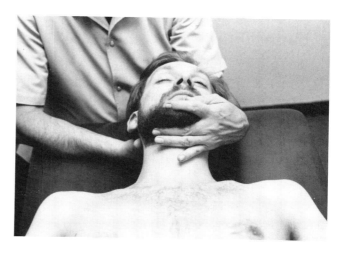

**Figure 13.33.** C0-C1 thrust procedure, starting position.

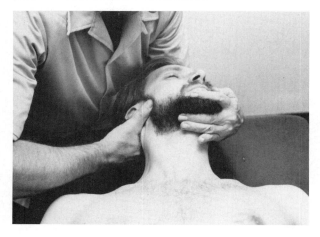

**Figure 13.34.** C0-C1 thrust procedure, engaging backward-bending, right sidebending, and left rotation barrier.

along the superior nuchal line. The operator's right hand cups the patient's chin with the index finger in front of the chin and with the right forearm along the right temporoparietal region (Fig. 13.35).

3. Forward-bending is introduced by rotating the head forward by the combined action of the operator's two hands.
4. Left sidebending is introduced by the operator's right forearm while maintaining the chin in the midline. This introduces right rotation as the coupled movement (Fig. 13.36).
5. The patient is instructed to push the head directly backward into the hand toward the table against resistance offered by the operator for 3–5 seconds of a mild isometric muscle energy contraction.
6. Following relaxation the operator increases the forward-bending and left sidebending to the new barrier.
7. Patient's isometric procedure repeated 3–5 times.
8. Retest.
   Note: An eye motion activating force can be utilized with instructions to the patient to look up toward the operator when the barrier is engaged and with the operator engaging a new barrier when the patient looks toward the feet.

A high-velocity, low-amplitude, low-force thrust procedure for occipitoatlantal junction in which the occiput resists forward-bending is as follows:

*Cervical spine*
Occipitoatlantal junction
    Diagnosis
        Position: Extended, sidebent right, rotated left
        Motion restriction: Flexion, sidebending left, rotation right

1. Patient supine on table, operator sitting at head of table.
2. Operator's left hand cradles occiput with web of thumb and index finger on bone at insertion of spinal extensor muscles (not over posterior occipitalatlantal membrane).
3. Operator's right hand cradles patient's chin with right forearm along right side of patient's mandible and temporal region (Fig. 13.37).
4. Flexion is introduced to barrier sensed by operator's right hand.
5. Left sidebending of patient's head is introduced by operator's right forearm, (note that patient's chin remains in the midline, resulting in right rotation) (Fig. 13.38).
6. When barrier is engaged in flexion, left sidebending and right rotation, a high-velocity, low-amplitude, low-

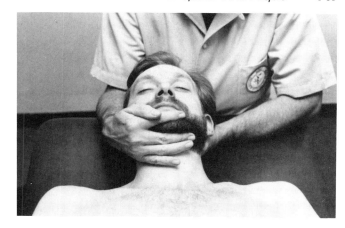

**Figure 13.35.** C0-C1 muscle energy, starting position.

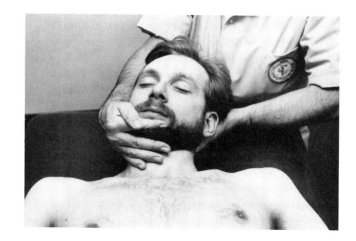

**Figure 13.36.** C0-C1 muscle energy, forward-bending, left side-bending, right rotation barrier.

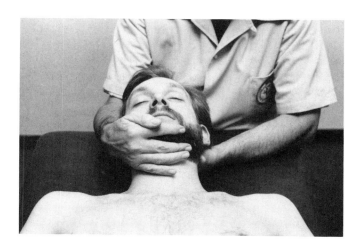

**Figure 13.37.** C0-C1 thrust procedure, starting position.

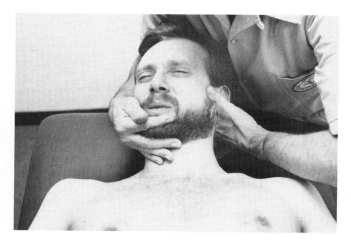

**Figure 13.38.**   C0-C1 thrust procedure, engaging forward-bending, left sidebending, right rotation barrier.

force thrust is applied in a cephalic direction with simultaneous action of operator's two hands.

7.   Retest.

In the craniocervical junction one frequently encounters muscle hypertonicity. Soft tissue inhibitory technique at the insertion of muscle to bone is frequently of value in this region with specific attention given to the hypertonic short and long muscles at the occiput. Another procedure of value in this region is a modified craniosacral technique described as occipital decompression. This condition is evaluated as follows:

—With the patient supine on the table and the operator sitting at the head, with the head cradled in the operator's hands, the middle finger of each hand palpates along the occipital bone in the suboccipital region as far forward as possible while staying on bone (Fig. 13.39).

—With flexion of the distal interphalangeal joint, the operator senses for equality or inequality of tissue tension in the region and particularly resiliency to the occipital bone on each side.

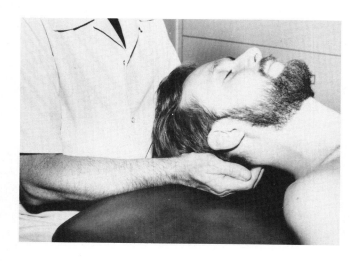

**Figure 13.39.**   Occipital decompression.

—A normal finding is of equal tension and resiliency in the region.

—A positive finding is interpreted when one side is more tense and less resilient than the other.

A modified direct action craniosacral technique for occipital decompression is as follows:

1. Patient supine on table with operator sitting at the head.
2. The palms of the operator's hands cradle the head with the middle finger extended along the inferior aspect of the occipital bone as far forward as possible in the direction of the foramen magnum.
3. The operator's forearms are placed on the table and the distal interphalangeal joints of the index fingers are flexed.
4. The operator's elbows are now brought together in the midline resulting in a posterolateral traction effort on the fingertip contact with the occiput.
5. The position is held until release is felt in the tense and nonresilient area.
6. It is occasionally useful to increase the fingertip tension on the dysfunctional side when the elbows are brought together.
7. The goal of treatment is to balance the tone and resiliency of the occiput and the suboccipital tissues.

The procedures described here can be useful in a myriad of head, neck, and upper extremity problems. These diagnostic and therapeutic procedures deal with all of the possible dysfunctions found in the region. There are many similar procedures that are variations on the theme, but the principles described here have been found to be highly effective in the manual medicine approach to the cervical spine.

# 14
## THORACIC SPINE TECHNIQUE

Twelve vertebrae comprise the thoracic spine and are noted for their posterior kyphosis. The thoracic spine is intimately related to the rib cage and essentially works as a single unit. Alteration in thoracic spine function influences the rib cage, and alteration in rib cage function alters the thoracic spine. Hence, from the respiratory-circulatory model of manual medicine, the thoracic spine assumes major importance in providing optimal functional capacity to the thoracic cage for respiration and circulation. The thoracic spine takes on additional importance from the neurologic perspective because of its relationship with the sympathetic division of the autonomic nervous system. All twelve segments of the thoracic spinal cord give origin to preganglionic sympathetic nerve fibers, which exit through the intervertebral canals of the thoracic vertebra and either synapse in, or traverse through, the lateral chain sympathetic ganglion lying on the anterior aspect of the costovertebral articulations. Recall that the preganglionic sympathetic nerve innervation to the soma and viscera above the diaphragm takes origin from the first four to five segments of the thoracic cord. All of the viscera and soma below the diaphragm receive their preganglionic sympathetic nerve fibers from the spinal cord below T5. Many of the tissue texture abnormalities used in the diagnosis of somatic dysfunction

appear to be manifestations of altered secretomotor, pilomotor, and vasomotor functions of the skin viscera. Because the sympathetic nervous system is segmentally organized, skin viscera and internal viscera share many sympathetic nervous system reflexes. It has been clinically noted that internal viscera sharing preganglionic innervation origin in the spinal cord with somatic segments demonstrating tissue texture abnormality, may be involved in dysfunctional or diseased states.

### FUNCTIONAL ANATOMY

The typical thoracic vertebra has a body roughly equal in its transverse and anteroposterior diameters. The vertebral bodies have demi-facets, located posterolaterally at the upper and lower margins of the body, which articulate with the head of the rib. These demi-facets are true arthrodial joints with an articular cartilage and capsule. The posterior arch of the thoracic vertebra has apophyseal joints on the superior and inferior articular pillars. The superior apophyseal joints face backward, laterally, and slightly superiorly, and the inferior apophyseal joints face just the reverse. Theoretically this facet facing would provide a great deal of rotation to the thoracic vertebra, but rotation is restricted by the attachment of the ribs. The transverse processes

**150**

are unique in that the anterior surface has a small articular facet for articulation with the posterior-facing facet of the tubercle of the adjacent rib. The relationship of the costovertebral and costotransverse articulations greatly influences the type and amount of rib motion. The posterior aspects of the transverse processes are valuable anatomical landmarks for structural diagnosis of thoracic spine dysfunction. The spinous processes project backward and inferiorly and, in the midportion, are severely shingled one upon the other (See rule of threes, Chapter 5).

The atypical thoracic vertebra are those that are transitional between the cervical and thoracic spines, and the thoracic and lumbar spines. T1 has long transverse processes, in fact, the longest transverse processes in the thoracic spine. The lateral portion of the vertebral body has a uni-facet for articulation with the head of the first rib. While the inferior apophyseal joint facing is typically thoracic, the superior apophyseal joint facing is transitional from the cervical spine and may have typical cervical characteristics. T1 is also the junction of the change in anteroposterior curve between the cervical and thoracic spine. Dysfunction of T1 profoundly affects the functional capacity of the thoracic inlet and related structures.

T12 is the location of transition to the lumbar spine. The superior apophyseal joint facing is usually typically thoracic, while the inferior apophyseal joint facing tends toward lumbar characteristics. The lateral body has a uni-facet for articulation with the twelfth rib. The transverse processes are quite short and rudimentary, and are difficult to palpate with certainty. T12 is the location for the change in the anteroposterior curve between the thoracic kyphosis and the lumbar lordosis, a location of change in mobility of two areas of the spine, and a point of frequent dysfunction.

The thoracic kyphosis is normally a smooth posterior convexity without severe areas of increased convexity or "flattening". The observation of "flat spots" within the thoracic kyphosis should alert the diagnostician to evaluate this area carefully for nonneutral, type II, vertebral somatic dysfunction. The thoracic kyphosis changes at its upper and lower extremities (at the transitional zones) to flow into the cervical and lumbar lordoses. Because of this, frequently the upper segments of the thoracic spine are viewed from the perspective of the cervical spine, while the lower thoracic segments are viewed as an extension of the lumbar spine. Many techniques for cervical dysfunction are highly appropriate and effective in the upper thoracic spine, and many lumbar techniques are effective in the lower thoracic spine.

## THORACIC SPINE MOTION

Motion in the thoracic spine is not great, primarily because of the restriction caused by the attachment of the rib cage. Thoracic segments have forward-bending and backward-bending movement, as well as coupled movements of sidebending and rotation to the same side and to opposite sides. There is considerable controversy about the normal coupling of sidebending and rotation to opposite sides as part of neutral spinal mechanics. While type I neutral sidebending and rotation to opposite sides is taught as the norm, the group behavior of thoracic segments depends upon where in the thoracic kyphosis the neutral curve is introduced, and whether sidebending or rotation is introduced first. Clinically, the thoracic vertebrae demonstrate neutral type I group behavior in some segments, and show single vertebral motion segment, type II, nonneutral behavior as well.

## Diagnosis of Thoracic Vertebral Somatic Dysfunction

If the screening and scanning examination leads one to pursue specific segmental definition in the thoracic spine, the following diagnostic procedures have been found to be useful. Layer palpation of the paravertebral tissues will elicit the characteristic soft tissue changes in areas segmentally related to the

vertebral dysfunction. Of prime importance is the palpation of muscle hypertonicity at the deepest muscle layer, primarily in
the levator costales.

The most useful test of vertebral motion and restriction in the thoracic spine is
described in Chapter 6, namely monitoring
change in the relationship of paired transverse processes through an arc of forward-
bending to backward-bending. For the
upper thoracic spine from T1 to T5 (and occasionally 6), the patient is seated with the
operator behind. The operator palpates the
posterior aspect of the transverse processes
of the suspected dysfunctional segment
(Fig. 14.1), and the patient is instructed to
actively look down at the floor (Fig.14.2)
and up at the ceiling (Fig. 14.3). In the presence of a nonneutral, type II, ERS restriction, the transverse process on one side will
become more prominent during the forward-bending movement, and the two
transverse processes will become more symmetrical during the backward-bending
movement. In a nonneutral, type II, FRS
restriction, one transverse process will
become more prominent during the backward-bending movement, and the transverse processes will become more sym-

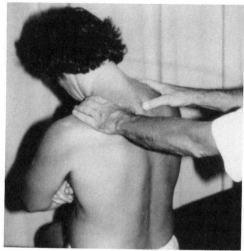

**Figure 14.2.** Motion testing upper thoracic
vertebra into forward-bending.

metric during forward-bending. Group
dysfunctions show three or more vertebra
to have prominent, transverse processes;
during the forward- to backward-bending
arc, the posterior characteristics of these
transverse processes may change, but they
never become symmetrical. Three-segment
group, type I dysfunctions are common in
the upper thoracic spine.

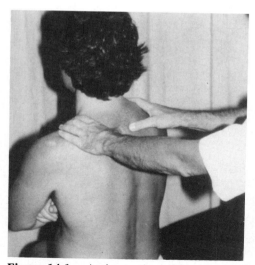

**Figure 14.1.** Active testing of function,
upper thoracic spine. Palpation of transverse
process of suspected dysfunctional segment.

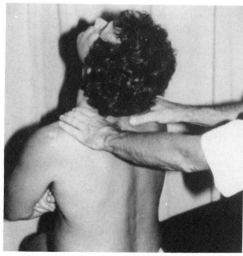

**Figure 14.3.** Motion testing of upper thoracic vertebra into backward- bending.

The lower thoracic to midthoracic region is evaluated with the patient assuming the three positions of full forward-bending while sitting (Fig. 14.4), neutral position while prone on the table (Fig. 14.5), and full backward-bending from the prone position by the elevation of the head and shoulders (Fig. 14.6). The diagnostic criteria for nonneutral, type II, FRS and ERS dysfunctions, as well as group, neutral, type I dysfunctions are as described above.

In the presence of a primary, structural scoliosis of the thoracic spine, structural diagnosis becomes quite difficult. The group of segments involved in the primary scoliosis behave as a neutral, type I dysfunction. It is interesting that patients with this condition have minimal symptomatology until a minor traumatic event occurs. Then this vertebral area becomes extremely symptomatic. What is frequently found in this situation is the presence of nonneutral type II dysfunction(s) within the primary scoliotic curve. It is quite difficult to identify these nonneutral, type II dysfunctions but if the examiner makes a diligent search from one segment to the other, observing the behavior of single vertebral motion units rather than the total curve, one can frequently identify the symp-

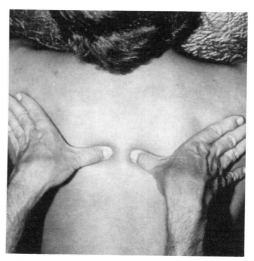

**Figure 14.5.**  Motion testing, mid to lower thoracic region. Neutral position.

tomatic and aggravating nonneutral dysfunction in the primary scoliotic curve.

## Manual Medicine Techniques for Thoracic Spine Dysfunction

The muscle energy procedures for thoracic spine somatic dysfunction are usually accomplished with the patient in the sitting position, but all of the procedures to be de-

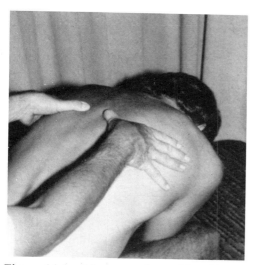

**Figure 14.4.**  Motion testing, mid and lower thoracic region. Forward-bent position.

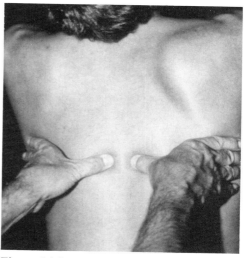

**Figure 14.6.**  Motion testing, mid and lower thoracic region. Backward- bending position.

scribed can be modified to have the patient in the horizontal position either supine, lateral-recumbent, or prone.

### T1 to 5
### Sitting
### Diagnosis

> Position: Flexed (forward-bent), sidebent left, rotated left ($FRS_{Lt}$)
> Motion restriction: Extension (backward-bending), right sidebending, right rotation

1. Patient sits upright with operator standing behind.
2. Operator palpates the transverse process of the dysfunctional segment and the spinous process of the segment below to monitor motion.
3. Operator's left hand and forearm controls patient's head and neck (Fig. 14.7).
4. A small amount of right rotation is introduced and then the segment is taken into backward-bending.
5. Right sidebending and right rotation are introduced to the barrier and the patient is instructed to side-bend the head to the left or flex the head forward (Fig. 14.8).
6. Following contraction and relaxation the operator increases the extension, right sidebending and right rotation to the barrier and the patient's left sidebending effort is repeated.
7. Step 6 is repeated two or three times.
8. Retest.

### T1 to T5
### Sitting
### Diagnosis

> Position: Extended (backward-bent), left sidebent, left rotated ($ERS_{Lt}$)
> Motion restriction: Flexion (forward-bending), right sidebending, right rotation

1. Patient sits with the operator standing behind.
2. Operator's left hand palpates left transverse process of dysfunctional segment and spinous process of segment below.

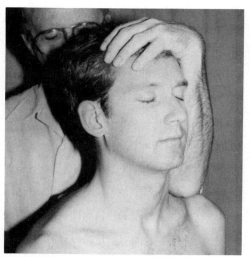

**Figure 14.7.** Seated, muscle energy technique. Nonneutral dysfunction ($FRS_{left}$). Right hand palpates at dysfunctional segment, left hand and forearm contact head and neck.

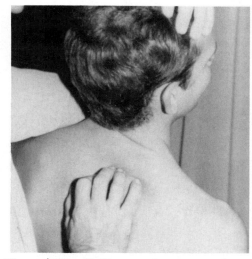

**Figure 14.8.** Sitting, muscle energy technique for nonneutral dysfunction ($FRS_{left}$), engagement of extension, right sidebending, and right rotation barrier.

3. Operator's right hand controls patient's head and neck.
4. Flexion of the head and neck is introduced by posterior translation of the patient's upper body (Fig. 14.9).
5. Right sidebending and right rotation are introduced by the operator introducing some right-to-left translation through the shoulder girdle (Fig. 14.10).
6. Patient is instructed to move the head backward or to left sidebend. (Note that the head may be encircled with the operator's right hand in a "turban" fashion).
7. Following contraction and subsequent relaxation, operator increases forward-bending, right sidebending, and right rotation to next restrictive barrier.
8. Repeat step 7 two to three times.
9. Retest.

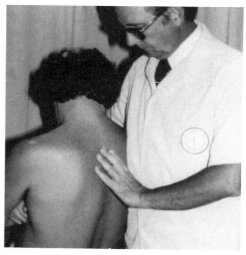

**Figure 14.10.** Sitting, muscle energy technique for upper thoracic spine nonneutral dysfunction (ERS$_{left}$). Right sidebending and right rotation barrier introduced by left translation.

T1 to T5
Sitting
Diagnosis: Group Dysfunction
       Position: Neutral, sidebent left, rotated right (NS$_L$R$_R$) or (EN Rt)
       Motion restriction: Sidebending right, rotation left.

1. Patient sits erect with operator standing behind.
2. Operator monitors group particularly at the apex (Fig. 14.11).
3. The operator's right hand controls head and neck.
4. Right sidebending is introduced by translating the shoulders from right to left and the face is rotated left to barrier sense (Fig. 14.12).
5. Patient is instructed to sidebend head to the left against resistance.
6. Increased right sidebending and left rotation are made.
7. Patient again sidebends head to the left.
8. Steps 6 and 7 are repeated two to three times.
9. Retest.

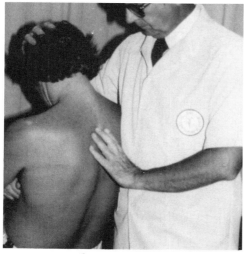

**Figure 14.9.** Sitting, muscle energy technique for upper thoracic spine nonneutral dysfunction (ERS$_{left}$) while palpating dysfunctional segment forward-bending introduced by posterior translation.

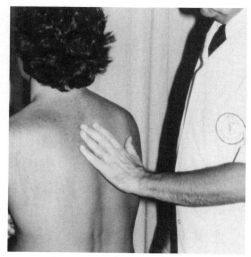

**Figure 14.11.** Sitting technique, upper thoracic spine, neutral dysfunction ($EN_{right}$), operator monitors at apex with right hand controlling head and neck.

T5 to T12
Sitting
Diagnosis

> Position: Extended (backward-bent), right rotated, right side-bent ($ERS_{Rt}$)
> Motion restriction: Flexion (forward-bending), left sidebending, left rotation

1. Patient sitting with operator behind.
2. Patient's right hand grasps the right side of the neck and the left hand the right elbow.
3. Operator places left arm above patient's left shoulder grasping the patient's right shoulder.
4. Operator's right hand monitors right transverse process of the dysfunctional segment and the spinous process of the segment below (Fig. 14.13).
5. Forward-bending (flexion) is introduced down to the dysfunctional

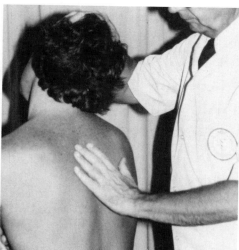

**Figure 14.12.** Sitting, muscle energy technique, upper thoracic spine, neutral dysfunction ($EN_{right}$). While in neutral, translation left introduces right sidebending and left rotation to barrier.

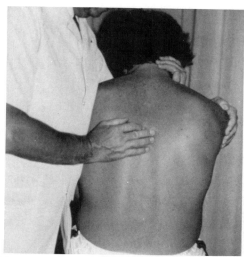

**Figure 14.13.** Sitting, muscle energy technique, mid and lower thoracic region, nonneutral dysfunction ($ERS_{right}$). Operator grasps right shoulder with left arm and monitors dysfunctional segment with right hand.

segment by anterior-to-posterior translation of the trunk at the level of the dysfunctional segment (Fig. 14.14).

6. Left sidebending and left rotation are introduced through the operator's control of the patient's shoulders and with translation from left to right of the patient's trunk at the level of the dysfunctional segment (Fig. 14.15).

7. Patient is instructed to sidebend trunk to the right isometrically.

8. Increased forward-bending, left sidebending, and left rotation are taken up to the next barrier.

9. Patient repeats right sidebending or right rotation or extension movement isometrically 2 to 3 more times.

10. Retest.
    Note: This technique can be adapted for use in the lumbar spine.

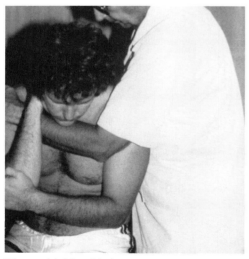

**Figure 14.14.** Sitting, muscle energy technique, mid to lower thoracic region, nonneutral dysfunction (ERS$_{right}$). Forward-bending barrier engaged by posterior translation.

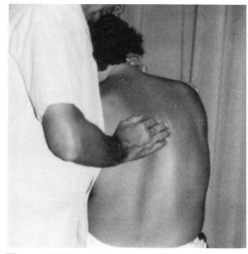

**Figure 14.15.** Sitting, muscle energy technique, mid to lower thoracic region, nonneutral dysfunction (ERS$_{right}$). Left sidebending and left rotation barriers engaged by right translation.

T5 to T12
Diagnosis
  Position: Flexed (forward-bent), rotated right, sidebent right (FRS$_{Rt}$)
  Motion restriction: Extension (backward-bending), sidebending left, rotation left

1. Patient seated with operator behind.

2. Operator's left hand controls patient's left shoulder and operator's right hand monitors right transverse process of dysfunctional segment and the spinous process of the segment below (Fig. 14.16).

3. Right sidebending is introduced by asking the patient to drop the right shoulder while the operator introduces left rotation (Fig. 14.17). (Note the translation from right to left at the dysfunctional segment.)

4. The patient provides a left sidebending effort against resistance. This procedure uses neutral me-

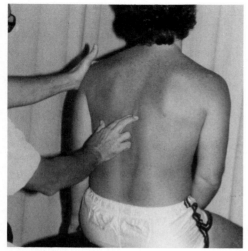

**Figure 14.16.** Sitting, muscle energy technique, mid to lower thoracic region, nonneutral dysfunction (FRS$_{right}$). Operator monitors transverse process dysfunctional segment.

chanics to introduce left rotation at the dysfunctional segment.

5. Left sidebending is now introduced by asking the patient to raise the right shoulder while the opera-

tor depresses the left shoulder, maintaining left rotation. Simultaneously the patient is instructed to move the abdomen forward introducing extension (Fig. 14.18).

6. Operator resists patient effort of right sidebending or right rotation.

7. Increase backward-bending, left sidebending, and left rotation to the new barrier.

8. Operator again resists patient's effort of right sidebending, or right rotation (Fig. 14.19).

9. Following 3 to 5 repetitions, the operator's left hand slides across the patient's chest and returns shoulders to neutral while maintaining extension.

10. Operator's right hand blocks segment below the dysfunctional segment and left hand resists patient's effort to pull the chest forward. This maneuver fully closes facet joints bilaterally at the dysfunctional segment (Fig. 14.20).

11. Retest.

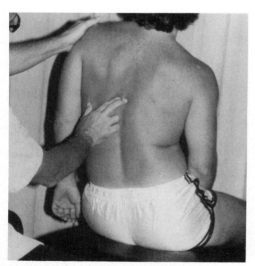

**Figure 14.17.** Sitting, muscle energy technique, mid to lower thoracic region, nonneutral dysfunction (FRS$_{right}$). Right sidebending and left rotation introduced by left translation (step 1).

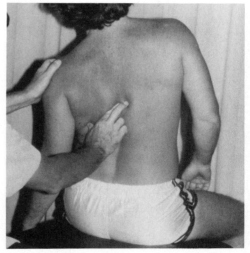

**Figure 14.18.** Sitting, muscle energy technique, mid to lower thoracic region, nonneutral dysfunction (FRS$_{right}$). Left sidebending and extension introduced while maintaining left rotation (step 2.)

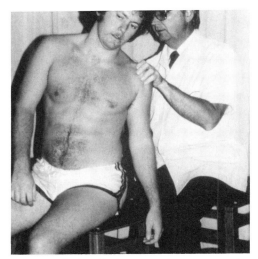

**Figure 14.19.** Sitting, muscle energy technique, mid to lower thoracic region, nonneutral dysfunction (FRS$_{right}$). Operator resists right sidebending and right rotation.

T5 to T12
Group Dysfunction
Diagnosis
    Position: Neutral, sidebent right, rotated left (NS$_{Rt}$R$_{Lt}$) or (ENLt)

    Motion restriction: Neutral, sidebending left, rotation right

1. Patient sitting with right hand holding left shoulder.
2. Operator stands behind patient and threads right hand under patient's right upper arm and grasps the left shoulder.
3. Operator's left hand (thumb) monitors group dysfunction primarily at the apex (Fig. 14.21).
4. With the patient sitting erect the operator introduces left sidebending and right rotation until barrier sense is encountered (Fig. 14.22).
5. Patient is instructed to sidebend to the right (pull right shoulder down to table).
6. Operator increases left sidebending and right rotation and maintains thumb—blocking force near apex of group dysfunction.
7. Patient repeats right sidebending effort against resistance.
8. Steps 6 and 7 are repeated two to three times.
9. Retest.

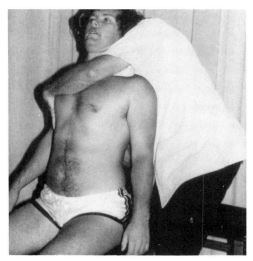

**Figure 14.20.** Sitting, muscle energy technique, mid to lower thoracic region, nonneutral dysfunction (FRS$_{right}$). Operator blocks lower segment and resists patient's forward bending effort (step 3).

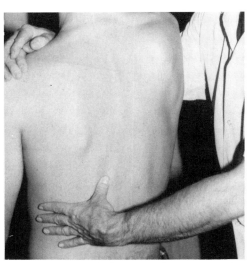

**Figure 14.21.** Sitting, muscle energy technique, mid to lower thoracic region, neutral dysfunction (EN$_{left}$). Operator monitors at apex of group dysfunction.

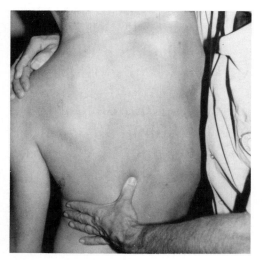

**Figure 14.22.** Sitting, muscle energy technique, mid to lower thoracic region, neutral dysfunction (EN$_{left}$). Operator engages left sidebending and right rotation barrier.

High-velocity, low-amplitude, low-force thrust procedures for the thoracic spine are accomplished primarily in the supine and seated positions. The prone position is used sparingly and mainly for those restrictions which have a major extension restriction component. These procedures usually apply a fulcrum on the inferior vertebra at the dysfunctional level. The principle is to hold one segment and move the other upon it. Usually the procedure is to hold the inferior segment and move the superior

dysfunctional segment on it. High-velocity, low-amplitude thrust procedures (mobilization with impulse) for the thoracic spine are as follows:

Prone
  Diagnosis: Group dysfunction ( 3 or more segments), (Type I)
  Position: Neutral, sidebent left, rotated right (NS$_L$R$_R$) or (EN$_{Rt}$)
  Motion restriction: Sidebending right, rotation left

1. Patient prone on table with operator at head of table.
2. Patient's chin is maintained in midline and controlled by operator's right hand.
3. Operator's left thumb is placed at the intertransverse process area directed toward the articular pillar on the inferior side of the segment at the apex of the group curve (Fig. 14.23).
4. Right sidebending and left rotation of the patient's neck and upper thoracic spine is introduced by the operator's right hand and takes up all of the slack to the dysfunctional group segments.
5. A high-velocity, low-amplitude, low-force thrust is applied through the combined activity of the holding of the head by the right hand and the exaggeration of the group by the

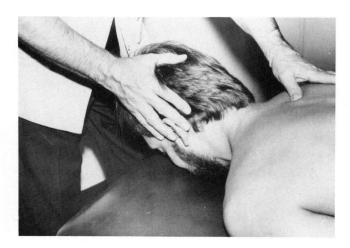

**Figure 14.23.** Prone, high-velocity/low-amplitude thrust technique, upper thoracic region, neutral dysfunction (EN$_{right}$). Operator's left thumb at group curve apex and directed towards articular pillar.

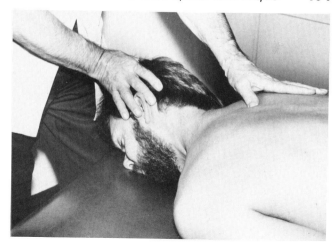

**Figure 14.24.** Prone, high-velocity/low-amplitude thrust technique, upper thoracic region, neutral dysfunction (EN$_{right}$). Thrust applied through the thumb in a ventral and left translatory direction.

thumb of the operator's left hand (Fig. 14.24).

6. Retest.

T1 to T5
Prone technique
Diagnosis: Nonneutral dysfunction (type II)
    Position: Flexed, rotated left, sidebent left (FRS$_{Lt}$)
    Motion restriction: Extension, right rotation, right sidebending

1. Patient prone on table with operator standing at left side of head of table, palpating at level of segmental dysfunction.

2. Operator's right hand moves patient's chin to the right (introducing right sidebending) and rotates the face to the right (Fig. 14.25).

3. Physician's pisiform bone makes contact on the right transverse process of the inferior segment of the vertebral motor unit.

4. A high-velocity, low-amplitude, low-thrust force is applied by the operator's left hand on the transverse process of the inferior vertebra while the operator's right hand maintains right sidebending and right rotation of the superior vertebral segment. The thrust of the left

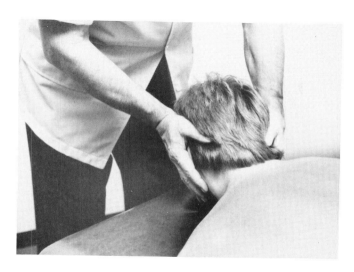

**Figure 14.25.** Prone, high-velocity/low-amplitude thrust technique, upper thoracic region, nonneutral dysfunction (FRS$_{left}$). Right sidebending, right rotation introduced.

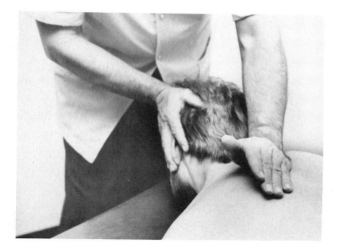

**Figure 14.26.** Prone, high-velocity/low-amplitude thrust technique, upper thoracic region, nonneutral dysfunction (FRS$_{left}$). Operator's right hand introduces extension. Left rotation thrust on inferior segment.

hand introduces extension and left rotation of the inferior segment resulting in closure of the right facet joint (Fig. 14.26).

5.  Retest.

T1 to T5
Sitting
Diagnosis: Group dysfunction (type I)
    Position: Neutral, sidebent left, rotated right (NS$_L$R$_R$) or (EN$_{Rt}$)
    Motion restriction: Sidebending right, rotation left

1.  Patient sitting on table with operator behind. Operator's left hand and forearm controls patient's head and left side of the neck.
2.  Operator's right thumb is between transverse processes at the apex of the dysfunctional segments directed toward the inferior facet joint of the segment at the apex of the curve (Fig. 14.27).
3.  Operator introduces right sidebending and left rotation of the patient's head (Fig. 14.28).
4.  Operator's right thumb localizes all motions to the apex of the dysfunctional group by a left translatory movement.
5.  When all of the right sidebending and left rotational restriction barriers are engaged, a high-velocity,

low-amplitude, low-force thrust is introduced by exaggerating the patient's position primarily through the application of force through the operator's right thumb.

6.  Retest.

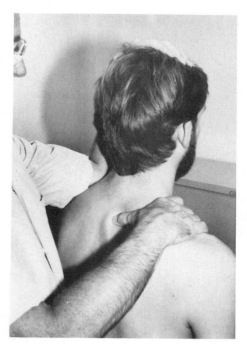

**Figure 14.27.** Sitting, high-velocity/low-amplitude thrust technique, upper thoracic region, neutral dysfunction (EN$_{right}$). Operator's right thumb directed toward inferior facet at apex of curve.

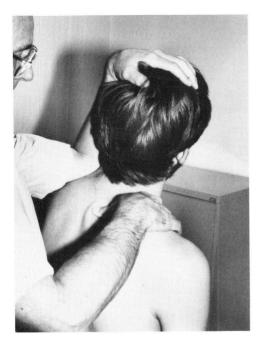

**Figure 14.28.** Sitting, high-velocity/low-amplitude thrust technique, upper thoracic region, neutral dysfunction ($EN_{right}$). Right sidebending, left rotation barrier engaged and followed by thrust through operator's thumb.

T1 to T5
Sitting
Diagnosis: Nonneutral dysfunction (type II)
      Position: Extended, left rotated, left sidebent ($ERS_{Lt}$)

Motion restriction: Flexion, right rotation, right sidebending

1. Patient sitting on table with operator standing behind patient.
2. Operator's left hand and forearm controls the head and left side of the patient's neck and the operator's right hand placed over the patient's right shawl area with the thumb in contact with the right side of the spinous process of the superior segment of the dysfunctional vertebral motion unit (Fig. 14.29).
3. Operator's left hand introduces flexion, right rotation, right sidebending of the patient's head and neck down to the dysfunctional segment while the operator's right thumb introduces left translatory movement localizing at the dysfunctional segment (Fig. 14.30).
4. When the flexion, right sidebending and right rotational barriers are all engaged, a high-velocity, low-amplitude, low-force thrust is introduced by exaggerating the patient's position by the operator's right thumb against the spinous process of the superior segment of the dysfunctional vertebral motion unit.
5. Retest.

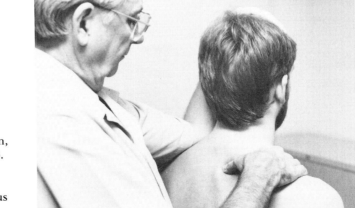

**Figure 14.29.** Sitting, high-velocity/low-amplitude thrust technique, upper thoracic region, nonneutral dysfunction ($ERS_{left}$). Operator controls left side patient's head and neck and right thumb contacts right side spinous process dysfunctional segment.

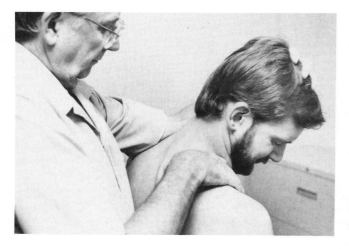

**Figure 14.30.** Sitting, high-velocity/low-amplitude thrust technique, upper thoracic region. Forward-bending, right rotation, right sidebending barrier engaged and followed by thrust with operator's right thumb.

T1 to T5
Sitting
Diagnosis: Nonneutral dysfunction (type II)

    Position: Flexed, sidebent left, rotated left (FRS$_{Lt}$)

    Motion restriction: Extension, right sidebending, right rotation

1. Patient sitting on table, operator standing behind, patient's left arm over operator's left thigh with operator's left foot on table.
2. Patient's head and neck controlled by operator's left hand and forearm with operator's right hand overlying the patient's right shawl area with thumb in contact with the right side of the spinous process of the superior segment of the dysfunctional vertebral motor unit (Fig. 14.31).
3. Operator's left hand introduces extension, right sidebending, right rotation of the patient's head and neck down to the dysfunctional segment while the operator's right hand introduces translation movement to the left at the dysfunctional segment (Fig. 14.32).
4. When all of the extension, right sidebending, and right rotational barriers are engaged, a high-velocity, low-amplitude, low-force thrust is introduced through the thumb against the spinous process of the dysfunctional segment.
5. Retest.

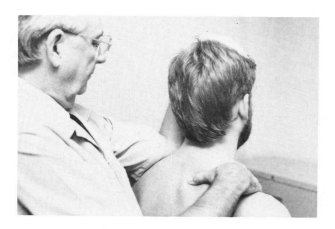

**Figure 14.31.** Sitting, high-velocity/low-amplitude thrust technique, upper thoracic region, nonneutral dysfunction (FRS$_{left}$). Operator controls patient's head and neck with right thumb contacting right side spinous process dysfunctional segment.

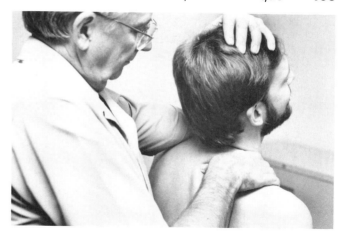

**Figure 14.32.** Backward-bending, right sidebending, right rotation barrier engaged and thrust applied by operator's left thumb.

T5 to T10
Supine
Diagnosis: Group dysfunction (type I)
    Position: Neutral, sidebent right, rotated left
    Motion restriction: Sidebending left, rotation right

1. Patient supine on table, operator standing on right side.
2. Patient's arms crossed across torso with each hand holding the opposite shoulder and the arm opposite the operator superior to the other.
3. Operator's right hand placed under the patient's thoracic spine stabilizing the thoracic segment with the thenar eminence on the most posterior transverse processes of the dysfunctional segments (Fig. 14.33).
4. Patient's body returned to midline and slack taken up by operator's torso on the patient's crossed arms.
5. Operator's left hand introduces left sidebending and right rotation of the head, neck and upper trunk down to the dysfunctional segments (Fig. 14.34).
6. When slack is taken out a high-velocity, low-amplitude, low-force thrust is accomplished by the operator through the crossed arms of the patient to the group dysfunctional segments.
7. Retest.

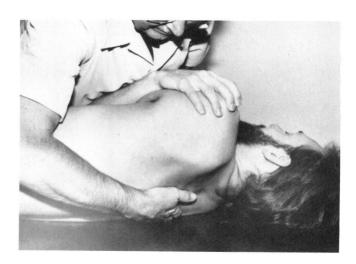

**Figure 14.33.** Supine and high-velocity/low-amplitude thrust technique, mid to lower thoracic region, neutral dysfunction ($EN_{left}$). Operator's right hand under thoracic convexity.

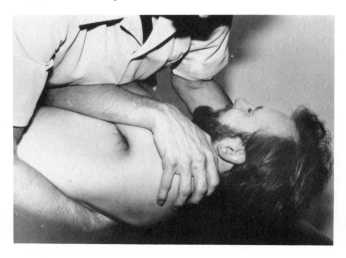

**Figure 14.34.** Supine, high-velocity/low-amplitude thrust technique, mid to lower thoracic region, neutral dysfunction ($EN_{left}$). Left sidebending and right rotation barrier engaged down to operator's right hand fulcrum.

T5 to T10
Supine
Diagnosis
    Position: Segment bilaterally extended (both facets in the closed position)
    Motion restriction: Sagittal plane flexion

1. Patient supine on table with operator standing on one side.
2. Patient's arms are crossed over the chest, one arm above the other, with patient holding the opposite shoulder with each hand.
3. The operator places the right hand under the patient's torso localizing to the inferior segment of the dysfunctional vertebral motor unit.
4. With the patient returned to the midline, the operator's left forearm and hand lifts the patient's head, neck and upper trunk to forward-bending (Fig. 14.35).
5. With the operator's torso in contact with the crossed arms, localization is made toward the localizing operator's right hand underneath the patient.
6. When the flexion barrier is engaged, exaggeration is made by a high-velocity, low-amplitude, low-force thrust applied by the

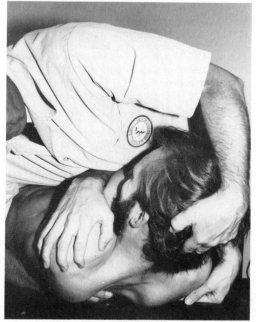

**Figure 14.35.** Supine, high-velocity/low-amplitude thrust technique, mid to lower thoracic region, midplane dysfunction bilaterally extended. With fulcrum placed by operator's right hand under inferior segment, forward-bending to barrier introduced by operator's left hand. Thrust follows toward fulcrum.

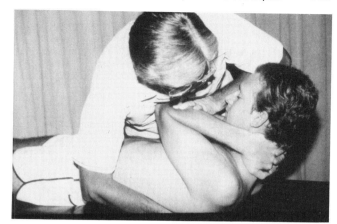

**Figure 14.36.** Supine, high-velocity/low-amplitude thrust technique, mid to lower thoracic region. Variation of arm placement particularly useful in mid to lower thoracic region.

operator's body to the patient's crossed arms while the operator's left hand increases the flexion moment.

7. A variation can be the use of the patient's hands clasped behind the neck and both elbows brought together for control of the patient's upper trunk. This variation is useful in the mid to lower thoracic region (Fig. 14.36).

8. Retest.

T5 to T10
Supine
Diagnosis
> Position: Bilateral flexed (both facets don't close)
> Motion restriction: Bilateral extension in sagittal plane

1. Patient supine on table with both arms crossed in front of the chest with the hands grasping the shoulder. The arm opposite the operator being superior.
2. Operator's right hand placed underneath the patient stabilizing the lower segment of the two segment dysfunction.
3. Patient returned to midline and operator controls the patient's upper trunk, neck, and head with the left arm.

4. Patient's upper trunk taken into extension over the fulcrum of the operator's right hand and a thrust is applied of high velocity, low amplitude, low force *above* the fulcrum introducing extension of the superior segment over the inferior (Fig. 14.37).
5. Variation of both hands clasped behind the neck can be utilized in this technique (Fig. 14.36).
6. Retest.

T5 to T10
Supine
Diagnosis: Non neutral dysfunction (type II)
> Position: Extended, rotated left, sidebent left (ERS$_{Lt}$)
> Motion restriction: Flexion, right rotation, right sidebending

1. Patient supine on table with operator standing on patient's right side.
2. Patient's left arm across chest holding the right shoulder.
3. Operator's right hand stabilizes the lower segment of the two segment dysfunctional vertebral motion unit.
4. Patient returned to midline position and left elbow placed in the operator's right axilla (Fig. 14.38).

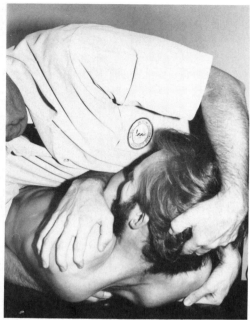

**Figure 14.37.** Supine, high-velocity/low-amplitude thrust technique, mid to lower thoracic region, midplane dysfunction, bilaterally flexed. With trunk into extension, thrust applied above the fulcrum, enhancing extension.

5. Operator's left hand grasps patient's head and introduces forward-bending, right rotation and right sidebending down to the superior segment of the dysfunctional vertebral motor unit (Fig. 14.39).

6. The high-velocity low-amplitude thrust is applied by the operator's right shoulder through the patient's left arm with simultaneous exaggeration of the patient's head, neck, and upper torso into flexion, right sidebending, and right rotation.

7. Retest.

In the supine thoracic spine techniques there are two principles necessary for success. The first is to always return the patient to the neutral position after placing the hand as the fulcrum under the patient. There are three different hand positions that can be used. They are

1) Hand flat with spinous processes placed in palm (Fig. 14.40);

2) All fingers flexed so that distal interphalangeal joints contact transverse processes on one side with the thenar eminence in contact with the opposite transverse processes (Fig. 14.41);

3) Index finger flexed tightly with the remaining fingers straight so that the flexed distal interphalangeal joint is on one transverse process and the metacarpophalangeal joint of the thumb is in contact with the opposite transverse process (Fig. 14.42).

The second principle is that the operator localizes force through the crossed arms

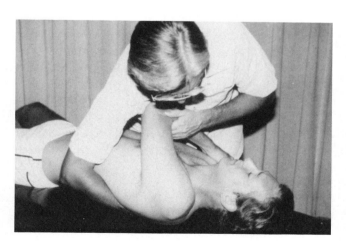

**Figure 14.38.** Supine, high-velocity/low-amplitude thrust technique, mid to lower thoracic region, nonneutral dysfunction ($ERS_{left}$). Operator's right hand under lower vertebra and patient returned to neutral.

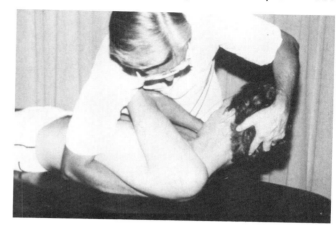

**Figure 14.39.** Supine, high-velocity/low-amplitude thrust technique, mid to lower thoracic region, nonneutral dysfunction (ERS$_{left}$). Operator introduces forward-bending, right rotation, and right sidebending to upper vertebra, thrust applied.

and chest wall directed appropriately toward the fulcrum hand (Fig. 14.43).

> T5 to T10
> Prone
> Diagnosis: Nonneutral dysfunction (type II)
>> Position: Flexed, rotated right, sidebent right (FRS$_{Rt}$)
>> Motion restriction: Extension, left rotation, left sidebending

1. Patient prone on table. Operator standing at side.

2. Operator's left hand with pisiform contact on the superior aspect of the left transverse process puts tension in a caudad direction (Fig. 14.44).

3. The operator's right hand with pisiform contact on the right transverse process of the dysfunctional segment of the patient pressing anteriorly introduces left rotation of the involved segment (Fig. 14.45).

4. Slack is taken out with caudad direction of the operator's left hand and anterior rotation with the operator's right hand.

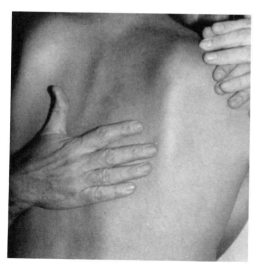

**Figure 14.40.** Supine, high-velocity/low-amplitude thrust technique, hand placement. Spinous processes are in palm.

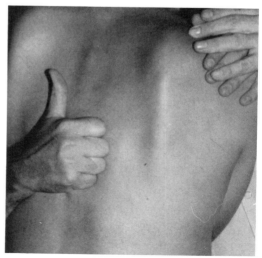

**Figure 14.41.** Supine, high-velocity/low-amplitude thrust technique, hand placement. Flexion of all fingers with thenar eminence.

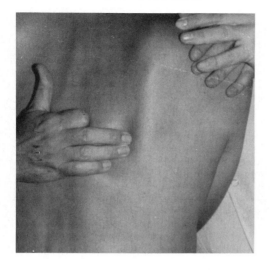

**Figure 14.42.** Supine, high-velocity/low-amplitude thrust technique, hand placement. Tightly flexed index finger and metacarpal phalangeal joint.

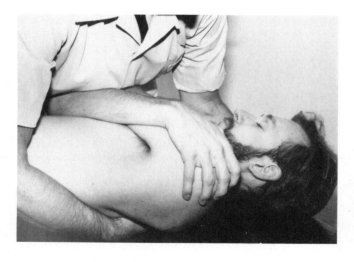

**Figure 14.43.** Supine, high-velocity/low-amplitude thrust technique, thoracic spine. Crossed arms, lever directed toward fulcrum.

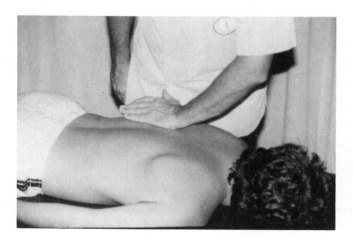

**Figure 14.44.** Prone, high-velocity/low-amplitude thrust, mid to lower thoracic region, nonneutral dysfunction ($FRS_{right}$). Left pisiform contact, left transverse process.

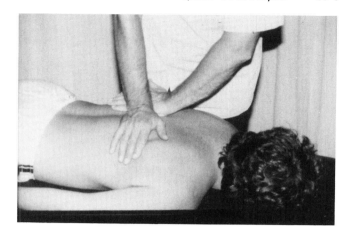

**Figure 14.45.** Prone, high-velocity/low-amplitude thrust, mid to lower thoracic region, non-neutral dysfunction (FRS$_{right}$). Right pisiform contact, right transverse process of dysfunctional segment.

5. When slack is taken up, a high-velocity, low-amplitude, low-force thrust is made introducing extension, left rotation, and left side-bending of the dysfunctional segment.
6. Retest.

T5-10
Seated
Diagnosis
     Position: Bilateral extended
     Motion restriction: Bilateral flexion

1. Patient seated on a stool with hands clasped behind neck.
2. Operator palpates level of dysfunction and places knee on the spinous process of the inferior vertebra of the vertebral motion segment (Fig. 14.46).
3. Operator threads both hands over the arms and grasps each forearm of the patient.
4. Flexion is introduced until all slack is taken out (Fig. 14.47).
5. High-velocity low-amplitude thrust is made by pulling the operator's hands directly posterior enhancing flexion from above against the fixed lower vertebra.
6. Retest.

T5-10
Sitting
Diagnosis
     Position: Bilateral flexed
     Motion restriction: Bilateral extension

1. Patient sitting with hands clasped behind neck.

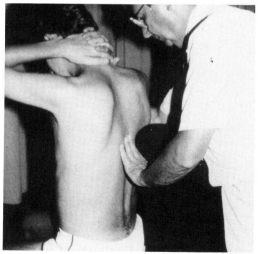

**Figure 14.46.** Seated, high-velocity/low-amplitude thrust technique, mid to lower thoracic region, bilateral extended dysfunction. Knee placed on spinous process inferior vertebra.

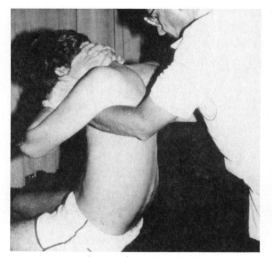

**Figure 14.47.** Seated, high-velocity/low-amplitude thrust technique, mid to lower thoracic region, bilateral extended dysfunction. Flexion barrier engaged to upper segment, and thrust by pulling into flexion.

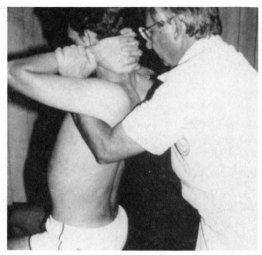

**Figure 14.48.** Sitting, high-velocity/low-amplitude thrust, mid to lower thoracic region, bilateral flexed dysfunction. With knee on spinous process lower vertebra thrust by lifting trunk into extension over fulcrum.

2.  Operator stands behind patient with knee on spinous process of inferior vertebra of motion unit.
3.  Operator threads both forearms under patient's upper arm bilaterally and grasps patient's wrist.
4.  All slack taken out into trunk extension and a high-velocity low-amplitude thrust is accomplished by lifting the patient's upper body into extension over the fulcrum of the operator's knee (Fig. 14.48).
5.  Retest.

T5-10
Sitting
Diagnosis: Nonneutral dysfunction (type II)

> Position: Extended, rotated left, sidebent left ($ERS_{Lt}$)
> Motion restriction: Flexion, right rotation, right sidebending, (left facet will not open)

1.  Patient sitting with hands clasped behind neck.

2.  Operator stands behind patient with knee on the right transverse process of the lower segment of the vertebral motion unit (Fig. 14.49).
3.  Operator threads arms under patient's axilla and grasps each wrist.
4.  Operator introduces forward bending, right sidebending, right rotation down to the involved segment (Fig. 14.50).
5.  A high-velocity low-amplitude thrust is accomplished by the operator pulling the patient's upper trunk into forward bending, right sidebending, and right rotation with a posterior pull through operator's arms.
6.  Retest.

T5-10
Sitting
Diagnosis: Nonneutral dysfunction (type II)

> Position: Flexed, rotated left, sidebent left ($FRS_{Lt}$)

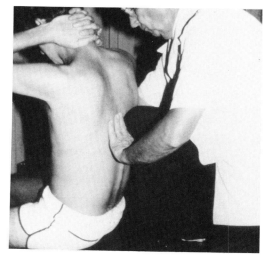

**Figure 14.49.** Sitting, high-velocity/low-amplitude thrust technique, mid to lower thoracic spine, non-neutral dysfunction (FRS$_{\text{left}}$). Knee contact on right transverse process, lower segment.

Motion restriction: Extension, rotation right, sidebending right, (right facet will not close)

1. Patient sits on table with arms clasped behind neck.
2. Operator stands behind patient with knee on the right transverse process of the inferior segment of the vertebral motion unit (Fig. 14.51).
3. Operator threads arms under patient's axilla and grasps patient's wrist.
4. Operator introduces extension, right sidebending, right rotation down to the involved segment. (Fig. 14.52).
5. When all slack is taken up, a high-velocity low-amplitude thrust is made by the operator exaggerating the extended, right sidebent, right rotated position of the patient's upper trunk in a lifting and posterior translation direction over the fulcrum placed by the operator's right knee.
6. Retest.

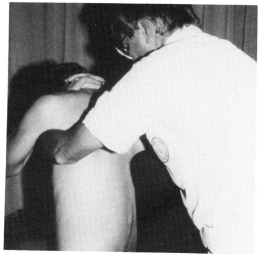

**Figure 14.50.** Sitting, high-velocity/low-amplitude thrust technique, mid to lower thoracic spine, non-neutral dysfunction (FRS$_{\text{left}}$). Forward-bending, right sidebending, right rotation to upper vertebra and thrust applied.

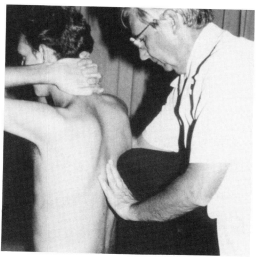

**Figure 14.51.** Sitting, high-velocity/low-amplitude thrust technique, mid to lower thoracic spine, non-neutral dysfunction (FRS$_{\text{left}}$). Knee on right transverse process, inferior vertebra.

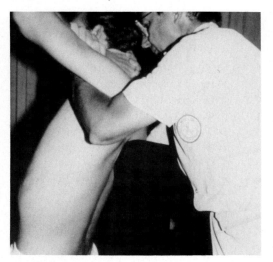

**Figure 14.52.** Sitting, high-velocity/low-amplitude thrust technique, mid to lower thoracic spine, neutral dysfunction (FRS $_{left}$). Extension, right sidebending, right rotation introduced to superior vertebra and thrust applied.

In the seated thoracic high-velocity, low-amplitude, low-force techniques, the knee may be placed in an alternative fashion. Instead of being placed on the transverse process of the inferior vertebra of the motion segment as a holding force, the knee may be placed on the posterior transverse process of the superior vertebra of the dysfunctional motion segment. An anterior thrusting force by the knee on the transverse process causes rotation of the dysfunctional vertebra to the opposite side. It is also possible to use a small pillow or a rolled-up towel as a fulcrum instead of the knee.

In the treatment sequence, the thoracic spine should be evaluated and treated before evaluation of rib function. Only occasionally is it found useful to treat major rib dysfunction first to better evaluate and treat the thoracic spine.

# 15

## *RIB CAGE TECHNIQUE*

The thoracic cage consists of the 12 thoracic vertebra, the paired 12 ribs, the sternum, and the related ligaments and muscles. The 12 paired ribs maintain the contour of the thoracic cage, much like a cylinder, to house the thoracic viscera, primarily the heart and great vessels, the lungs, trachea, and esophagus. The thoracoabdominal diaphragm functions as the piston within the cylinder of the thoracic cage to change the relative negative interthoracic pressure for respiratory activity. The diaphragm is the main muscle of respiration and also is of significance as a major "pump" of the low pressure venous and lymphatic systems.

At the cephalic end of the thoracic cage is the thoracic inlet which is bounded by the body of T1, the medial margins of the right and left first rib, the posterior aspect of the manubrium of the sternum, and the medial end of the right and left clavicle. It is through the thoracic inlet that the esophagus, trachea, and major vessels of the neck and upper extremity pass. Of particular importance is the fact that the lymphatic system for the total body drains into the venous system immediately posterior to the medial end of the clavicle and first rib bilaterally at the thoracic inlet. Alteration in rib cage function can influence respiratory activity, circulatory activity (arterial, venous, and lymphatic), and neural activity (particularly of the intercostal nerves and the brachial

plexus superior to rib one bilaterally). It should be noted that the thoracic lateral chain ganglia of the symphathetic division of the autonomic nervous system lie just anterior to the capsule of the costovertebral articulations bilaterally and are intimately connected to the posterior thoracic wall by heavy, dense fascia.

In many instances, rib cage dysfunction is a major component of dysfunction in the musculoskeletal system and yet it is frequently painless. Certain rib dysfunctions accompany pain along an intercostal space, frequently described as intercostal neuralgia. However, intercostal neuralgic symptoms in the absence of the dysfunctions to be described, should alert the physician to look for organic causes of intercostal neuralgia, e.g., herpes zoster, cord tumor, and primary or secondary inflammatory or neoplastic disease of the thoracic viscera.

### *FUNCTIONAL ANATOMY*

Ribs can be described as typical or atypical. The atypical ribs are those with the numbers one and two, namely rib 1, 2, 11, and 12. The first rib is quite broad and flat and articulates with T1 by a unifacet. It forms the lateral portion of the thoracic inlet and is subject to multiple types of dysfunction. The second rib articulates by two demifacets with T1 and T2. Anteriorly it articu-

**175**

lates by a strong cartilaginous attachment with the manubriogladiolar junction of the sternum at the angle of Louis. Alteration in function of the second rib has a profound influence on the function of the sternum within the thoracic cage. Ribs 11 and 12 are short and articulate by unifacets with the respective 11th and 12th thoracic vertebra. The quadratus lumborum muscle is attached to the inferior margin of rib 12. The anterior extremities of the 11th and 12th ribs are buried into the posterior abdominal wall. There is no osseous or cartilagenous attachment at the anterior extremity of these ribs and they are frequently asymmetrical in length.

The typical ribs are ribs 3 through 10, with three articulations, two posteriorly and one anteriorly. The posterior articulations are the costovertebral, where the rib head attaches to demifacets of the vertebral body above and below, and, through a strong ligamentous attachment, to the annulus of the intervertebral disk. For example, rib 3 attaches to the inferior demifacet of T2, the superior demifacet of T3, and the intervening intervertebral disk. The second articulation posteriorly is the costotransverse. This synovial joint is between the anterior surface of the transverse process and the articular surface on the posterior aspect of the rib. The anterior articulation is the costochondral and each rib attaches to the sternum either directly or through the costal arch. Normal rib motion requires mobility at the costovertebral, costotransverse, and costochondral articulations. The typical ribs also have a rib angle which is the most posterior aspect of the rib shaft and is the location for the attachment of the iliocostalis muscles.

The diaphragm is the primary inspiratory muscle of respiration and exhalation is, in large measure, a passive activity due to the recoil of the thoracic cage. Other inspiratory muscles include the external intercostals, the sternocostalis, and the accessory muscles of inspiration. The accessory muscles of inspiration are the sternomastoid, the scalenes, the pectoralis major

and minor, occasionally the serratus anterior and latissimus dorsi, serratus posterior superior, and the superior fibers of the iliocostalis. The primary expiratory muscles are the internal intercostals and the accessory expiratory muscles which are the abdominals, the lower fibers of the iliocostalis, the serratus posterior inferior, and the quadratus lumborum. While the internal and external intercostal muscles are viewed as inspiratory and expiratory muscles, in large measure their role is to maintain the contour of the thoracic cage cylinder and to prevent invagination of tissue into the thoracic cylinder with increasing negative intrathoracic pressure.

The motion characteristics of ribs are of inhalation and exhalation. During inhalation the anterior extremity of a rib goes superiorly in a pump-handle fashion and the lateral aspect of the rib go superiorly in a bucket-handle fashion. During exhalation, both pump-handle and bucket-handle movements occur in the caudad direction. All ribs have both pump-handle and bucket-handle motion, but the more cephalic ribs have more pump-handle movement, and the lower ribs have more bucket-handle movement. In large measure the type of movement of a rib is determined by the axis of the costovertebral to the costotransverse articulation. In the upper ribs, this axis is more transverse providing for more pump-handle activity, while in the lower ribs this axis is more anteroposterior in direction, providing for more bucket-handle-type movement. It should be noted that the anterior end of the rib is not as fixed as the posterior so that the bucket-handle movement described is only relative. To be truly bucket-handle, both the anterior and posterior ends of the rib should be fixed.

A third rib movement is that described as caliper. This movement occurs at the 11th and 12th ribs in which inhalation takes the rib posteriorly and laterally, and exhalation more anteriorly and medially, like the caliper action of ice tongs.

A fourth movement of ribs called rib torsion accompanies the rotation of the thoracic spine. When two thoracic vertebra to which typical ribs are attached are involved in rotational movement, there is resultant torsional movement in the attached ribs. For example, when T5 rotates to the right in relation to T6, the posterior aspect of the right 6th rib turns externally and the posterior aspect of the left 6th rib turns internally. This torsional movement continues around the rib cage to the sternal attachment, and the anterior extremity of the right 6th rib is somewhat flattened and the anterior extremity of the left 6th rib is somewhat accentuated. Upon return to neutral, the bilateral rib torsional movement should return to bilateral symmetry.

### Structural Diagnosis of the Rib Cage

As in all other structural diagnostic procedures designed to elicit somatic dysfunction, we look for asymmetry, altered range of motion, and tissue texture abnormality. The rib cage is palpated for contour anteriorly, posteriorly, and laterally. Palpation of the posterior rib cage concentrates on the rib angles and their participation in the bilateral, symmetrical, posterior contour of the rib cage. The rib angles of the typical ribs are divergent from above downward and each rib angle should participate in that contour. Palpation is carried out in the prone and sitting positions (Figs. 15.1, 15.2). If one rib angle appears to be more or less prominent in the posterior contour than its fellow on the opposite side and in relation to the ribs above and below, there is high likelihood of rib dysfunctions termed subluxations, either anterior or posterior. The anterior portion of the rib cage is palpated for symmetry at the anterior extremity of the rib just lateral to the costochondral articulation (Fig. 15.3). Again one notes the participation of each rib in the anterior convexity of the rib cage. If one rib is more or less prominent than the one above and below, and in comparison to the one on the opposite side, suspicion of an anterior or posterior rib subluxation is high. In palpating the rib cage one is interested in the posterior contour of each rib, the upper and lower margin of the rib, and the interspace above and below each rib. Normally the posterior aspect of the rib is convex with the superior border being less easily palpable (less sharp) than the inferior margin (more sharp). The interspace above and below each rib should be symmetrical and the right and left comparable interspaces should likewise be symmetrical. Alteration in the characteristics of the superior and inferior margin of the rib, together with alteration in intercostal space, should raise the suspicion of torsional rib dysfunction.

As one palpates the rib cage for contour, one also searches for the presence of tissue texture abnormality, primarily hypertonicity and tenderness of muscle attachment to ribs. The iliocostalis muscle group

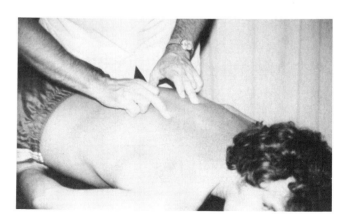

**Figure 15.1.** Diagnostic palpation of rib angles, prone.

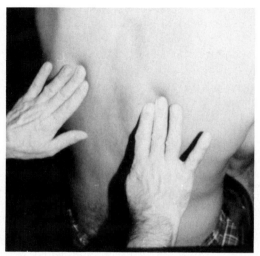

**Figure 15.2.** Diagnostic palpation of rib angles, sitting.

attaches to the rib angle, and is frequently tender and tense in the presence of rib dysfunction at that level. Tension and tenderness of the intercostal muscle throughout the intercostal space is also sought. It is frequently noted that tenderness and tension of intercostal muscles is present in the interspace above a rib which has exhalation restriction and on the interspace below the

rib that has inhalation restriction. Palpation of the costochondral articulation of ribs often identifies one or more as exquisitely tender. This is frequently described as costochondritis (Tietze's syndrome) but is more usually associated with dysfunction of that rib.

Assessment of rib cage range of motion is accomplished by symmetrically placing the hands over the rib cage and following an inhalation and exhalation effort, both quiet and forced respiration. One elicits motion of ribs by groups, upper and lower, as well as individually. The lower ribs are tested for bucket-handle movement by palpating laterally (Fig. 15.4), and for pump-handle activity by palpating anteriorly (Fig. 15.5). The midribs are palpated laterally (Fig. 15.6) and anteriorly, (Fig. 15.7) for bucket-handle and pump-handle motion respectively. The upper ribs are evaluated for pump-handle and bucket-handle activity (Fig. 15.8). The first rib is followed by paired fingers palpating the first costal cartilage just inferior to the medial end of the sternum, and again inhalation and exhalation effort is evaluated (Fig. 15.9). To test for the caliper movement of the 11th and 12th ribs, the patient is prone on the table with the thumbs just lateral to the spinous

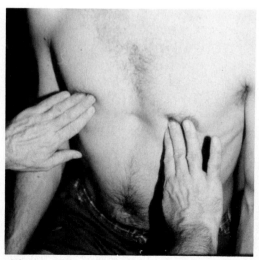

**Figure 15.3.** Diagnostic palpation of rib at costochondral articulation.

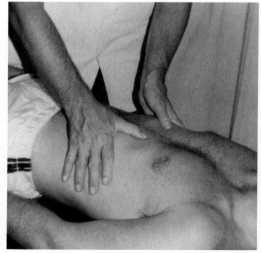

**Figure 15.4.** Motion palpation lower ribs for bucket-handle movement.

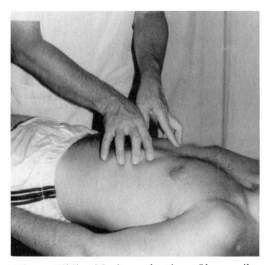

**Figure 15.5.** Motion palpation of lower ribs for pump-handle movement.

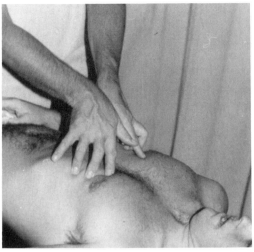

**Figure 15.7.** Motion palpation of middle ribs for pump-handle movement.

process overlying the posterior-medial aspect of the rib and the index and middle fingers overlying the 11th and 12th ribs laterally (Fig. 15.10). Inhalation and exhalation movement is tested. It is important that the fingers be in contact with symmetrical portions of the 11th and 12th ribs which may not necessarily be at the tip of each.

## Rib Cage Somatic Dysfunction

Rib dysfunctions are classified as structural and respiratory. The structural rib dysfunctions include anterior and posterior subluxation, and, in the instance of the first rib, a superior subluxation. A second structural rib dysfunction is rib torsion which usually accompanies nonneutral dysfunctions of

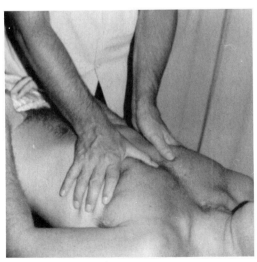

**Figure 15.6.** Motion palpation of middle ribs for bucket-handle movement.

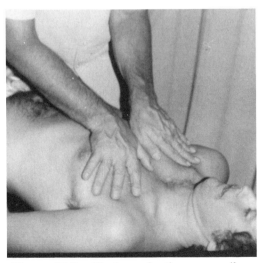

**Figure 15.8.** Motion palpation upper ribs.

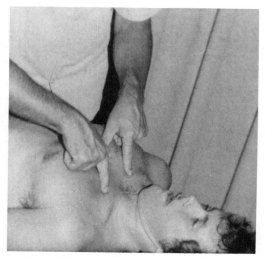

**Figure 15.9.** Motion palpation of 1st rib at costal cartilage.

the thoracic spine. Usually these dysfunctions resolve when the nonneutral thoracic spine dysfunction has been successfully treated. The third structural rib dysfunction is traumatic in nature and is called a rib compression. An anteroposterior compression of the rib cage results in narrowing of the AP diameter of a rib and prominence of that same rib laterally. These rare dysfunctions are usually traumatic and follow such accidents as a driver striking the steering wheel of a car or AP compression of a rib cage during a sporting activity. A fourth nonphysiologic or structural rib dysfunc-

tion is a variant of the physiologic bucket-handle movement. In this dysfunction the rib behaves as though both the anterior and posterior ends were fixed and the rib flexes upward and downward laterally. The hypothetical axis of motion is straight anteroposterior rather than having the bucket-handle physiologic movement determined by the axis formed by the costovertebral and costotransverse articulations. This dysfunction can occur with the rib either laterally flexed up (superiorly) or down (inferiorly). This dysfunction has also been termed "bucket-bail". The diagnostic criteria for the structural rib dysfunctions are as follows:

Anterior subluxation:

1. Rib angle less prominent in posterior rib cage contour.
2. Rib angle tender with tension of iliocostalis muscle.
3. Anterior extremity of the rib more prominent in anterior rib cage contour.
4. Marked motion restriction of inhalation and exhalation.
5. Frequent complaint of "intercostal neuralgia" at adjacent interspace.

Posterior subluxation:

1. Rib angle more prominent in posterior contour of rib cage.

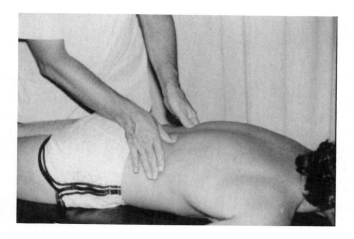

**Figure 15.10.** Motion palpation of 11th and 12th ribs.

2. Rib angle tender with tension of iliocostalis muscle.
3. Anterior extremity of the rib less prominent in anterior rib cage contour.
4. Marked restriction of rib in inhalation and exhalation movement.
5. Frequent complaint of "intercostal neuralgia" in adjacent interspace.

Superior first rib subluxation:

1. Palpation superior aspect of first rib just anterior to the trapezius muscle shows dysfunctional rib to be approximately 5 mm cephalic in relation to contralateral side.
2. Marked tenderness of superior aspect of first rib.
3. Restriction of motion in respiratory activity.
4. Hypertonicity of scalene muscles on ipsilateral side.

External rib torsion:

1. Superior border of dysfunctional rib more prominent.
2. Inferior border of dysfunctional rib less prominent.
3. Tension and tenderness at iliocostalis muscle attachment at rib angle.
4. Widened intercostal space above, and narrowed intercostal space below, dysfunctional rib.
5. Respiratory motion restriction.

Note: Internal torsional dysfunction has reverse findings and is usually found on contralateral side. External torsion dysfunction are most common and relate to nonneutral ERS dysfunction to the ipsilateral side.

Rib compression:

1. Flattening of the contour of the rib cage at the anterior and posterior extremity of the dysfunctional rib.
2. Prominence of the rib shaft in the midaxillary line.
3. Frequent tenderness of intercostal space above and below dysfunc-

tional rib and complaint of "intercostal neuralgia".
4. Motion restriction variable.

Lateral flexed rib (bucket-bail):

1. Marked respiratory rib restriction.
2. Prominence of rib shaft in midaxillary line.
3. Asymmetry of interspace above and below dysfunctional rib.
4. Frequent pain and tender interspace.
5. Present in typical ribs and frequently seen in ribs 2, 3, and 4.
6. Usual dysfunction is superior position (flexed up).

Respiratory rib dysfunctions occur either singly or in groups and demonstrate restriction of either inhalation or exhalation movement. In group respiratory rib dysfunctions we speak of the *key rib*. The key rib is the one at the upper or lower end of the group dysfunction. The key rib is the major restrictor of the group's ability to move into either inhalation or exhalation. In exhalation group rib dysfunction, the key rib is at the bottom of the dysfunctional group. In inhalation group rib dysfunction, the key rib is at the upper end of the group. It is important to identify the key rib in a group respiratory inhalation or exhalation restriction as it is that rib to which manual medicine therapy is initially addressed (Fig. 15.11).

*Exhalation Restriction:*

1. The rib or group of ribs that ceases moving first during exhalation effort.
2. The key rib is at the bottom of the group.

*Inhalation Restriction:*

1. The rib or group of ribs that ceases moving first during inhalation effort.
2. The key rib is at the bottom of the group.

In determining respiratory rib dysfunction, not only is one interested in the inhala-

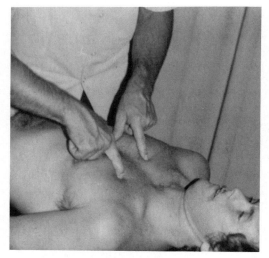

**Figure 15.11.** Diagnosis of key rib.

tion or exhalation motion restriction and the identification of the key rib, but also whether the bucket-handle or pump-handle component of movement demonstrates the most restriction. Within group rib dysfunction, there may be more one key rib. After successfully treating one key rib in a group (either the top or the bottom), reexamination should be made to see if there are other single ribs within the group which are dysfunctional in the same direction.

## Treatment of Rib Cage Dysfunction

In treating dysfunction of the rib cage there are principles of treatment sequence which should be followed for the best result. Almost without exception, one should make structural diagnosis and manual medicine treatment to the thoracic spine prior to addressing the ribs individually or in groups. In most instances, rib torsional dysfunction responds simultaneously with treatment of the nonneutral dysfunction of the related thoracic vertebra. Before looking for and treatment of dysfunction of ribs 1 and 2, it is most important that evaluation and appropriate treatment be made to T1. This is particularly important for the influence of the unifacet for the 1st rib on each side of T1. The second major principle of treatment of

rib dysfunction is to treat structural rib dysfunction prior to the treatment of respiratory rib dysfunction. Frequently the key rib of a group of respiratory rib dysfunction has a structural rib dysfunction. Treatment of the structural rib dysfunction frequently results in restoration of normal movement to the members of the group. When there is no longer evidence of structural rib dysfunction, then respiratory rib dysfunction can be addressed with the goal of restoration of maximal, symmetrical, inhalation-exhalation movement.

The following techniques are direct action, combined muscle energy, respiratory assist, and operator guiding techniques.

## Structural Rib Dysfunction

*First rib*
Diagnosis: Superior subluxation, left 1st rib

1. Patient sitting with operator behind.
2. Operator places fingerpads of second, third and fourth finger anterior to the left trapezius muscle, pulling it posteriorly, and placing fingerpads on superior aspect of left 1st rib.
3. Operator's right hand and forearm control the right side of the patient's head and neck.
4. Left sidebending and left rotation of the patient's head and neck are accomplished and followed by caudad force on the superior aspect of the 1st rib by the operator's left fingerpads.
5. Patient exerts a right sidebending effort of the head and neck against equal and opposite resistance of the operator's right hand and forearm activating the right scalene muscles and resulting in inhibition of the left scalene muscles.
6. Following relaxation of the left scalenes, and with caudad traction on the 1st rib, the superior subluxation can be felt to release and be re-

stored to symmetry with the opposite side.

7. Reexamine.

*Typical ribs*

Diagnosis: Anterior subluxation (example: right 5th rib)

1. Patient sitting with right hand holding opposite (left) shoulder.
2. Operator stands behind patient with right thumb placed upon the shaft of the dysfunctional rib medial to the rib angle, and with left hand holding the patient's right elbow (Fig. 15.12).
3. Operator places a posterolateral "pull" force on the rib shaft, while,
4. Patient is instructed to "pull" the right elbow laterally, (Fig. 15.13) or "pull" the right elbow caudally (Fig. 15.14).
5. Three to five repetitions are made until release is sensed under the operator's right thumb and restoration of symmetry occurs.
6. Occassionally it is useful to place the patient's left fist overlying the anterior extremity of the dysfunctional rib so that during the pulling motion

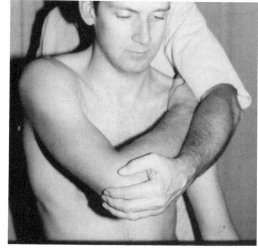

**Figure 15.13.** Combined technique for typical rib anterior subluxation. Patient pulls right elbow laterally.

in the caudad direction, there is a anterior to posterior force directed upon the dysfunctional rib (Fig. 15.15).

7. Reexamine.

*Typical Ribs*

Diagnosis: Posterior subluxation (example: right 5th rib)

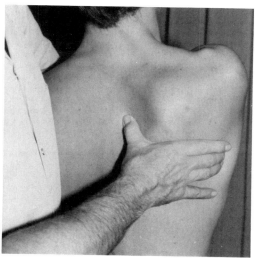

**Figure 15.12.** Combined technique for typical rib anterior subluxation. Thumb on rib shaft medial to angle.

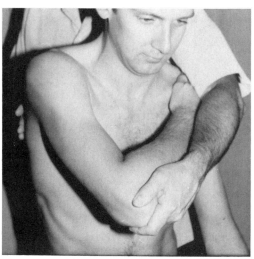

**Figure 15.14.** Combined technique for typical rib anterior subluxation. Patient pulls right elbow caudally.

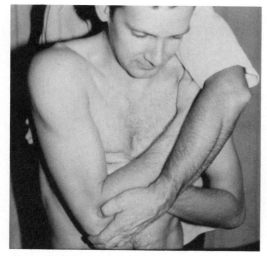

**Figure 15.15.** Combined technique for typical rib anterior subluxation. Variation with left fist overlying anterior end dysfunctional rib.

1. Patient sitting with right hand grasping opposite left shoulder.
2. Operator stands behind patient with right thumb placed along shaft of the dysfunctional rib lateral to the rib angle, and with left hand holding patient's right elbow (Fig. 15.16).
3. An anteromedial "push" force is placed along the shaft of the dys-

functional rib while the patient is instructed to "push" the elbow to the left into the operator's hand, (Fig. 15.17) or "push" the right elbow toward the ceiling (Fig. 15.18).
4. Three to five repetitions are made until release is felt and symmetry restored.
5. Reexamine.

Rib subluxations are hypermobile and following correction, stabilization of the rib cage by either strapping or a rib belt is frequently useful.

*Typical Ribs*
Diagnosis: Rib torsion (example: right 5th rib)

1. Patient sits on table with right hand holding the left shoulder.
2. Operator stands behind patient with right thumb in contact with the rib angle of dysfunctional rib, and with left hand holding patient's right elbow (Fig. 15.19).
3. In the presence of external torsional restriction, the thumb exerts a rotary force anteriorly on the superior border of the dysfunctional rib while the patient is instructed to lift

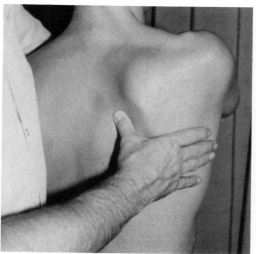

**Figure 15.16.** Combined technique, typical rib, posterior subluxation. Thumb on rib shaft lateral to rib angle.

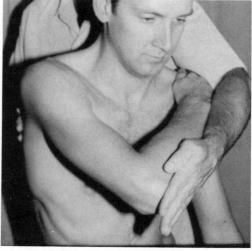

**Figure 15.17.** Combined technique, typical rib, posterior subluxation. Patient pushes elbow to the left.

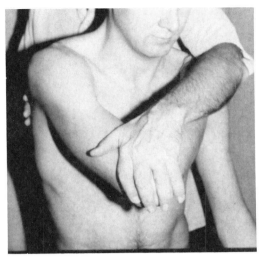

**Figure 15.18.** Combined technique, typical rib, posterior subluxation. Patient pushes elbow to the ceiling.

the right elbow in a cephalic direction against the resistance of the operator's left hand.

4. In the presence of internal torsion the operator's right thumb puts a posterior rotational force on the inferior margin of the dysfunctional rib while the patient is instructed to pull the right elbow in a caudad di-

rection against resistance by the operator's left hand (Fig. 15.20).

5. Three to five repetitions are made until release is felt and contour reestablished.
6. Reexamine.

*Typical Rib*
Diagnosis: AP rib compression (example: right 6th rib)

1. Patient sits with operator standing at side.
2. Operator puts middle finger of right and left hand over the prominent rib in the patient's midaxillary line.
3. Patient sidebends to the right while the operator puts medial compressive force on the dysfunctional rib (Fig. 15.21).
4. Patient inhales and exhales and holds breath at the point of minimal rib tension, usually in exhalation.
5. Operator maintains medial compressive force on dysfunctional rib while patient is instructed to sidebend left against resistance offered by operator's body (Fig. 15.22).
6. Three to five repetitions are made.
7. Reexamine.

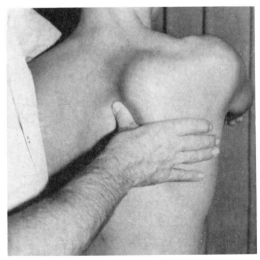

**Figure 15.19.** Combined technique, typical rib, torsional dysfunction. Thumb contacts rib angle and exerts superior or inferior pressure.

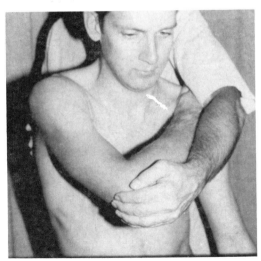

**Figure 15.20.** Combined technique, typical rib, torsional dysfunction. Patient lifts elbow cephalad or caudad as instructed.

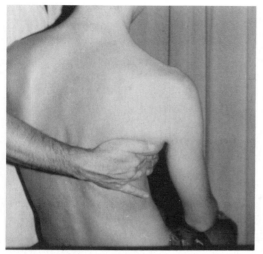

**Figure 15.21.** Combined technique, typical rib, AP compression. With patient right sidebent, operator puts medial compressive force on rib.

*Typical Rib*
Diagnosis: Rib laterally flexed superior (up) (example: left 3rd rib)

1. Patient supine on table with operator standing on side of dysfunction, facing cephalically.

2. Operator places right hand along rib cage in midaxillary line with finger pads above the dysfunctional rib.

3. Operator's left hand introduces left sidebending of the head and trunk down to dysfunctional rib (Fig. 15.23).

4. Patient instructed to exhale and reach down toward left knee increasing left sidebending (Fig. 15.24).

5. After several respiratory efforts and increased sidebending, the operator holds superior aspect of dysfunctional rib and left hand straightens head and neck (Fig. 15.25).

6. Retest.

### Inhalation Restriction: Principles of Treatment

1. **Operator pulls rib angle lateral and caudad.**
2. **Patient inhalation effort.**
3. **Contraction of muscle.**
   **Rib 1 and 2—scalenes**
   **Rib 3,4,5—pectoralis minor**
   **Rib 3-9—serratus anterior**

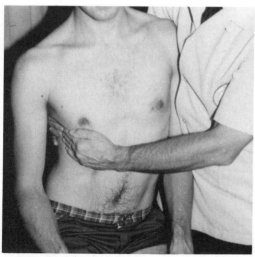

**Figure 15.22.** Combined technique, typical rib, AP compression. With patient right sidebent, patient sidebends left against resistance.

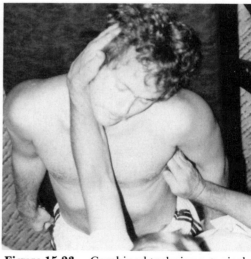

**Figure 15.23.** Combined technique, typical rib, laterally flexed superior. Operator introduces left sidebending.

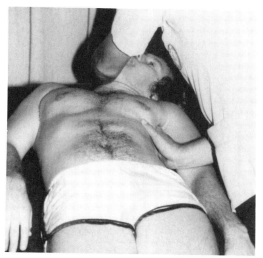

**Figure 15.24.** Combined technique, typical rib, laterally flexed superior. Patient increases left sidebending and exhales.

*Ribs 1 and 2*
Diagnosis: Inhalation restriction (right side example)

1.  Patient supine on table with operator standing on left side.
2.  Operator's fingers of left hand grasp right 1st and 2nd ribs medial

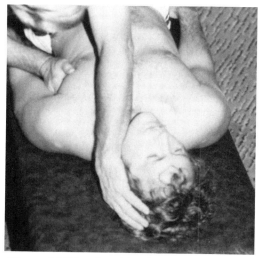

**Figure 15.25.** Combined technique, typical rib, laterally flexed superior. Operator holds superior aspect of dysfunctional rib and returns trunk to neutral.

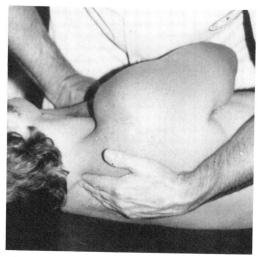

**Figure 15.26.** Combined technique for inhalation restriction, ribs 1 and 2. Operator pulls 1st and 2nd ribs laterally and caudad.

to the angle and pull laterally and caudad (Fig. 15.26).

3.  Patient's head is sidebent and rotated left to put the scalene muscles on stretch.
4.  Patient is instructed to take a deep breath and at maximal inhalation to lift the head from the table and sidebend it to the right energizing the right scalene muscles (Fig. 15.27).
5.  Operator's right hand offers resistance to patient's head and neck.
6.  Three to five repetitions are made.
7.  Reexamine.

An alternative method utilizes the elevation of the patient's right arm with the forearm held against the patient's head (Fig. 15.28). This reduces caudad traction on the 1st and 2nd rib from the fascia of the right upper extremity.

*Ribs 3, 4, 5*
Diagnosis: Inhalation restriction (right side example)

1.  Patient supine on table with operator standing on patient's left side.
2.  Operator's fingers of left hand grasp ribs 3, 4 and 5 medial to the

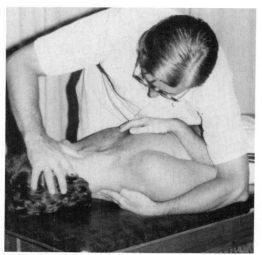

**Figure 15.27.** Combined technique for inhalation restriction, ribs 1 and 2. At maximal inhalation patient flexes and sidebends head right, activating right scalenes.

rib angle and pull laterally and caudad (Fig. 15.29).
3. Patient's right arm is elevated and abducted putting the pectoral muscle on stretch and with operator's left hand controlling patient's right elbow.

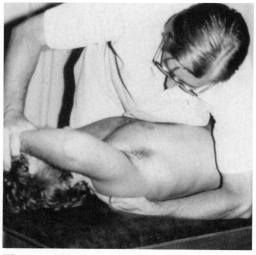

**Figure 15.28.** Combined technique for inhalation restriction, ribs 1 and 2. Alternative position to resist patient flexion and right sidebending effort.

4. Patient instructed to take deep inhalation.
5. Patient then instructed to push right elbow anteriorly (Fig. 15.30) against operator's resistance for pumphandle component of restriction, or laterally for bucket-handle component of restriction (Fig. 15.31).
6. Three to five repetitions are made.
7. Reexamine.

*Ribs 6, 7, 8, 9*
Diagnosis: Inhalation restriction (right side example)

1. Patient supine on table with operator standing on patient's left side.
2. Operator's fingers of the left hand contact the 6th, 7th, 8th and 9th ribs medial to the angles and pull laterally and caudad (Fig. 15.32).
3. Operator's right hand grasps patient's right wrist and carries the patient's right arm above and over the head putting the upper extremity on stretch (Fig. 15.33).
4. Patient instructed to take a deep breath.
5. Patient instructed to pull the right elbow to the right, energizing the serratus anterior muscle to elevate the ribs.
6. Three to five repetitions.
7. Reexamine.

## Exhalation Restriction: Principles of Treatment

1. **Patient position (sidebending and flexion as appropriate).**
2. **Operator holds rib into exhalation position.**
3. **Patient exhalation effort.**
4. **Return patient position to neutral while holding rib in exhalation position.**

*Lower Ribs*
Diagnosis: Exhalation restriction (left side example)

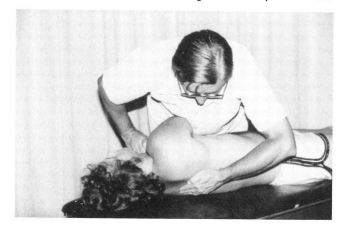

**Figure 15.29.** Combined technique, inhalation restriction, ribs 3, 4, 5. Operator pulls ribs 3, 4 and 5 laterally and caudad.

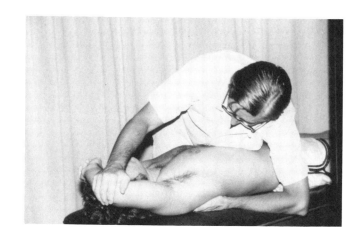

**Figure 15.30.** Combined technique, inhalation restriction, ribs 3, 4, 5. Operator resists arm flexion for pump-handle restriction.

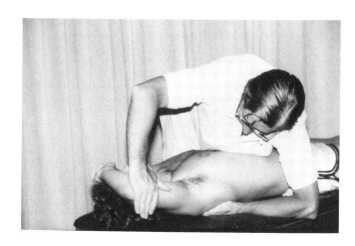

**Figure 15.31.** Combined technique, inhalation restriction, ribs 3, 4, 5. Operator resists arm adduction for bucket-handle restriction.

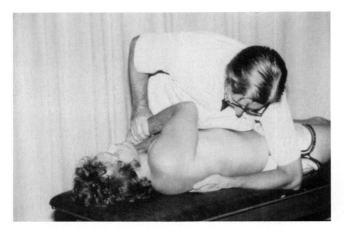

**Figure 15.32.** Combined technique, inhalation restriction, ribs 6, 7, 8, 9. Operator pulls ribs 6, 7, 8, and 9 laterally and caudad.

1. Patient supine on table with operator standing at the left side of the head of the table.
2. Operator's left thumb and thenar eminence placed along superior aspect of dysfunctional key rib spanning the costochondral junction (Fig. 15.34).
3. Operator's right hand under patient's head, neck, and upper thoracic spine to control patient's body position (Fig. 15.35).
4. Operator introduces left sidebending and flexion down to key rib (Fig. 15.36).
5. Patient instructed to take short breath in and exhale completely.
6. Operator follows rib into exhalation and *holds* in that position.
7. Patient's respiratory effort is repeated with operator holding the key rib in the previously obtained exhalation position.
8. Increasing sidebending and flexion of patient's trunk by operator's right hand follows each exhalation effort (Fig. 15.37).
9. When maximum exhalation has been obtained, patient's head, neck, and upper trunk are returned to neutral while key rib is held in exhalation position.
10. The operator's left thumb is released from the key rib *slowly.*
11. Reexamine.

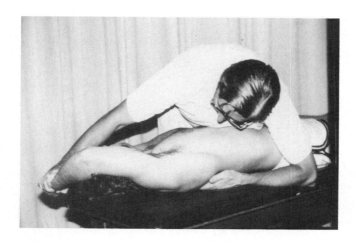

**Figure 15.33.** Combined technique, inhalation restriction, ribs 6, 7, 8, 9. Operator resists adduction effort of patient's right arm.

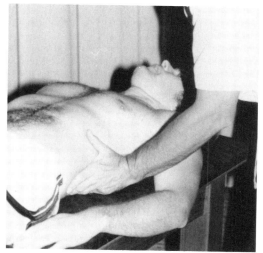

**Figure 15.34.** Combined technique, exhalation restriction, lower ribs. Thumb and thenar eminence span costochondral junction of dysfunctional rib.

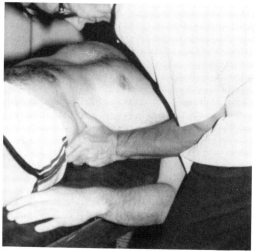

**Figure 15.36.** Combined technique, exhalation restriction, lower ribs. Left sidebending and flexion introduced to key rib.

*Upper Ribs*
Diagnosis: Exhalation restriction (left side example)
1. Patient supine on table with operator standing at left side of head of table.

2. Operator's left thumb and thenar eminence is in contact with the superior aspect of the shaft of the dysfunctional key rib spanning the costochondral junction. (Note that the more cephalic the rib the more

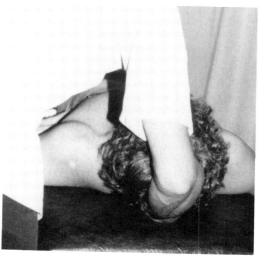

**Figure 15.35.** Combined technique, exhalation restriction, lower ribs. Operator controls patient's neck and trunk.

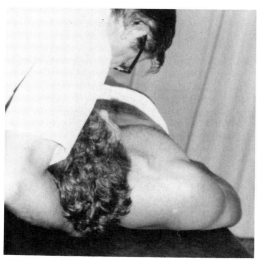

**Figure 15.37.** Combined technique, exhalation restriction, lower ribs. Left sidebending and flexion increased following exhalation effort.

medial the costochondral junction becomes) (Fig. 15.38).

3.  Operator's right hand controls patient's head, neck, and upper thoracic spine.

4.  Operator introduces flexion and sidebending to side of exhalation restriction with more flexion for pump-handle component and sidebending for bucket-handle component (Fig. 15.39).

5.  Patient instructed to take in small breath and exhale completely.

6.  Operator's thumb follows rib into exhalation position and *holds* there.

7.  Increased flexion and sidebending are introduced from above.

8.  Three to five repetitions of exhalation effort are introduced with operator's left thumb holding rib in exhalation position and right arm increasing flexion and sidebending.

9.  When maximum exhalation effort has been achieved, patient's head and neck are returned to neutral

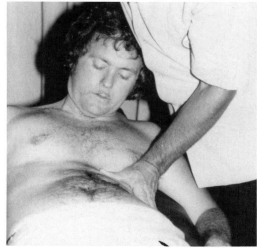

**Figure 15.39.** Combined technique, exhalation restriction, upper ribs. Flexion and sidebending introduced to engage pump-handle or bucket-handle component.

while operator holds dysfunctional rib in exhalation position (Fig. 15.40).

10.  Operator's left thumb is released *slowly*.

11.  Reexamine.

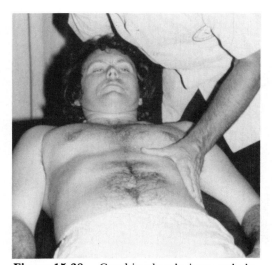

**Figure 15.38.** Combined technique, exhalation restriction, upper ribs. Thumb contacts superior aspect dysfunctional rib.

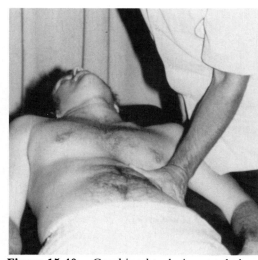

**Figure 15.40.** Combined technique, exhalation restriction, upper ribs. Operator holds dysfunctional rib and returns trunk to neutral.

*First Rib*

Diagnosis: Exhalation restriction, bucket-handle component (left side example)

1. Patient supine on table with operator standing at head of table.
2. Operator's left thumb placed on the superior aspect of the shaft of the left 1st rib, posterior to the neurovascular bundle (Fig. 15.41).
3. Operator's right hand cradles patient's head and controls flexion and sidebending left.
4. Patient instructed to take small breath in and exhale completely while operator sidebends head to the left and left thumb follows 1st rib into exhalation (Fig. 15.42).
5. While holding left 1st rib in exhalation, patient instructed to repeat minimal inhalation and maximal exhalation.
6. Operator increases sidebending during exhalation effort (Fig. 15.43).

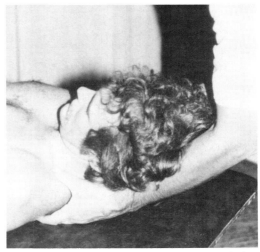

**Figure 15.42.** Combined technique, exhalation restriction, 1st rib (bucket- handle component). Head flexed and sidebent left with thumb following exhalation effort.

7. When maximum exhalation effort has been achieved, operator holds 1st rib in exhalation position and returns head to neutral.

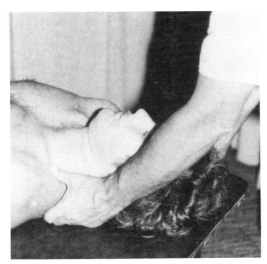

**Figure 15.41.** Combined technique, exhalation restriction, 1st rib (bucket- handle component). Left thumb on first rib shaft posterior to neurovascular bundle.

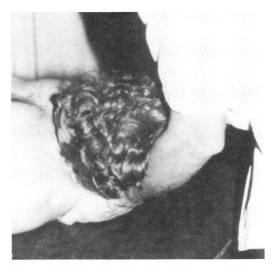

**Figure 15.43.** Combined technique, exhalation restriction, 1st rib (bucket- handle component). Head flexed and sidebent left with thumb following exhalation effort. Operator increases left sidebending with successive exhalation efforts.

8. Operator's left thumb releases patient's left 1st rib *slowly.*
9. Reexamine.

*First Rib*
Diagnosis: Exhalation restriction pump-handle motion (left side example)

1. Technique is the same as for bucket-handle restriction with the exception of step 2, operator's left thumb placed on superior aspect of 1st rib anterior to the neurovascular bundle (Fig. 15.44) and step 3, operator introduces more flexion than side-bending of the patient's head and neck (Fig. 15.45).

*Ribs 11 and 12*
Diagnosis: Exhalation restriction (right side example)

1. Patient prone on table with arm at side reaching toward feet.
2. Operator stands on left side of patient.

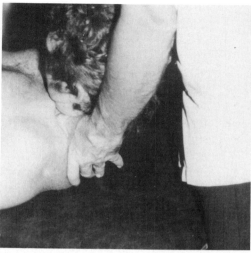

**Figure 15.45.** Combined technique, exhalation restriction in the 1st rib (pump-handle component). Operator induces flexion of head and neck.

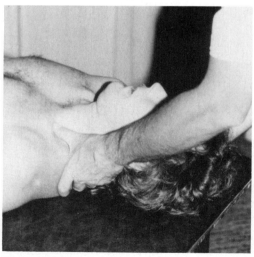

**Figure 15.44.** Combined technique, exhalation restriction in the 1st rib (pump-handle component). Left thumb on 1st rib anterior to neurovascular bundle.

3. Operator's heel of left hand, medial to the angle of the 11th and 12th ribs, exerts a lateral, and **slightly caudad force (Fig. 15.46).**
4. Operator's right hand grasps the patient's right anterior superior iliac spine (Fig. 15.47).
5. Patient instructed to inhale slightly and exhale maximally.
6. Operator's left hand carries the 11th and 12th ribs in a caudad direction.
7. Operator's right hand lifts patient's right pelvis off the table (Fig. 15.48).
8. Following complete exhalation effort of the patient, instruction is given to pull the anterior superior iliac spine down toward the table against resistance offered by the operator's right hand.
9. Three to five repetitions are made.
10. Reexamine.

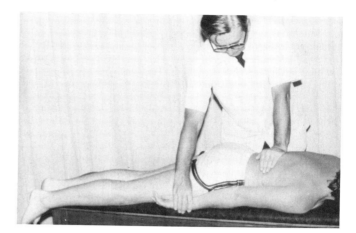

**Figure 15.46.**  Combined technique, exhalation restriction, ribs 11 and 12. Operator's hand exerts lateral force on angles of ribs 11 and 12.

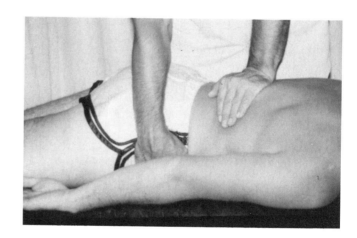

**Figure 15.47.**  Combined technique, exhalation restriction, ribs 11 and 12. Right hand grasps patient's ASIS.

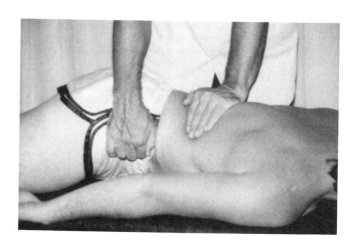

**Figure 15.48.**  Combined technique, exhalation restriction, ribs 11 and 12. Right hand lifts pelvis off the table.

*Ribs 11 and 12*
Diagnosis: Inhalation restriction (right side example)

1.  Patient prone on table with right arm over the head reaching cephalically.
2.  Operator stands at left side of patient.
3.  Operator's heel of left hand in contact with patient's right 11th and 12th ribs medial to the angle, exerting a lateral and slightly cephalic force (Fig. 15.49).
4.  Operator's right hand grasps the patient's right anterior superior iliac spine (Fig. 15.50).
5.  Patient instructed to take a maximal inhalation effort and hold.
6.  Operator lifts patient's right pelvis off table.
7.  Patient instructed to pull the right anterior superior iliac spine down to the table.
8.  Three to five repetitions are made.
9.  Reexamine.

## Direct Action High-Velocity Thrust (Mobilization with Impulse): Rib Technique

High-velocity thrusting technique can be used to treat respiratory restriction of ribs, both single rib and key rib for groups, as well as rib torsion dysfunction. High-velocity thrusting procedures are contrain-

dicated in the rib subluxations. The treatment sequence is the same as described above. In the presence of an inhalation or exhalation group dysfunction, the key rib is identified and treated individually with high-velocity thrust technique. Exhalation restrictions are treated from below upward and inhalation restrictions from above downward.

In the presence of rib torsional dysfunction the high-velocity thrusting procedure is a variation of that described for ERS non-neutral dysfunction of the thoracic spine in the supine position (see Chapter 14). The technique is modified by the addition of use of the thenar eminence of the operator's thumb on the inferior aspect of the rib that is externally torsioned, and a cephalic pressure is placed upon the rib at the time of the thrust. Frequently two cavitation pop sounds occur in rapid sequence when the thrust is applied.

*Rib 1*
Diagnosis: Inhalation or exhalation restriction

1.  Patient supine on table.
2.  Operator stands at opposite side of dysfunctional rib and slides arm under patient with hand grasping dysfunctional rib (Fig. 15.51).
3.  Operator's fingerpads contact the superior aspect of the shaft of the 1st rib.

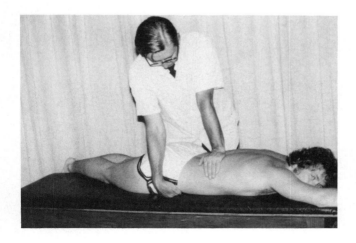

**Figure 15.49.** Combined technique, inhalation restriction, ribs 11 and 12. Operator's hand exerts lateral and slightly cephalic force on 11 and 12 ribs.

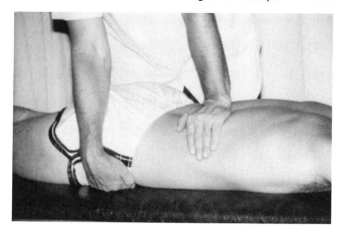

**Figure 15.50.** Combined technique, inhalation restriction, ribs 11 and 12. Right hand grasps patient's ASIS.

4.  With exhalation restriction operator depresses anterior aspect of shaft of rib. With inhalation restriction operator's fingers depress posterior aspect of 1st rib.

5.  Operator's opposite hand sidebends patient's head and neck toward and rotates the head away from the dysfunctional rib taking up all slack at the dysfunctional rib (Fig. 15.52).

6.  A high-velocity low-amplitude thrust is accomplished with the operator's hand in contact with the first rib in the axis of the forearm while the operator's opposite hand

exaggerates the head and neck position.

7.  Reexamine.

*Typical ribs - supine*
Diagnosis: Inhalation or exhalation restriction

1.  Operator's thumb and thenar eminence make contact with the dysfunctional rib (Fig. 15.53). With exhalation restriction the thumb and thenar eminence are below the posterior aspect of the shaft of the rib exerting a force superiorly (Fig. 15.54). With inhalation restriction the thumb and thenar eminence are

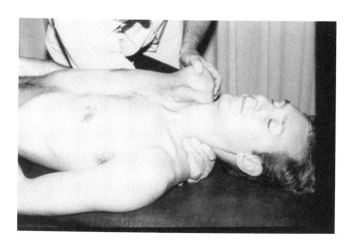

**Figure 15.51.** High-velocity, low-amplitude thrust technique, respiratory rib restriction, rib 1. Operator contacts superior aspect rib 1 directing toward inhalation or exhalation.

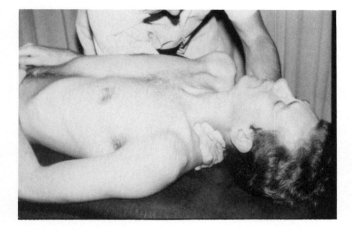

**Figure 15.52.** High-velocity, low-amplitude thrust technique, respiratory rib restriction, rib 1. Patient's head and neck sidebent toward and rotated away from dysfunctional rib and followed by thrust by hand on rib.

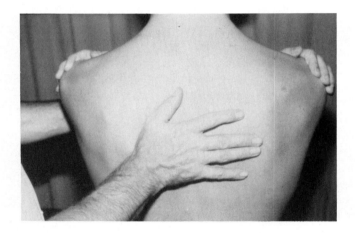

**Figure 15.53.** Supine, high-velocity, low-amplitude thrust technique, typical rib inhalation or exhalation restriction. Thenar eminence contacts functional rib.

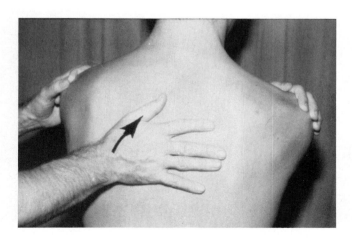

**Figure 15.54.** Supine, high-velocity, low-amplitude thrust technique, typical rib, inhalation or exhalation restriction. For exhalation restriction, thenar eminence below rib shaft.

on the superior aspect of the posterior shaft of the rib and are carried caudad (Fig. 15.55).

2. The patient's arm on the side of dysfunction is brought across the rib cage grasping the shoulder on the opposite side (Fig. 15.56).

3. The operator places his thumb and thenar eminence on the dysfunctional rib either at the inferior aspect for exhalation restriction or the superior aspect for inhalation restriction (Fig. 15.57).

4. The patient's elbow is contacted by the operator's chest or abdomen and a localizing force is directed toward the operator's thumb and thenar eminence on the dysfunctional rib (Fig. 15.58).

5. With inhalation restriction the patient makes a deep inhalation effort and the operator thrusts through the patient's arm while concurrently taking the thumb inferiorly on the posterior contact of the rib shaft. With exhalation restriction the patient makes a deep exhalation effort and the operator's thumb on the inferior aspect of the posterior shaft moves cephalically at the time of the high-velocity low-amplitude thrust.

6. Reexamine.

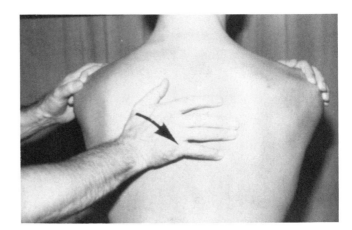

**Figure 15.55.** Supine, high-velocity, low-amplitude thrust technique, typical rib, inhalation or exhalation restriction. For inhalation restriction, thenar eminence above rib shaft.

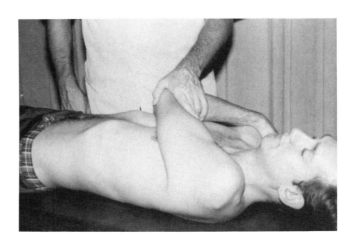

**Figure 15.56.** Supine, high-velocity, low-amplitude thrust technique, typical rib, inhalation or exhalation restriction. Lever arm formed by patient's arm grasping opposite shoulder.

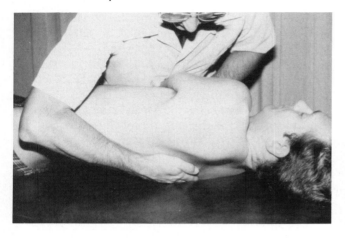

**Figure 15.57.** Supine, high-velocity, low-amplitude thrust technique, typical rib, inhalation or exhalation restriction. Operator's thenar eminence on dysfunctional rib.

*Atypical ribs 11 and 12*
Diagnosis: Inhalation or exhalation restriction

1.  Patient prone on table with operator standing opposite to dysfunctional rib.
2.  Operator's hand overlying the medial aspect of the angle of the 11th and 12th ribs.
3.  With exhalation restriction the patient's body is sidebent toward the side of restriction with the arm at the side pointing down toward the patient's knee on the side of restriction (Fig. 15.59).
4.  The operator's opposite hand grasps the anterior superior iliac spine on the side of rib dysfunction and takes up all the slack by a rotary movement of the pelvis.
5.  When all of the slack is taken out, a high-velocity, low-amplitude thrust is exerted through the hand in contact with the dysfunctional ribs in a lateral and caudad direction.
6.  For inhalation restriction the operator's hand contact remains the same but the patient moves the arm on the involved side over the head encouraging inhalation direction. With this dysfunction, the operator's thrust is laterally and superiorly after all slack has been taken up from rotation of the pelvis from below by the hand contact with

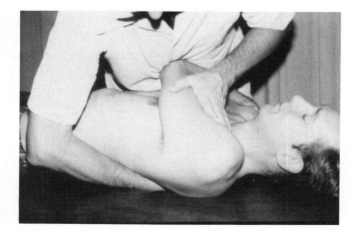

**Figure 15.58.** Supine, high-velocity, low-amplitude thrust technique, typical rib, inhalation or exhalation restriction. Thrust applied toward thenar eminence on dysfunctional rib.

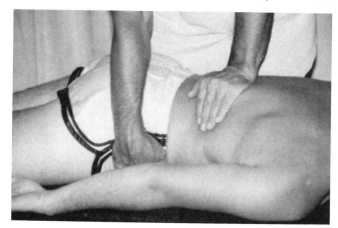

**Figure 15.59.** Prone, high-velocity, low-amplitude thrust technique, ribs 11 and 12, inhalation or exhalation restriction. With operator's hand on 11 and 12 ribs, patient sidebend toward exhalation restriction of rib.

the anterior superior iliac spine (Fig. 15.60).

7. Reexamine.

*Rib 1 - sitting*
Diagnosis: Inhalation and exhalation restriction

1. Patient sitting on the table.
2. Operator standing behind patient with the thumb, web of the hand, and index finger overlying the 1st rib on the dysfunctional side (Fig. 15.61).
3. The patient's axilla opposite to the dysfunctional rib is placed on top of the operator's knee with foot on table (Fig. 15.62).

4. Operator's hand opposite of that in contact with the dysfunctional rib sidebends the patient's head and neck toward the side of dysfunctional rib, with some left translation, until all slack is taken out (Fig. 15.63).

5. A high-velocity low-amplitude thrust is directed medially and caudad through the operator's hand in contact with the dysfunctional rib which exaggerates the patient's head and neck body posture into sidebending toward the side of the dysfunction.

6. Reexamine.

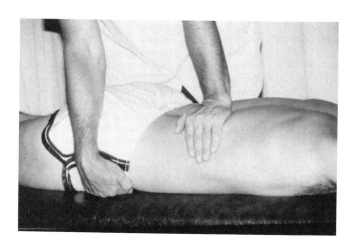

**Figure 15.60.** Prone, high-velocity, low-amplitude thrust technique, ribs 11 and 12, inhalation or exhalation restriction. For inhalation restriction, patient's arm above head and operator's thrust laterally and superiorly.

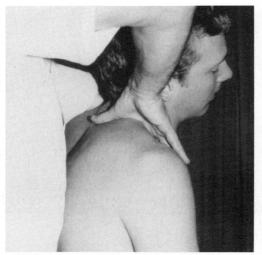

**Figure 15.61.** Sitting, high-velocity, low-amplitude thrust technique, rib 1. Thumb and index finger overlay 1st rib.

*Lower typical ribs and atypical 11th and 12th ribs, lateral recumbent*

Diagnosis: Inhalation or exhalation restriction

1. Patient in the lateral recumbent position on the table with the dysfunctional rib up (Fig. 15.64).

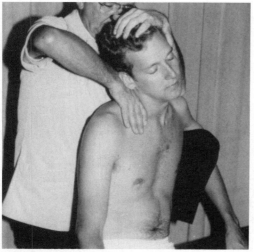

**Figure 15.62.** Sitting, high-velocity, low-amplitude thrust technique, rib 1. Operator's knee supports patient's trunk.

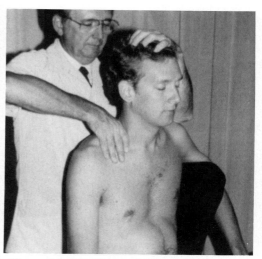

**Figure 15.63.** Sitting, high-velocity, low-amplitude thrust technique, rib 1. Operator sidebends patient's head and neck toward dysfunctional rib and thrust applied medially and caudad.

2. Operator stands in front of patient with the pisiform of the caudad hand in contact with the medial aspect of the dysfunctional rib.
3. Operator's cephalic hand contacts the anterior aspect of the patient's uppermost shoulder on the side of the dysfunctional rib (Fig. 15.65).
4. All slack is taken out down to the dysfunctional rib by posterior rotation of the patient's trunk by the operator's cephalic hand.
5. A high-velocity thrust is accomplished through the axis of the operator's forearm and hand in contact with the dysfunctional rib either into an inhalation or exhalation direction.
6. Reexamine.

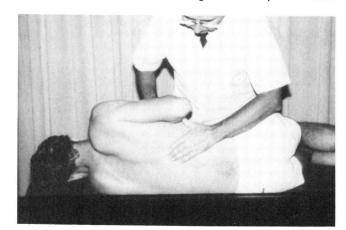

**Figure 15.64.** Lateral recumbent, high-velocity, low-amplitude thrust technique, lower ribs. Patient in lateral recumbent position, dysfunctional rib up.

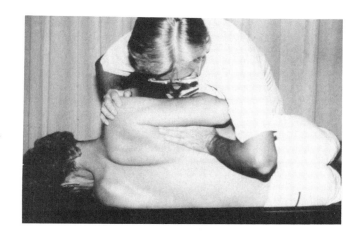

**Figure 15.65.** Lateral recumbent, high-velocity, low-amplitude thrust technique, lower ribs. With pisiform contact on dysfunctional rib, operator's cephalic hand controls upper trunk. Thrust applied through pisiform contact.

# 16

## LUMBAR SPINE TECHNIQUE

The lumbar spine and its relationship to the pelvic girdle (see Chapter 17) originate many of the structures incriminated in patients' complaints of "low back pain". Since the classic report of Mixter and Barr in 1934, the lumbar intervertebral disk and its pathologies have received a great deal of attention from physicians in many disciplines. The differential diagnosis of 'low back pain' continues to be a dilemma for the examining physician and 60 to 80% of cases are still classified as idiopathic. After the exclusion of organic and pathological conditions by orthodox orthopedic and neurologic testing, the examiner is left with the difficulty of determining any other treatable source for the back pain. It is in these patients that the ability to identify and to treat functional abnormalities of the musculoskeletal system has been found clinically effective. It is strongly recommended that the structural diagnostic procedures identified here and in Chapter 17, be used concurrently with orthopedic and neurologic testing of the lower trunk and lower extremities. Including functional diagnosis in these patients greatly reduces the number that need be classified as idiopathic. Much more clinical research is needed on the origin of pain in dysfunctions of the lumbar spine and pelvis and the efficacy and mechanisms of manual medicine therapeutic applications.

## FUNCTIONAL ANATOMY

The five lumbar vertebra are the most massive in the vertebral column. The vertebral bodies are kidney shaped and are solidly constructed to participate in weight bearing of the superincumbent vertebral column. The posterior arches are also strongly developed with large spinous processes which project almost directly posterior from the vertebral bodies. The transverse processes are quite large and those at L3 are usually the broadest in the lumbar column. The lumbar lordosis has an anterior convexity with L3 usually being the most anterior segment. L4 and L5 have limited motion because of the strong attachments of the iliolumbar ligaments to the osseous pelvis, so L3 becomes the first lumbar segment that is freely movable.

The articular pillar has a superior apophyseal joint which faces posteriorly and medially, and an inferior apophyseal joint which faces laterally and anteriorly. The superior facet is somewhat concave and the inferior facet somewhat convex. The facing of the lumbar apophyseal joint is variable and asymmetry is quite common. Because of the shape of the apophyseal joints, only a small amount of axial rotation movement is present individually or as a group. When the plane of the apophyseal joints is more sagittal, there appears to be increased stability of the lumbar spine. The more coronal facing the lumbar apophyseal joints are, the more mobility and potential hypermobility appears to be present. In the presence of asymmetry, with one apophyseal joint being sagittal and the other being coronal, there appears to be an increase in the risk of disc degeneration and herniation, with a tendency toward herniation to the side of the coronal facing facet. Asymmetrical apophyseal joints also appear to influence the motion characteristics of the segment and are frequently found in patients with recurrent and refractory dysfunctional problems in the lumbar spine. Between the superior and inferior apophyseal joints lies the structure called the pars interarticularis. When disruption occurs at this level, for whatever reason, the condition is called spondodylolysis. If there is separation at this level, the body, pedicle, and superior articular pillar can slide anteriorly while the spinous process, laminae, and inferior articular pillar are held posteriorly, resulting in the condition called spondylolisthesis.

The lower lumbar region is frequently the site of developmental variations. In addition to asymmetrical development of the apophyseal joints, other variations in the posterior arch occur resulting in unilateral and bilateral changes in size and shape of the transverse process, culminating in a transitional lumbosacral vertebra which may have more lumbar or more sacral characteristics, (referred to in the past as lumbarization and sacralization). Failure of closure of the posterior arch is not infrequently seen and occasionally the spinous process of L5 is missing. Absence of these structures must result in alteration of the usual ligamentous and muscular attachments in the region.

The motions available in the lumbar spine are primarily flexion and extension. There is a small amount of right and left sidebending and a minimal amount of rotation. The coupled movements of sidebending and rotation available in the lumbar spine are both neutral, type I, and nonneutral, type II. In the neutral and backward-bending position of the lumbar spine, sidebending and rotation are coupled to opposite sides. When the lumbar spine is in the forward-bending position, sidebending and rotation couple to the same side. Because of the intimate attachments of the iliolumbar ligaments from L4 and L5 to the osseous pelvis, these two segments have less mobility than the upper three lumbar vertebrae. The lumbosacral junction has distinctive motion characteristics in which L5 and the sacrum normally move in opposite directions to each other. For instance, with sidebending right and rotation left of the sacrum between the innominates, L5 normally adapts by sidebending left and rotating right. As the sacrum goes into anterior nutation (flexion of the sacrum between the innominates), L5 moves into backward-bending (extension) in relation to the sacrum. With the reverse motions, just the opposite occurs. Absence of this normal motion relationship of L5 to the sacrum is of great clinical significance and is termed "nonadaptive lumbar response" to sacral function. It is for this reason that, in the application of manual medicine procedures to the lower back, the lumbar spine dysfunctions must be diagnosed and treated before those at the two sacroiliac joints, so that the normal relationship of L5 to the sacrum can occur.

### Structural Diagnosis of Lumbar Spine Dysfunction

The lumbar spine can have neutral, type I, dysfunctions of three or more segments. The upper lumbar segments are frequently involved in group dysfunctions along with the lower segments of the thoracic spine. Nonneutral, type II, dysfunctions of both the ERS- and FRS-type occur in the lumbar spine. If, during the screening and scanning procedure, one finds flattening of the lumbar lordosis, the probability of FRS dysfunction with extension restriction is high. Alternately, if the lumbar lordosis is increased, the likelihood of ERS-type flexion restriction is high.

In diagnosing segmental definition the examiner is again most interested in the tissue texture characteristics of the deeper layers of paravertebral muscle, particularly hypertonicity of the multifidi, rotatores, and intertransversariae. To evaluate specific segmental motion restriction, one again utilizes the relationship of the posterior aspect of the transverse processes in three positions. Starting from below and working upward, one looks for the first pair of transverse processes which are asymmetric, and then the relative relationship is evaluated with the patient forward-bent (Fig. 16.1), neutral prone on the table (Fig. 16.2), and backward-bent in the sphinx position (Fig. 16.3). If one transverse process is more posterior in the fully forward-bent position and becomes symmetric in the sphinx position, then a nonneutral, type II, ERS dysfunction is present at that level. If one transverse process is more prominent in the sphinx position, but is symmetric in the fully forward-bent position, then a nonneutral, type II, FRS restriction is present. If three or more transverse processes remain prominent throughout all three positions, a neutral, type I, dysfunction is present in those segments. Nonneutral, type II, dysfunctions are commonly identified at the top and bottom of group dysfunctions. It is fre-

quently difficult to evaluate the functional capacity of the upper segments in the lumbar spine until those identified in the lower regions are successfully treated. There is a great deal of carryover effect into the mid and upper lumbar spine from nonneutral, type II, dysfunctions at L4 and L5. L4 and L5, as described above, do not have a great deal of mobility because of the ligamentous attachments, but as in other areas of the musculoskeletal system which normally have small amounts of movement, when that movement is lost, it seems to have a disproportionately great clinical significance. Nonneutral dysfunctions of L4 and L5 are frequently encountered in association with dysfunction of the two sacroiliac joints.

## Manual Medicine Procedures for Dysfunctions of Lumbar Spine

With the possibility of both group, type I dysfunctions, and FRS and ERS nonneutral, type II dysfunctions, techniques for all three diagnoses are needed by the treating physician. One should be able to treat a patient either in the erect sitting or in the lateral recumbent, supine, or prone positions to meet the patient's need.

Muscle energy procedures for lumbar spine dysfunction are as follows:

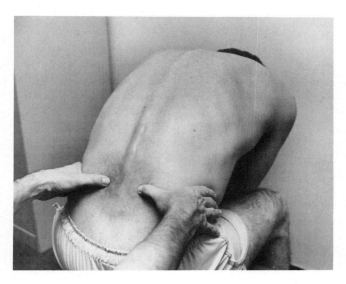

**Figure 16.1.** Lumbar diagnosis, forward-bent position.

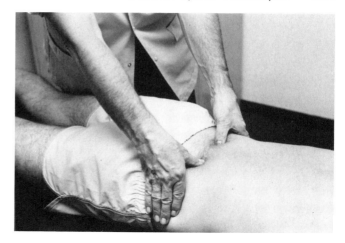

**Figure 16.2.** Lumbar diagnosis, prone neutral position.

*Lumbar spine*
Sitting
Neutral group dysfunction
   Position: Neutral, sidebent left, rotated right ($NS_L R_R$) or (EN Rt)
   Motion restriction: Neutral, sidebending right, rotation left

1. Patient seated with operator standing to the right side.
2. Patient's left hand on right shoulder and operator's right arm grasps upper trunk with the patient's right shoulder in the operator's right axilla, and with the operator's right hand grasping the patient's left shoulder.
3. Operator's thumb (or pisiform) is in contact with the apex of the right-sided convexity preparing to exert a translatory force from right to left (Fig. 16.4).
4. Operator introduces right sidebending and left rotation through the shoulders while translating from right to left with the contact at the apex (Fig. 16.5).
5. Patient attempts to sidebend to the left against operator's equal and opposite resistance for 3 to 5 seconds.
6. Following patient relaxation, operator increases right sidebending and left rotation and patient again introduces left sidebending effort.
7. Repeat 2 or 3 times.
8. Reexamine.

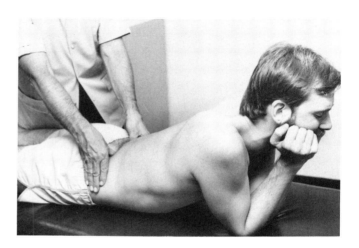

**Figure 16.3.** Lumbar diagnosis, backward-bent position.

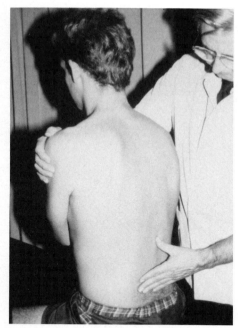

**Figure 16.4.** Sitting, muscle energy technique, neutral, group dysfunction. Operator's thumb contacts apex of convexity.

*Lumbar spine*
Sitting
      Position: Bilateral flexed
      Motion restriction: Bilateral extension

1. Patient sits with each hand holding the opposite shoulder.
2. Operator stands behind and with left hand grasps patient's elbows (Fig. 16.6).
3. Heel of operator's right hand is placed on spinous process of inferior segment exerting anterior translatory force.
4. Patient's upper trunk is extended over the fulcrum applied by the operator's right hand (Fig. 16.7).
5. Patient is instructed to forward-bend upper trunk against equal and opposite resistance offered by operator's left hand.
6. Following relaxation of patient, increased anterior translation with the right hand and backward-bending

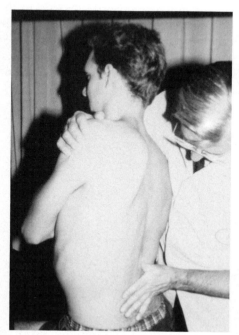

**Figure 16.5.** Sitting, muscle energy technique, neutral, group dysfunction. Operator introduces right sidebending and left rotation and resists patient's left sidebending effort.

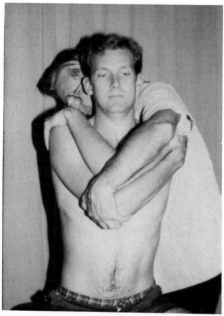

**Figure 16.6.** Sitting, muscle energy technique, lumbar spine, bilateral flexed. From behind operator's left hand grasps patient's elbows.

of the trunk is accomplished and patient's effort repeated.

7. Repeat 2 to 3 times.
8. Reexamine.

*Lumbar spine*
Sitting
Position: Forward bent (flexed), right rotated, right sidebent (FSR$_{Rt}$)
Motion restriction: Backward bending (extension), left sidebending, left rotation

1. Same as technique for lower thoracic spine (Chapter 14, Figs. 14.16–14.20) adapted for localization to appropriate lumbar segment.

*Lumbar spine*
Sitting
Position: Backward bent (extended), right rotated, right sidebent (ERS$_{Rt}$)

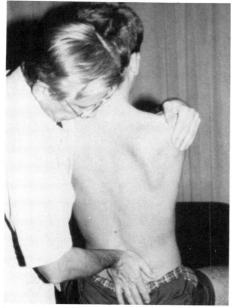

**Figure 16.7.** Sitting, muscle energy technique, lumbar spine, bilateral flexed. Patient's trunk extended over fulcrum applied by operator's right hand. Operator resists trunk forward-bending.

Motion restriction: Forward bending (flexion), left sidebending, left rotation

1. Same procedure as for thoracic spine (Chapter 14, Figs. 14.13–14.15) adapted for localization to dysfunctional lumbar segment.

*Lumbar spine*
Sitting
Nonneutral, type II, ERS dysfunction, variation 2
Position: Backward bent (extended), left sidebent, left rotated (ERS$_{Lt}$)
Motion restriction: Forward-bending (flexion), right sidebending, right rotation

1. Patient sits on stool with left hand holding the right shoulder and the right arm dropped at the side.
2. Operator stands at left side of patient with left hand grasping the patient's right shoulder and controlling the left shoulder with the left axilla (Fig. 16.8).
3. Forward-bending, right sidebending, and right rotation are introduced from above downward to the dysfunctional segment by the operator and the patient is instructed to reach gently toward the floor with the right hand (Fig. 16.9).
4. When the first barrier is reached the patient is instructed to sidebend to the left against the left axilla providing equal resistance for 3 to 5 seconds.
5. Following relaxation by the patient, increased forward-bending, right sidebending and right rotation is made until the new barrier is engaged.
6. Left sidebending or left rotation of the patient is again made against equal and opposite resistance by the operator.
7. When all right sidebending and right rotation restriction is removed

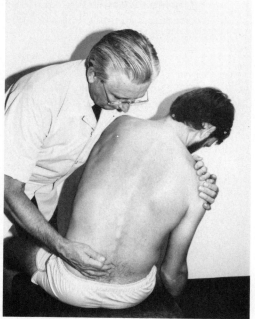

**Figure 16.8.** Sitting, muscle energy technique, lumbar spine, nonneutral dysfunction (ERS_left). Operator controls patient's trunk by grasping right shoulder with left shoulder in operator's axilla.

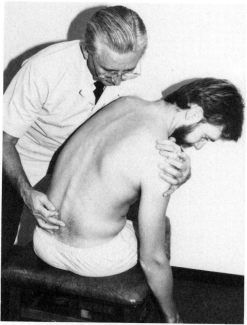

**Figure 16.9.** Sitting, muscle energy technique, lumbar spine, nonneutral dysfunction (ERS_left). Forward-bending, right sidebending, and right rotation introduced to dysfunctional segment.

the patient is carried forward into full forward-bending without losing the right rotation and right sidebending until the patient is fully forward-bent (Fig. 16.10).

8.  Patient is now instructed to lift the shoulders toward the ceiling which fully forward-bend the segment opening both facets (Fig. 16.11).
9.  Reexamine.

The following are muscle energy techniques in the recumbent position:

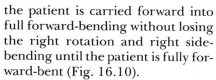

*Lumbar spine*
Lateral recumbent (Sims position)
   Position: Backward-bent (extended), left sidebent, left rotated (ERS_Lt).
   Motion restriction: Forward-bending (flexion), right sidebending, right rotation

1.  Patient lies on the table with both knees and feet together, knees and hips flexed slightly, and lying on the right hip. The patient's left arm dangles over the side of the table and the right arm is at the side of the patient on the table (right lateral Sims position).
2.  Operator stands in front of patient and controls the patient's flexed knees by the operator's anterior right thigh.
3.  Operator's right hand palpates at interspinous level at the dysfunctional segment and flexes the knees and hips up until the lower segment first begins to move.
4.  Right rotation is introduced by asking the patient to reach the floor with the left hand while the operator increases downward pressure on the patient's left shoulder until the

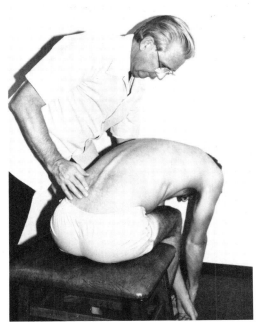

**Figure 16.10.** With all right sidebending and right rotation restriction removed, patient carried to full forward-bending.

upper segment first moves (Fig. 16.12).

5.  Localization having been made, the patient's feet are dropped over the edge of the table introducing right sidebending at the dysfunctional segment (Fig. 16.13).
6.  Patient is instructed to lift the feet toward the ceiling against resistance applied by the operator's right arm and hand. The operator's left hand monitors at the dysfunctional level (Fig. 16.14).
7.  A slight amount of flexion from below and right sidebending from below are introduced until the next barrier is engaged.
8.  Patient repeats the effort of lifting the feet to the ceiling.
9.  Two to 3 repetitions of steps 7 and 8 are made until restoration of function is achieved.
10.  Reexamine.

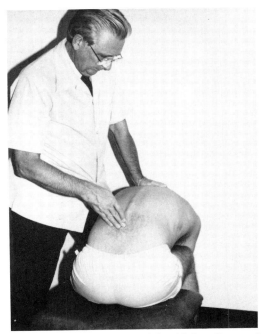

**Figure 16.11.** With all right sidebending and right rotation restriction removed, patient carried to full forward-bending. Operator resists patient's lift of shoulders to ceiling.

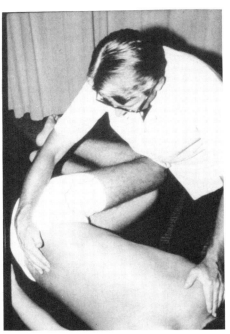

**Figure 16.12.** Lateral recumbent (Sims' position), muscle energy technique, lumbar spine, nonneutral dysfunction ($ERS_{left}$). Operator introduces right rotation by downward pressure on patient's left shoulder.

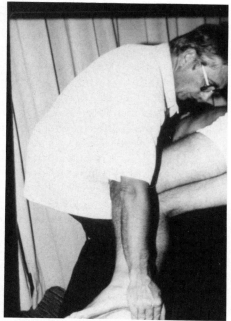

**Figure 16.13.** Lateral recumbent (Sims' position), muscle energy technique, lumbar spine, nonneutral dysfunction ($ERS_{left}$). Right sidebending introduced by dropping patient's feet off table.

*Lumbar spine*
Lateral recumbent
    Position: Forward bent (flexed), left rotated, left sidebent ($FRS_{Lt}$)
    Motion restriction: Backward-bending (extension), right rotation, right sidebending

1.  Patient lies on left side with knees and feet together and slightly flexed and with the shoulders perpendicular to the table.

2.  Operator stands in front and grasps the patient's lumbar area with the thumbs at the level of the dysfunctional segment, The operator "pulls" the segment forward by anterior translation localizing a backward-bending movement at the dysfunctional segment (Fig. 16.15).

3.  Further backward-bending is introduced from above downward by the operator pushing the patient's lower shoulder posteriorly. (Note: Do not allow the patient's lower shoulder to rotate. This maintains right sidebending of the trunk.)

4.  Backward-bending movement is introduced from below upward to the bottom segment of the dysfunctional level by extending the lower leg (Fig. 16.16). (Note: Do not allow the pelvis to rotate.)

5.  Right rotation is introduced from above downward to the superior vertebra at the dysfunctional level by asking the patient to reach backward and caudad with the right arm. The patient is instructed to hold the edge of the table for stability (Fig. 16.17).

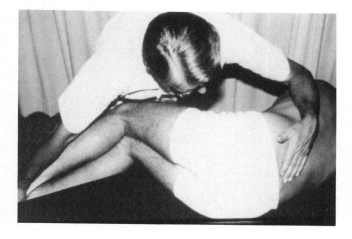

**Figure 16.14.** Lateral recumbent (Sims' position), muscle energy technique, lumbar spine, nonneutral dysfunction ($ERS_{left}$). Operator resists patient lifting feet to ceiling.

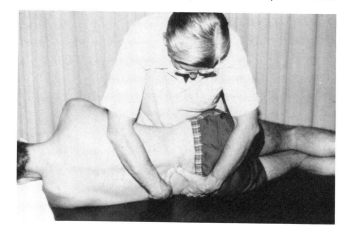

**Figure 16.15.** Lateral recumbent, muscle energy technique, lumbar spine, nonneutral dysfunction (FRS$_{left}$). Extension of dysfunctional segment by anterior translation.

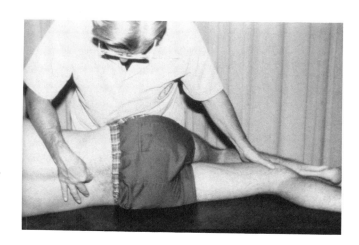

**Figure 16.16.** Lateral recumbent, muscle energy technique, lumbar spine, nonneutral dysfunction (FRS$_{left}$). Barrier engaged from below by extending lower leg.

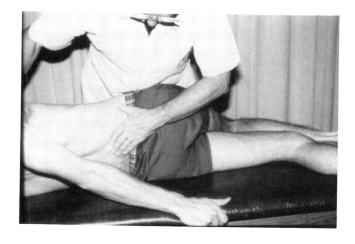

**Figure 16.17.** Lateral recumbent, muscle energy technique, lumbar spine, nonneutral dysfunction (FRS$_{left}$). Barrier engaged from below by extending lower leg. Right rotation from above to dysfunctional segment with patient grasping edge of table.

6. The operator grasps the patient's right ankle and abducts and internally rotates the lower extremity, introducing right sidebending from below (Fig. 16.18).
7. Patient is instructed to pull the right ankle to the left knee against equal and opposite resistance.
8. Increasing extension and right rotation can be engaged by asking the patient to reach further down along the edge of the table, while increased right sidebending occurs by the operator lifting the right leg toward the ceiling.
9. Patient repeats effort of pulling foot toward the left knee two to three times.
10. Reexamine.

*Lumbar spine*
Lateral recumbent
  Position: Neutral sidebent right, rotated left ($NS_R R_L$) or ($EN_{Lt}$)
  Motion restriction: Neutral, sidebending left, rotation right

1. Patient lies on the right side with the shoulders and hips perpendicular to the table and with the feet and knees together in a slightly flexed position.
2. Operator stands in front of patient monitoring the group dysfunctional

convexity with the fingers of the left hand (Fig. 16.19).
3. Operator's right hand controls the patient's lower extremity and flexes and extends the hips and knees until maximum ease (no flexion or extension restriction) is palpable at the site of the group dysfunction (Fig. 16.20).
4. Operator introduces left sidebending by lifting the feet toward the ceiling (Fig. 16.21).
5. Instruction is given to the patient to pull the feet down to the table against equal and opposite resistance for 3 to 5 seconds.
6. Left sidebending is increased by the operator lifting the feet.
7. Patient repeats effort of pulling feet to table (right sidebending).
8. Repeat 2 to 3 times.
9. Reexamine.

High-velocity, low-amplitude thrust manual medicine procedures (mobilization with impulse) are accomplished both in the sitting and recumbent positions. These procedures require localization precision so that a minimal amount of force is necessary for mobilization of the dysfunctional segment. All of the techniques described can be modified to become muscle energy procedures by asking the patient to move in the opposite direction at the position of localiza-

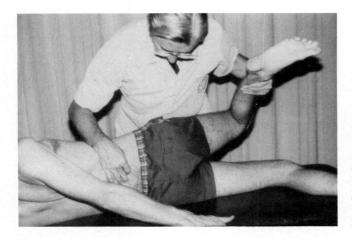

**Figure 16.18.** Lateral recumbent, muscle energy technique, lumbar spine, nonneutral dysfunction (FRS$_{left}$). Barrier engaged from below by extending lower leg. Operator introduces right sidebending from below and resists patient's effort to pull to table.

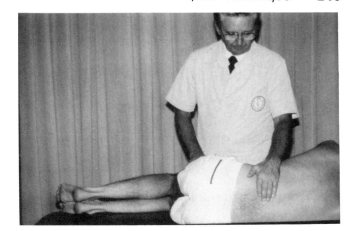

**Figure 16.19.** Lateral recumbent, muscle energy technique, lumbar spine, neutral dysfunction (EN$_{left}$). Operator monitors group convexity.

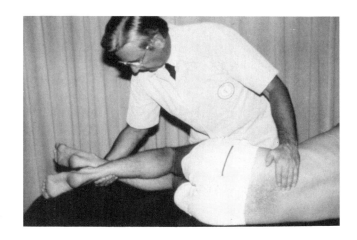

**Figure 16.20.** Lateral recumbent, muscle energy technique, lumbar spine, neutral dysfunction (EN$_{left}$). Neutral position found.

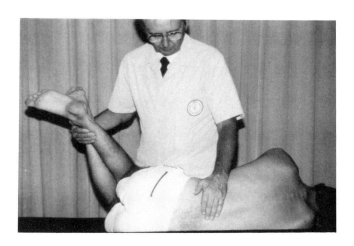

**Figure 16.21.** Lateral recumbent, muscle energy technique, lumbar spine, neutral dysfunction (EN$_{left}$). Left sidebending introduced while lifting feet to ceiling and operator resists patient's pull of feet to table.

tion against resistance offered by the operator. Both muscle energy and high-velocity thrust procedures identified here are direct action against the resistant barrier. Frequently two or three muscle energy efforts are used before the high-velocity, low-amplitude thrust.

*Lumbar spine*
L1 to L5
Lateral recumbent
Diagnosis: Group dysfunction (3 or more segments) (type I)
    Position: Neutral, sidebent right, rotated left ($NS_RR_L$) or ($EN_{Lt}$)
    Motion restriction: Sidebending left, rotation right

1. Patient lying in lateral recumbent position, operator in front, most posterior transverse processes toward the table.
2. Superior knee and thigh flexed so that the superior foot lies in the popliteal space of the inferior leg. Flexion and extension of lower extremities are accomplished to attain "neutral" (of flexion-extension in lumbar spine) (Fig. 16.22).
3. Patient's lower shoulder is pulled anterior and caudad (trunk no longer supported by shoulder) with rotation down to the involved segments (Fig. 16.23).

4. Operator's caudad arm controls the osseous pelvis and rotates it toward the operator with operator's cephalic arm controlling the shoulders and rotating the trunk away from the operator (Fig. 16.24).
5. All slack is taken out and localization of all forces from above and below occur at the apex of the curvature, with apex segment being perpendicular to the table (x-axis).
6. A high-velocity, low-amplitude, low-force thrust occurs with the operator dropping the weight down upon the pelvis by the caudad arm being "incorporated" as part of the operator's body.
7. Retest.

*Lumbar spine*
L1 to L5
Lateral recumbent
Diagnosis: Nonneutral dysfunction (type II)
    Position: Forward-bent (flexed), rotated left, sidebent left ($FRS_{Lt}$)
    Motion restriction: Backward-bending (extension), rotation right, sidebending right

1. Patient lying in the left lateral recumbent position (most posterior transverse process down).
2. With the patient's right foot hooked in the left popliteal space, the left

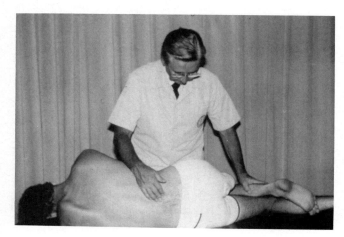

**Figure 16.22.** Lateral recumbent, high-velocity, low-amplitude thrust, lumbar spine, neutral group dysfunction ($EN_{left}$). With patient in lateral recumbent position, neutral obtained.

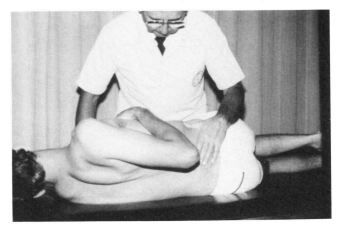

**Figure 16.23.** Lateral recumbent, high-velocity, low-amplitude thrust, lumbar spine, neutral group dysfunction (EN$_{left}$). Left sidebending and right rotation introduced by pulling shoulder anterior and cauded.

lower extremity is extended to incorporate the pelvis up to the inferior segment of the vertebral motion unit (Fig. 16.25).

3. With the shoulders perpendicular to the table, they are taken backward into extension from above downward to the superior segment of the vertebral motion unit (Fig. 16.26).

4. The operator's right hand rotates the patient's trunk to the right from above downward incorporating the superior segment. The operator's left forearm rotates the pelvis anteriorly with the arm incorporated as part of the operator's body (Fig. 16.27).

5. A high-velocity low-amplitude thrust is made with rotation of the pelvis to enhance extension at the dysfunctional segment.

6. Retest.

*Lumbar spine*
L1 to L5
Lateral recumbent
Diagnosis: Nonneutral dysfunction (type II)

      Position: Backward-bent (extended), rotated left, sidebent left (ERS$_{Lt}$)

      Motion restriction: Forward-bending (flexion), rotation right, sidebending right

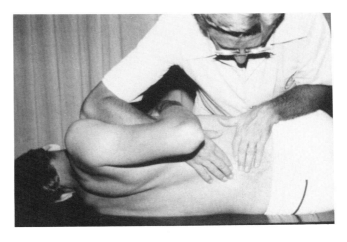

**Figure 16.24.** Lateral recumbent, high-velocity, low-amplitude thrust, lumbar spine, neutral group dysfunction (EN$_{left}$). Slack taken out from above and below by rotation and thrust applied.

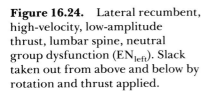

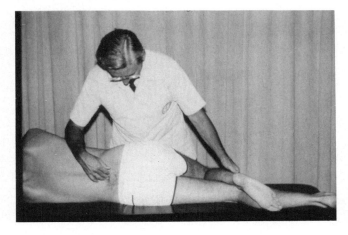

**Figure 16.25.**   Lateral recumbent, high-velocity, low-amplitude thrust, lumbar spine, nonneutral dysfunction ($FRS_{left}$). Barrier engaged from below by extending lower leg.

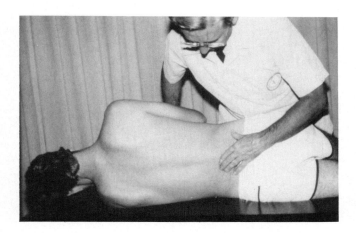

**Figure 16.26.**   Lateral recumbent, high-velocity, low-amplitude thrust, lumbar spine, nonneutral dysfunction ($FRS_{left}$). Barrier engaged from above by extension of trunk.

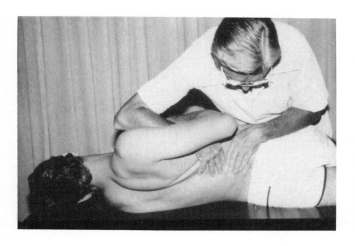

**Figure 16.27.**   Lateral recumbent, high-velocity, low-amplitude thrust, lumbar spine, nonneutral dysfunction ($FRS_{left}$). Right rotation from above, and thrust made from below at dysfunctional segment.

1. Patient lying in left lateral recumbent position with most posterior transverse process closest to the table, operator standing in front. Patient's shoulders and pelvis are perpendicular to the table (introducing right sidebending).
2. Flexion of the lower extremities at knee and thigh, incorporating the pelvis occurs until all of the slack is taken up to the inferior segment of the vertebral motion unit. Fixation of this position is made with the patient's right foot being hooked in the left popliteal area (Fig. 16.28).
3. With the patient's shoulders perpendicular to the table, the operator flexes the trunk until the superior vertebra of the vertebral motion segment first starts to move (Fig. 16.29).
4. Rotation to the right is introduced from above downward with the operator's right hand monitoring at the superior segment of the vertebral motion unit.
5. Slack is taken up by rolling the patient's pelvis anteriorly with the operator's left arm incorporated into his body and with the right arm rotating downward from above. The segment under treatment has its x-axis perpendicular to the table. A high-velocity, low-amplitude low-force thrust occurs with the operator rotating the pelvis anteriorly and cephalically (Fig. 16.30).
6. Retest.

*Lumbar spine*
L1 to L5
Sitting
Diagnosis: Group dysfunction (3 or more segments) (type I)
>    Position: Neutral, sidebent left, rotated right ($NS_L R_R$) ($EN_{RT}$)
>    Motion restriction: Sidebending right, rotation left

1. Patient sitting astride table, operator to right side, most posterior transverse processes toward the operator.
2. Patient's left arm holds right shoulder, operator reaches across the chest with right shoulder in right axilla and right hand on patient's left shoulder.
3. Operator's thumb placed at apex, or area of major restriction, of dysfunction between transverse processes acting as a fulcrum (Fig. 16.31).
4. Alternative method utilizes pisiform contact at same location (Fig. 16.32).
5. Patient is sidebent right while in the upright (neutral) position.

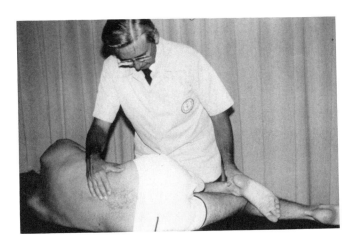

**Figure 16.28.** Lateral recumbent, high-velocity, low-amplitude thrust, lumbar spine, nonneutral dysfunction ($ERS_{left}$). Flexion from below to dysfunctional segment.

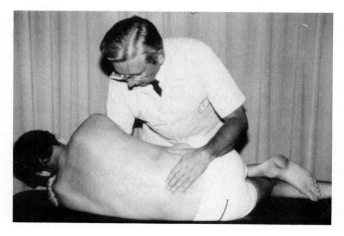

**Figure 16.29.** Lateral recumbent, high-velocity, low-amplitude thrust, lumbar spine, nonneutral dysfunction ($ERS_{left}$). Flexion from above to dysfunctional segment.

6. With all slack taken out, a high-velocity, low-amplitude thrust occurs simultaneously with exaggeration of sidebending by the operator dropping down with his right axilla and translating with the vertebral contact to the left, introducing right sidebending at the time of the thrust (Fig. 16.33). (Note: The extended forearm is blocked at the elbow against the operator's body).
7. Retest.

*Lumbar spine*
L1 to L5
Sitting
Diagnosis:
   Position: Bilaterally flexed (forward-bent)

Motion restriction: Bilateral extension (backward-bending)

1. Patient sitting astride table with both arms crossed in front with each hand holding the opposite shoulder.
2. Operator stands at side of patient with heel of hand overlying the spinous process and both transverse processes of the inferior vertebral of the dysfunctional vertebral motion unit (Fig. 16.34).
3. Operator grasps elbows of patient and extends trunk from above downward taking out all slack (Fig. 16.35).
4. With a combined movement of anterior translatory movement with the

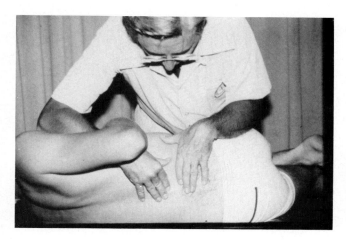

**Figure 16.30.** Lateral recumbent, high-velocity, low-amplitude thrust, lumbar spine, nonneutral dysfunction ($ERS_{left}$). Rotation to right from above, thrust applied by operator from below.

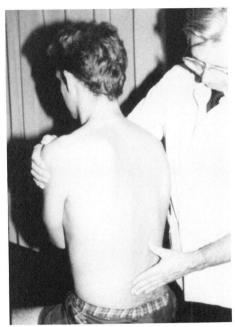

**Figure 16.31.** Sitting, high-velocity, low-amplitude thrust, lumbar spine, neutral dysfunction (EN$_{right}$). Operator's thumb placed at apex of group dysfunction.

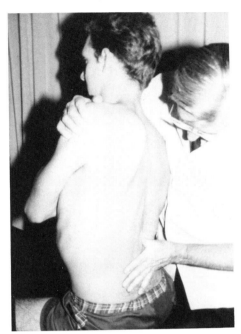

**Figure 16.33.** Sitting, high-velocity, low-amplitude thrust, lumbar spine, neutral dysfunction (EN$_{right}$). Barrier engaged by right sidebending and left rotation, and thrust applied by exaggeration of sidebending.

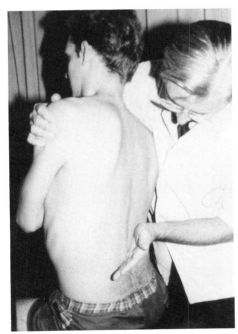

**Figure 16.32.** Sitting, high-velocity, low-amplitude thrust, lumbar spine, neutral dysfunction (EN$_{right}$). Alternative pisiform contact.

hand on the spinous process, and with extension of the trunk from above by the contact point on the elbow, a high-velocity, low-amplitude, low-thrust extends the superior vertebra over the inferior (Fig. 16.36).

5. Retest.

*Lumbar spine*
L1 to L5
Sitting
Diagnosis: Nonneutral dysfunction (type II)
    Position: Backward-bent (extended), rotated left, sidebent left (ERS$_{Lt}$)
    Motion Restriction: Forward-bending (flexion), rotation right, sidebending right

1. Patient sitting astride table with left hand holding right shoulder.
2. Operator stands at right side of patient, grasping patient's left shoul-

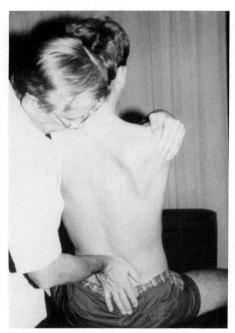

**Figure 16.34.** Sitting, high-velocity, low-amplitude thrust technique, lumbar spine, bilateral flexed. Heel of hand on lower vertebra.

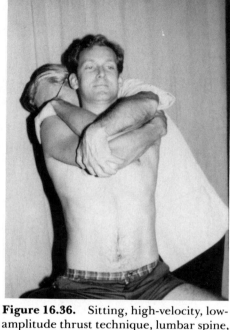

**Figure 16.36.** Sitting, high-velocity, low-amplitude thrust technique, lumbar spine, bilateral flexed. Thrust applied by extending superior vertebra over fulcrum.

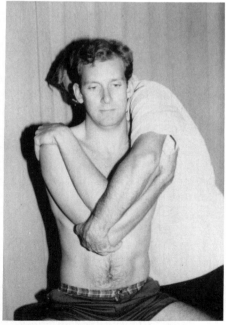

**Figure 16.35.** Sitting, high-velocity, low-amplitude thrust technique, lumbar spine, bilateral flexed. Operator grasps patient's elbows and extends trunk.

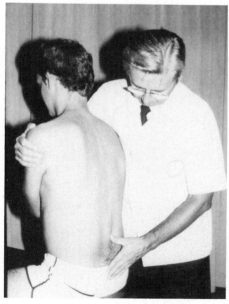

**Figure 16.37.** Sitting, high-velocity, low-amplitude thrust technique, lumbar spine, nonneutral dysfunction (ERS$_{left}$). Thumb on right side of spinous process.

der with right hand, right axilla on superior aspect of patient's right shoulder.

3. Thumb placed on right side of spinous process of dysfunctional segment (Fig. 16.37).
4. Operator uses forward-bending, right sidebending, and right rotation down to dysfunctional segment being contacted by operator's left thumb.
5. All slack is taken out and a high-velocity, low-amplitude, low-force thrust occurs simultaneously with the operator exaggerating the flexion, right sidebending, and right rotation of the patient's trunk and a left translatory movement of the thumb contact on the right side of the spinous process of the dysfunctional segment (Fig. 16.38).
6. Retest.

*Lumbar spine*
Sitting
Diagnosis: Nonneutral dysfunction (type II)

> Position: Forward-bent (flexed), rotated left, sidebent left ($FRS_{Lt}$) Motion restriction: Backward-bending (extension), rotation right, sidebending right.

1. Patient sitting astride table with the left hand on the right shoulder.
2. Operator stands to the right side of the patient with the right hand grasping the left shoulder and the right axilla on the superior aspect of the patient's right shoulder.
3. Thumb in contact with the right side of the spinous process of the dysfunctional segment (Fig. 16.39).
4. Patient's trunk is extended, right sidebent, and right rotated taking out all slack down to the dysfunctional segment (Fig. 16.40).

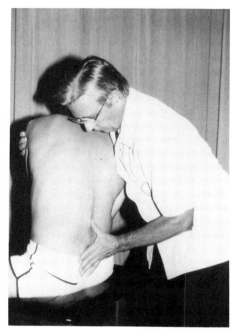

**Figure 16.38.** Sitting, high-velocity, low-amplitude thrust technique, lumbar spine, nonneutral dysfunction ($ERS_{left}$). When forward-bending, right sidebending, and right rotation barrier engaged, thrust applied by exaggeration of position and left translation by thumb contact.

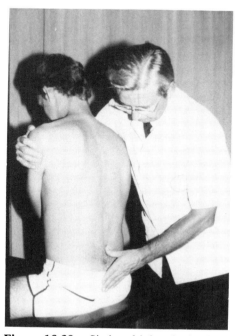

**Figure 16.39.** Sitting, high-velocity, low-amplitude thrust technique, lumbar spine, nonneutral dysfunction ($FRS_{left}$). Thumb contact on right side spinous process.

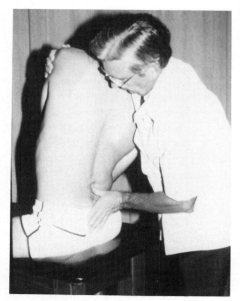

**Figure 16.40.**   Sitting, high-velocity, low-amplitude thrust technique, lumbar spine, nonneutral dysfunction (FRS$_{left}$). Barrier engaged by extension, right sidebending, and right rotation.

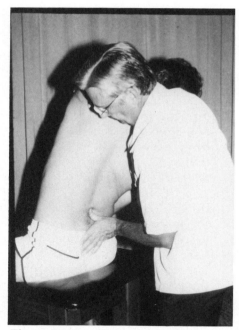

**Figure 16.41.**   Sitting, high-velocity, low-amplitude thrust technique, lumbar spine, nonneutral dysfunction (FRS$_{left}$). Thrust applied by exaggeration of patient position and left translation of spinous process.

5.   A high-velocity, low-amplitude thrust occurs with the operator's right arm and shoulder exaggerating extension, right sidebending, and right rotation and the left thumb in contact with the right side of the spinous process of the dysfunctional segment translating the segment left and anteriorly (Fig. 16.41).

6.   Retest.

# 17
# PRINCIPLES OF DIAGNOSIS AND TREATMENT OF PELVIC GIRDLE DYSFUNCTION

The role of the sacroiliac joints in the production of musculoskeletal pain syndromes continues to be controversial. For many years authorities stated that there was no movement at the sacroiliac joints, so they were not considered clinically significant. This was despite the fact that motion at the sacroiliac joints has been reported in the medical literature since the mid-19th century. Now it is generally conceded that the sacroiliac joints do move, albeit only a small amount, and the controversy has shifted to the types of motion available and the axes of rotation around which certain motions occur. It is beyond the scope of this volume to review the many works on sacroiliac motion. What will be presented is a diagnostic and therapeutic system for pelvic girdle dysfunction which has enabled this author to specifically diagnose and treat all of the physical findings available in pelvic girdle dysfunctions. The system is based on current knowledge of the movement of the joints within the pelvic girdle and adds a theoretical construct and terminology, to describe the various physical findings encountered during examination of the pelvic girdle. Fortunately, biomechanical research into the pelvic girdle is increasing and, as new knowledge is acquired, the theoretical construct provided here may well need modification.

Structural diagnosis and appropriate management of the pelvic girdle is of great importance to the postural structural model of manual medicine. The pelvic girdle joins the highly mobile extremities with the trunk and permits the highly complex mechanism of ambulation. This author's goal in manual medicine management of the pelvic girdle is the restoration of functional symmetry to the three bones and joints of the pelvic girdle during the walking cycle. Because the superior surface of the body of the sacrum supports the vertebral column, alteration in the sacrum can, and clinically does, have a profound effect on vertebral function above.

The pelvic girdle is also important in the respiratory circulatory model of manual medicine because of its relationship to the pelvic and urogenital diaphragms. Alteration in the functional capacity of the osseous pelvis can alter the function of the muscles of these diaphragms just as alteration in the thoracic spine and rib cage can influence the function of the thoraco-abdominal diaphragm.

The pelvic girdle is of extreme importance within the craniosacral concept and system. The sacrum has an inherent mobility between the two innominates as part of the craniosacral rhythm. Alteration in biomechanical function of the pelvic girdle can negatively influence the craniosacral mechanism, and, vice versa, alteration in the craniosacral mechanism can influence biomechanical function within the osseous pelvis. Obviously, the pelvic girdle is highly relevant in patients with musculoskeletal dysfunction and warrants investigation and appropriate management in all patients.

## FUNCTIONAL ANATOMY

The pelvic girdle consists of three bones and three joints. The sacrum is formed by the fused elements of the sacral vertebra and articulates superiorly with the last lumbar vertebra and caudally with the coccyx. The sacrum should be viewed as a component part of the vertebral axis. In many instances, the sacrum functions as an atypical lumbar vertebra between the two innominate bones, with the sacroiliac joints as atypical apophyseal joints. The right and left innominate bones consist of the fused elements of the ilium, ischium, and pubis. The two innominates are joined anteriorly by the symphysis pubis joint. Each innominate bone articulates cephalically with the sacrum at the ipsilateral sacroiliac joint, and caudally with the femur at the hip joint. Functionally, the innominate bone should be viewed as a lower extremity bone and the two sacroiliac joints as the junction of the vertebral axis and the lower extremity.

The joints of the pelvic girdle consist of the symphysis pubis and the two sacroiliac joints. The symphysis pubis is an amphiarthrosis with strong superior and inferior ligaments and a thinner posterior ligament. The opposing surfaces can range from symmetrically flat to quite asymmetrical and interlocking. The minimal amount of motion available at this joint is strongly influenced by the shape of the joint, the ligamentous integrity of the joint (particularly under the influence of hormonal changes), and the action of the abdominal muscles from above and the adductor muscles of the lower extremity below.

The sacroiliac joints are true arthrodial joints with a joint space, articular capsule, and articular cartilage. They are L-shaped in contour with a shorter upper arm and a longer lower arm, the junction occurring approximately at S2. The articular cartilage on the sacral side is much thicker than that on the ilial side. The joint contour usually has a depression on the sacral side at approximately S2 and a corresponding prominence on the ilial side. The shape of the sacroiliac joint varies markedly from individual to individual and from side to side in the same individual. During the aging process, there is an increase in the grooves on the opposing surfaces of the sacrum and ilium which affects motion. The sacroiliac joint usually has change in antero-posterior bevelling at approximately the junction of the upper and lower arm. The plane of the upper portion is convergent from behind forward while the lower portion is divergent from behind forward, resulting in an interlocking mechanism centering at approximately S2. Occasionally the opposing joint surfaces are quite flat and do not have the interlocking joint bevel change at S2 or the ilial prominence within the sacral depression. This type of sacroiliac joint is much less stable and the possibility of superior and inferior translatory movement, or shearing, exists. Occasionally the sacral concavity is replaced by a convexity with the ilial side being more concave. This joint structure provides for increased mobility, primarily in rotation medially and laterally, around a vertical axis.

Much of the integrity of the sacroiliac joint depends on ligamentous structures. The iliolumbar ligaments attach superiorly to the transverse processes of L4 and L5, and laterally to the anterior surface of the iliac crest. The lower fibers extend inferiorly and blend with the anterior sacroiliac ligaments. The anterior sacroiliac ligaments are two relatively flat and thin bands. They can be viewed as providing a sling from the two innominate bones for the anterior surface of the sacrum. The posterior sacroiliac ligaments have three layers. The deepest layer consists of short interosseous ligaments running from the sacrum to the ilium. The intermediate layer runs from the posterior arches of the sacrum to the medial side of the ilium, occupying most of the space overlying the posterior aspect of the sacroiliac joint. The long posterior sacroiliac ligaments blend together and course vertically from the sacral crest to the ilium. Inferiorly these posterior sacroiliac ligaments blend with the accessory sacroiliac ligaments, the sacrotuberous and the sacrospinous. The sacrotuberous ligament attaches to the inferior lateral angle of the sacrum and to the ischial tuberosity and has a crescent-shaped medial border. The sacrospinous ligament lies under the sacrotuberous and runs from the inferior lateral angle of the sacrum to the ischial spine. These two accessory ligaments contribute to the formation of the greater and lesser sciatic notches which are divided by the sacrospinous ligament.

Muscular attachment to the pelvic girdle is extensive but muscles that directly influence sacroiliac motion are difficult to identify. Movement of the sacroiliac mechanism appears to be mainly passive, in response to muscle action in the surrounding areas. The abdominal muscles, including the two obliques, the intermedius, and the rectus abdominus, insert on the superior aspect of the pelvic girdle and are joined posteriorly by the quadratus lumborum, the lumbodorsal fascia, and the erector spinae mass. Six groups of hip and thigh muscles attach to the pelvic girdle and lower extremities. These hip muscles strongly influence the movement of the two innominates within the pelvic girdle. Anterior to the sacroiliac joints are two highly significant muscles, the psoas and piriformis. The psoas crosses over the anterior aspect of the sacroiliac joints in its travel from the lumbar region to insert into the lesser trochanter of the femur. The right and left piriformis muscles originate from the anterior surface of the sacrum, travel through the sciatic notch, and insert into the greater trochanter of the femur.

Muscle imbalance in any of these groups can profoundly affect pelvic girdle func-

tion. Imbalance in piriformis length and strength appears to strongly influence movement of the sacrum between the innominates. Imbalance of the pelvic and urogenital diaphragms is highly significant in patients with rectal, gynecological, and urological problems. The reader is strongly encouraged to review the anatomy of all these muscles in a standard anatomical text.

## MOTION IN THE PELVIC GIRDLE

The pelvic girdle functions as an integrated unit with all three bones moving at all three joints, influenced by the lower extremities below and the vertebral column and trunk above. This integration results in torsional movement, both left and right, around a vertical (y) axis. In torsional movement to the left, the symphysis turns left of the midline, the right innominate is carried forward, the left innominate is carried backward, and the sacrum turns somewhat to the left (counterclockwise pelvic rotation). Torsion to the right (clockwise rotation) is just the reverse. A simple screening test for this global torsional movement involves the patient in the supine position with the operator placing the palm of the hands over each anterior superior iliac spine. Alternate rocking of the osseous pelvis by pushing posteriorly on each anterior superior iliac spine results in a sensation of symmetry or asymmetry. If movement seems to be more restricted when pushing posteriorly on the right anterior superior iliac spine than with the left, one can presume that the pelvic girdle is torsioned to the left and that there is some restrictor in the mechanism which needs further evaluation.

The amount of movement present at the symphysis pubis and at both sacroiliac joints is certainly not great and more biomechanical research is needed to identify the specific motions available and to determine their axes. The descriptions which follow are based upon current biomechanical information and clinical observations. Many of the clinical observations cannot be adequately explained by current biomechanical information, and a theoretical construct is offered to explain some of the clinical observations and establish a vocabulary to describe both available normal motions and dysfunctions.

Movement at the symphysis pubis is quite small, but it occurs in one-legged standing and during the walking cycle. The normal integrity of the joint is maintained by strong ligaments, primarily superiorly and inferiorly. The ligaments become more lax as a result of hormonal change in females, particularly during pregnancy and delivery, and separation occurs to widen the internal pelvic diameter during delivery. In normal individuals standing on one leg, there is a slight superior shearing movement if the position is maintained for several minutes. After standing on the opposite leg, or with prolonged standing on both legs, the shearing movement returns to normal. During normal walking, the symphysis pubis serves as the axis for innominate rotation. Functional alteration of the symphysis pubis will affect the anterior and posterior rotational movement during walking.

Sacroiliac motion is movement of the sacrum between the two innominate bones, and requires the participation of both sacroiliac joints. Nutation and counternutation (anterior nutation—posterior nutation) is the sacral motion about which the most is known from biomechanical and radiographic research. Nutation is a nodding movement of the sacrum between the innominates, the sacral base moves anteriorly and inferiorly while the sacral apex moves posteriorly and superiorly. Counternutation occurs when the sacral base goes posteriorly and superiorly and the sacral apex goes anteriorly and inferiorly. This is the sacroiliac movement which occurs in two-legged standing and trunk forward and backward bends. Many other structures participate in trunk forward- and backward-bending, but the sacroiliac motion is described as nutation and counternutation. For the purposes of structural diagnosis, nutation is described as anterior or forward and counternutation is described as backward or posterior. The axis around which this anterior—posterior nutation occurs has been described differently by various investigators, but appears related to the upper and lower limbs of the sacroiliac joint and their junction somewhere around S2. Bilateral symmetry of anterior—posterior nutation depends on the symmetry of the two sacroiliac joints. With asymmetry of a patient's two sacroiliac joints being so common, asymmetry of this anterior—posterior nutation is also quite common. Anterior nutation is called sacral flexion in the biomechanical model and sacral extension in the craniosacral model. Posterior nutation is called sacral extension in the biomechanical model and sacral flexion in the craniosacral model.

Movement of the sacrum between the two innominates during walking is more complex and less well understood. If one palpates the right side of the sacral base with the right thumb, the right inferior lateral angle with the right index finger, and the left sacral base and left ILA with the left thumb and index finger, and follows movement of the sacrum during walking, the sacrum appears to have an oscillatory movement, first left, then right. The right base appears to move anteriorly while the left ILA moves posteriorly, and then the reverse occurs, with the left sacral base moving anteriorly and the right ILA moving posteriorly. This motion has been described as torsional movement because of the coupled sidebending and rotational sacral movement.

In one cadaveric study the coupling of sacral sidebending and rotation appeared to depend upon whether sidebending or rotation was introduced first. In the clinical observation of walking, it appears that sidebending and rotation of the sacrum always couple to opposite sides. In left torsional movement, the anterior surface of the sacrum rotates to face left (left rotation), while the superior surface of S1 (sacral base plane) declines to the right (right sidebending). Right rotation is the exact opposite.

For descriptive purposes, this complex, polyaxial, torsional movement is considered to occur around an oblique axis. By convention, the left oblique axis runs from the upper extremity of the left sacroiliac joint to the lower end of the right sacroiliac joint, and the right oblique axis runs from the upper end of the right sacroiliac joint to the lower extremity of the left sacroiliac joint. Although the exact biomechanics of the torsional movements of the sacrum are unknown, the hypothetical left and right oblique axes are useful for descriptive purposes.

In the normal walking cycle the sacrum appears to move with left torsion on the left oblique axis, return to neutral, rotate in right torsion on the right oblique axis, and then return to neutral. With left torsion on the left oblique axis, the sacrum rotates left and sidebends right, and the right sacral base moves into anterior nutation. In right torsional movement on the right oblique axis, the sacrum rotates right and sidebends left, and the left base moves into anterior nutational movement. Because the nutational component of this normal walking movement is anterior in direction, left torsion on the left oblique axis (L on L) and right torsion on the right oblique axis (R on R) are described as anterior torsional movements. In normal walking the nutational component of the anterior torsional movements is, ultimately, anterior on one side, return to neutral, anterior on the opposite side, and return to neutral. Posterior nutational movement does not appear to go beyond neutral in the normal walking cycle.

Since so much of the activity of the musculoskeletal system revolves around the walking cycle, maintenance of normal L-on-L and R-on-R sacral movement becomes an important therapeutic objective. Since walking occurs with the vertebral column in the neutral (neither flexed nor extended) position, the anterior torsional sacral movements are called neutral mechanics. During walking the thoracolumbar spine sidebends left and rotates right, then

sidebends right and rotates left with each step. This neutral movement of the vertebral column requires normal segmental mobility, and starts with the response of L5 at the lumbosacral junction. As the sacrum sidebends right and rotates left, L5 sidebends left and rotates right. Each vertebra above L5 should respond appropriately as part of a neutral group curve. A vertebra, particularly in the lower lumbar spine, with dysfunction of the nonneutral type gives a "nonadaptive" vertebral response to the sacrum. This is important because the lumbar spine is used as a lever during manual medicine treatment procedures for sacroiliac dysfunction. For this reason the lumbar spine should precede the sacroiliac in the treatment sequence.

A third sacral movement occurs when the trunk is forward-bent and sidebent or rotated to one side. This maneuver results in the nonneutral behavior of the lumbar spine with sidebending and rotation being coupled to the same side. The sacrum between the innominates participates in this maneuver by backward or posterior torsional movement. Posterior torsional movement can occur on either the left or right oblique axes, and the sidebending and rotational components appear to couple to opposite sides as in the anterior forward torsional movement during the normal walking cycle. In posterior torsional movement, however, one side of the sacral base goes into posterior nutation. In posterior torsional movement rotation is to the side opposite the axis (right on left and left on right). In posterior or backward torsion to the right on the left oblique axis, the sacrum rotates right, sidebends left, and the right base moves into posterior nutation. In backward or posterior torsion to the left on the right oblique axis, the sacrum rotates left, sidebends right, and the left base goes into posterior nutation. These posterior torsional movements can be described as nonneutral sacroiliac mechanics and are not part of the normal walking cycle.

The sacroiliac is at risk of injury (as is the lumbar spine) when the trunk is forward-bent and sidebending and rotation are introduced, resulting in nonneutral sacroiliac and lumbar mechanics. Simultaneous nonneutral dysfunction in the lower lumbar spine and a backward torsional dysfunction of the sacroiliac occurs in the well-known syndrome of "the well man bent over and the cripple stood up".

The sacroiliac region can also be viewed from the perspective of each innominate articulating with the sacrum at its respective sacroiliac joint. The motion can be described as the innominate moving on the sacrum (iliosacral movement). Since each innominate bone participates in the walking cycle by anterior and posterior rotation around the axis at the symphysis pubis, each innominate move with respect to its side of the sacrum. In anterior innominate rotation, the innominate rotates forward in relation to the sacrum with the anterior superior iliac spine being carried anterior and inferior; the posterior superior iliac spine being carried anterior and superior, and the ischial tuberosity being carried posterior and superior. In posterior innominate rotation, the anterior superior iliac spine is carried superior and posterior; the posterior superior iliac spine is carried posterior and inferior; and, the ischial tuberosity is carried anterior and superior. Anterior and posterior innominate rotation occurs in the presence of normal sacroiliac joint contour. If the opposing surfaces of the sacrum and ilium at the sacroiliac joint are altered, atypical movements appear clinically. A superior—inferior translatory shearing movement occurs when the opposing joint surfaces are flatter and more parallel. If the sacral side is more convex and the ilial more concave, then internal and external rotary movement around a vertical (y) axis appear to be clinically possible. These movements have been termed in-flare and out-flare.

Somatic dysfunction can occur with any of these motions within the pelvic girdle. Each of these motions is quite small, but when lost, each has a significant clinical effect. In dysfunctions within the pelvic gir-

dle, it is not uncommon to find restriction of several movements within the mechanism.

## STRUCTURAL DIAGNOSIS OF PELVIC GIRDLE SOMATIC DYSFUNCTION

As in all structural diagnosis, we look for the diagnostic triad of asymmetry, range of motion alteration, and tissue texture abnormality. In the pelvic girdle we specifically look for asymmetry of paired anatomical landmarks within the pelvic girdle and lower extremity; altered range of motion within the pelvic girdle (exemplified by the standing and seated flexion tests, the one-legged stork test of Gillet, and various springing or articulatory tests of movement at the sacroiliac joints); and, tissue texture abnormality primarily in the deep fascia and ligaments overlying the sacroiliac region, within the sacrotuberous ligament, and within the gluteal and perineal muscles. Various combinations of findings within the ART diagnostic triad lead to the diagnosis of somatic dysfunction of the pelvic girdle. The diagnostic process identifies dysfunction at the symphysis pubis (dysfunction between the two pubic bones), the sacroiliac joints (sacrum between the two innominates), and the iliosacral joints (each innominate as it articulates with its respective side of the sacrum).

The diagnostic sequence starts with the patient standing and proceeds to the patient sitting on a stool with the feet on the floor, or seated on a treatment table with the feet supported. The patient then assumes the recumbent position, supine, then prone, and finally back to the supine position.

### Standing

With the patient standing, the examiner looks for symmetry—asymmetry in the static position and performs motion tests (Figs. 2.12, 2.13).

—The patient stands with weight equally distributed on both feet, feet approximately acetabular distance apart.

—Examiner stands or sits behind patient.

—The examiner palpates the superior aspect of the iliac crest evaluating whether both are of equal height.

—The examiner palpates the superior aspect of the greater trochanter of each femur determining if they are level.

—If one crest and greater trochanter is higher than the other, there is presumptive evidence of anatomical shortening of one lower extremity.

—If one iliac crest is high but the greater trochanters are level, or if the iliac crests are level and one greater trochanter is high, there is presumptive evidence of bony asymmetry of the pelvic girdle (Figs. 2.16, 2.17).

The motion tests in the standing position are the standing flexion test and the one-legged (stork) test. The standing flexion test is as follows:

—The examiner palpates the inferior slope of each posterior superior iliac spine (Fig. 17.1).

—Patient is instructed to bend forward in a smooth fashion as far as possible without bending the knees (Fig. 17.2).

—The examiner follows the excursion of movement of each posterior superior iliac spine.

—The test is positive on the side in which the posterior superior iliac spine appears to move more cephalically and ventrally.

It is paradoxical that the side of the pelvis in which the posterior superior iliac spine moves the furthest is the side of pelvic girdle restriction. It is hypothesized that the downward and backward glide of the two limbs of the SI joint is lost, so the sacrum and the innominate move as a unit on the positive side. A false positive standing flexion test can occur with asymmetrical hamstring length and occurs with contralateral hamstring shortening.

The one-legged stork test is performed as follows:

—The examiner stands or sits behind the standing patient.

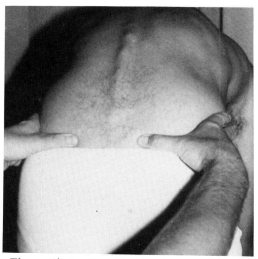

**Figure 17.1.** Standing flexion test. Palpate inferior slope PSIS.

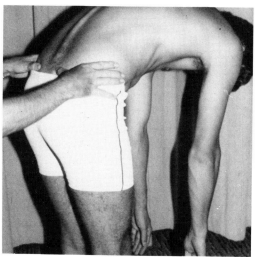

**Figure 17.2.** Standing flexion test. Patient forward-bends without bending knees.

—The examiner's left thumb is on the spinous process of S2 and the right thumb is on the right posterior superior iliac spine.

—The patient is asked to raise the right knee toward the ceiling, standing on the left leg.

—The normal response results in the thumb on the posterior superior iliac spine (PSIS) moving caudad in relation to the thumb on S2.

—The test is interpreted as positive when the thumb on the PSIS moves cephalically, occasionally accompanied by pelvic tilt toward the left side.

—Comparison is made with the opposite side by reversing the procedure.

—To test lower pole movement the left thumb is placed on the inferior end of the crest of the sacrum and the right thumb is placed on the right ischial tuberosity.

—Again the patient is requested to lift the right knee toward the ceiling.

—Test is interpreted as normal if the right thumb moves laterally and ventrally.

—The test is interpreted as restriction of the inferior pole of the right sacroiliac joint if the right thumb goes superiorly with an accompanying pelvic tilt to the left.

During the standing flexion test the examiner should also observe the response of the vertebral column, particularly the lower thoracic and lumbar spine, during the forward-bending motion challenge. One looks for the presence of altered lateral curvatures establishing a compensatory scoliosis, and also observes the segmental rhythm of the vertebra moving in the forward-bending direction. Is there loss of normal rhythm? Are there areas of block movement?

The standing flexion test is used to identify the side of dysfunction for the symphysis pubis and iliosacrum.

### Seated Examination

The patient is now placed in the seated position for the seated flexion test (Figs. 2.18, 2.19).

—The patient sits on an examination stool, feet on the floor and knees apart, or sits on the examining table with the feet supported.

—The examiner stands behind the patient and palpates the inferior slope of each posterior superior iliac spine (Fig. 17.3).

—The patient is requested to bend forward with the arms hanging freely between the knees (Fig. 17.4).

—The examiner follows the relative movement of each posterior superior iliac spine.

—The PSIS which moves the furthest cephalically and ventrally is interpreted as positive.

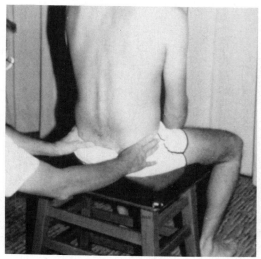

**Figure 17.3.**    Seated flexion test. Palpation PSIS.

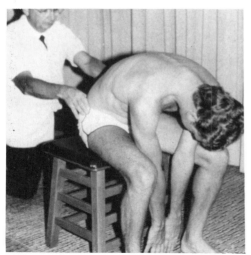

**Figure 17.4.** Seated flexion test. Patient forward-bends with arms hanging free.

lumbar dysrhythmia, and/or the introduced compensatory scoliosis is more aggravated during the standing flexion test, major restrictors in the lower extremities are suggested. If the vertebral dysrhythmia and compensatory scoliosis is worse during the seated flexion test, major restriction above the pelvic girdle is likely. This differentiation can help determine where additional diagnostic and therapeutic procedures will be most fruitful.

The relative position of the right and left inferior lateral angles and the right and left sacral base can be evaluated when the patient is fully forward-bent as in the seated flexion test. This can be most useful in identifying which of the sacroiliac dysfunctions is present.

The seated flexion test is used to determine the side of dysfunction in sacroiliac dysfunctions. A positive test on one side is indicative of unilateral sacroiliac restriction on that side or bilateral sacroiliac dysfunction across the opposite oblique axis.

The examiner again monitors the response of the vertebral column, particularly the lower thoracic and lumbar spine, for segmental dysrhythmia or a compensatory scoliotic curvature. Try to determine if the alteration in the vertebral mechanics is more severe during the standing flexion test or the seated flexion test. If there is greater

### Supine Position

The patient is asked to lie recumbent on the examining table in the supine position. To assure that the patient is lying symmetrically on the buttocks, ask the patient to bend the knees, lift the hips off the table, return the buttocks to the table, and then extend the lower extremities.

—The examiner stands on the side of the table which permits the dominant eye to be over the patient's midline.

—The examiner palpates the superior aspect of each iliac crest in relation to the horizontal plane (Fig. 17.5).

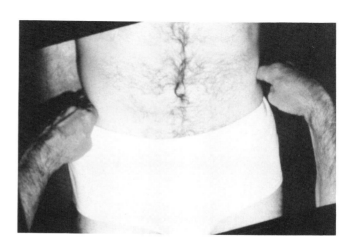

**Figure 17.5.** Supine position, palpation iliac crest height.

—If one crest is significantly higher than the other, the examiner's index of suspicion should be high that an innominate shear dysfunction is present. This must be verified and treated, if present, before proceeding with the remaining pelvic girdle examination.

The examiner now evaluates each pubic bone.

—The heel of the hand is placed on the lower abdomen and moved caudad until meeting the superior aspect of the pubic bones (Fig. 17.6).

—The examiner places the finger pads of a corresponding finger from each hand in the midline on the superior aspect of the symphysis pubis.

—Examiner moves each finger laterally approximately 1 to 1¼ inch and palpates symmetrical portions of each pubic bone, either on the superior aspect of the pubic ramus or the superior aspect of the pubic tubercle (Fig. 17.7).

—The examiner evaluates the position of each pubic bone in relation to the horizontal plane.

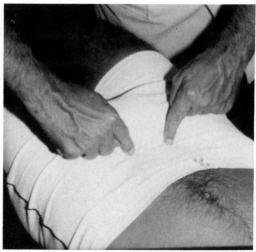

**Figure 17.7.**   Palpation superior aspect pubic tubercle bilaterally.

—The examiner evaluates tension and tenderness of the inguinal ligaments at their insertion on the pubic tubercle.

If the pubic bones are not level and the tension of the two inguinal ligaments is asymmetric, a pubic symphysis dysfunction is present which should be appropriately treated before proceeding with the diagnostic process.

The patient is now placed in the prone position to evaluate the position of the sacrum between the two innominates which are now triangulated on the examination couch by the symphysis pubis and the two anterior superior iliac spines. The examination starts distally and proceeds cephalically. The first anatomical landmark evaluated is the medial malleolus.

—The patient is prone on the table with the dorsum of the foot free and the distal tibia and fibula at the edge of the table.

—The examiner palpates the most inferior aspect of each medial malleolus determining which is longer or shorter (Fig. 17.8).

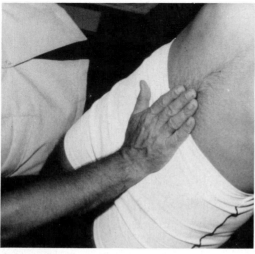

**Figure 17.6.**   Supine palpation, symphysis pubis. Heel of hand moves caudad.

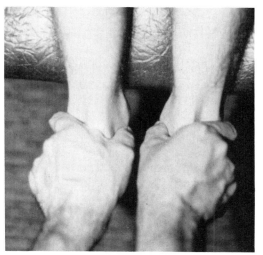

**Figure 17.8.** Prone evaluation of leg length at inferior aspect medial malleolus.

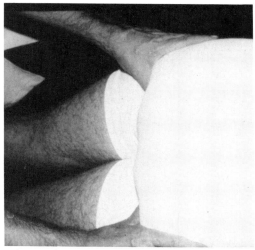

**Figure 17.9.** Palpation of inferior aspect of ischial tuberosity, bilaterally.

—A confirmatory test has the operator dorsiflex the feet and sight down (in a perpendicular fashion) to the pads of each heel. Determine which is longer or shorter.

In the prone position the length of the leg is a function of lumbar adaptation to sacral base declination. If the sacral base declines to the left (sidebent left), the normal adaptation of the lumbar spine is a convexity to the left. A left lumbar convexity appears to lengthen the left leg and shorten the right leg. Therefore, the prone examination of leg length at the medial malleolus is used in the evaluation of sacroiliac somatic dysfunction.

The next procedure evaluates the level of the two ischial tuberosities.

—The examiner uses each thumb to follow the fascia at the gluteal crease anteriorly and then superiorly until the pad of the thumb strikes the most inferior aspect of the ischial tuberosity (Fig. 17.9).

—Evaluation is made of the ischial tuberosities against the horizontal plane.

—A difference of approximately the width of the thumb (6 mm) in level is considered positive.

—Care must be exercised to be on the most inferior aspect of the ischial tuberosity as the posterior inferior aspect is large and rounded.

The examiner evaluates the tension of the inferior aspect of the sacrotuberous ligament.

—The examiner's thumbs proceed from the inferior aspect of the ischial tuberosity medially, then superiorly, then posterolaterally.

—Palpate the medial side of the sacrotuberous ligament on each side (Fig. 17.10).

—The normal finding is a firm, smooth, crescent-shaped structure, bilaterally.

—A positive finding is one sacrotuberous ligament being more lax or tense than the normal on the opposite side.

—Frequently, tenderness is elicited on the dysfunctional side.

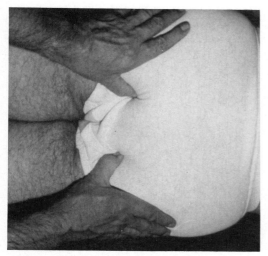

**Figure 17.10.** Palpation of medial aspect sacrotuberous ligament, bilaterally.

The level of the ischial tuberosity and tone of the sacrotuberous ligament are the two most important findings for a diagnosis of innominate shear dysfunction.

The inferior lateral angle (ILA) of the sacrum is now evaluated (Fig. 17.11). It is the most valuable diagnostic landmark for sacroiliac dysfunction. The examiner is interested in the relationship of each inferior lateral angle to both the coronal and horizontal planes. Determine whether one inferior lateral angle is more posterior or inferior than the other. To identify the inferior lateral angle

—The examiner palpates the caudal end of the sacral crest and identifies the sacral hiatus.

—Approximately ½ to ¾ inch lateral to the sacral hiatus is found the posterior aspect of the inferior lateral angle (Fig. 17.12).

—The palpating thumbs are placed symmetrically over the posterior aspect of the inferior lateral angle evaluating against the coronal plane (Fig. 17.13).

—The examiner's thumbs are then turned under the inferior lateral angle so that the thumb pads are on the inferior aspect to evaluate against the horizontal plane (Fig. 17.14).

In some cases the inferior lateral angle appears to be more posterior than inferior, and, occasionally, more inferior than posterior. However, if it is posterior, it is also inferior, and vice versa.

The posterior aspect of the inferior lateral angle is a valuable anatomical landmark to follow during a motion/position challenge. The posterior aspect of the inferior lateral angle can be viewed as the posterior aspect of the transverse process of S5 and can be utilized in the same fashion as is done for the vertebral segment motion test. The relationship of each inferior lateral angle is examined in

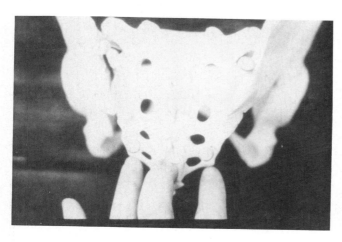

**Figure 17.11.** Palpation of sacral hiatus.

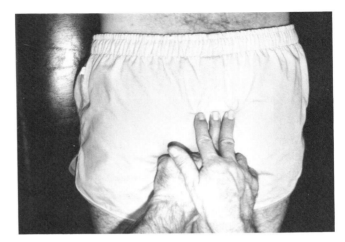

**Figure 17.12.** Identification of inferior lateral angle.

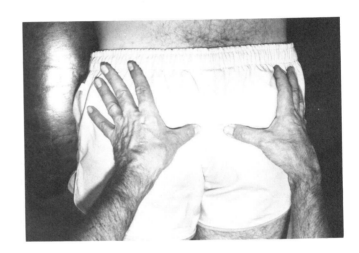

**Figure 17.13.** Palpation of posterior aspect of inferior lateral angle.

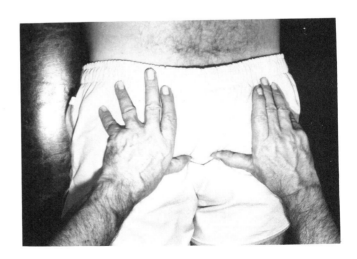

**Figure 17.14.** Palpation of inferior aspect of inferior lateral angle.

—Neutral position (prone on the table).

—The backward-bent position (prone on table, trunk elevated, patient resting on elbows, and the chin in the hands—sphinx position.) (Fig. 17.15).

—The forward-bent position (while seated doing the seated flexion test) (Fig. 17.16).

The behavior of the inferior lateral angle during this three-position test is most useful in the diagnosis of torsional dysfunction of the sacroiliac mechanism. When palpating the inferior lateral angle, one is also palpating the superior attachment of the sacrotuberous ligament, and any tissue texture abnormality, either tension or tenderness, should be ascertained. If the sacrum is dysfunctional in a position which places the sacrotuberous ligament on tension, it will be palpably tense and usually tender.

The next anatomical landmark to be palpated is the posterior superior iliac spine. This anatomical landmark has previously been used during the standing and seated flexion test and is now used to locate the base of the sacrum and sacral sulcus and the posterior aspect of L5.

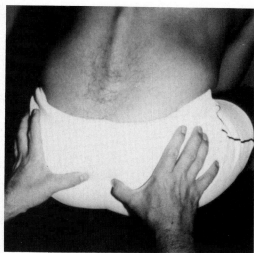

**Figure 17.16.** Palpation inferior lateral angle in trunk, forward-bent position.

—Each thumb is placed over the most posterior aspect of the posterior superior iliac spine (Fig. 17.17).

—By moving the thumbs medially and then superiorly at an angle of approximately 30°, one strikes the posterior arch of L5.

—If one moves medially and caudad at approximately 30° one moves to the base of the sacrum (posterior arch of S1).

The relationship of the base of the sacrum and the posterior arch of L5 is important to evaluate and identify if L5 is adaptive to changes of sacral base declination.

Having identified the posterior superior iliac spine, the examiner is interested in the level of the sacral base against the coronal plane. The sacral base is identified by

—Starting from the posterior aspect of the posterior superior iliac spine.

—Each thumb palpates medially and then caudally at approximately 30°.

—Depth evaluation is made with the tip of the thumb to see which side of the

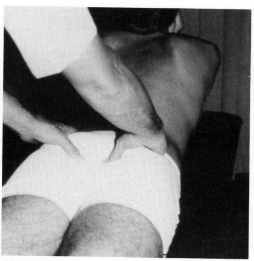

**Figure 17.15.** Palpation inferior lateral angle in trunk backward-bent position.

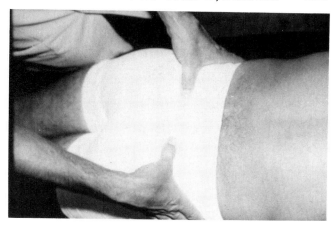

**Figure 17.17.** Palpation of posterior aspect PSIS.

sacral base appears to be more anterior or posterior (Fig. 17.18).

The level of the sacral base is frequently termed the "depth of the sacral sulcus." If one sacral base is more anterior than the other, the sacral sulcus is said to be "deep" on that side. This author prefers to describe the sacral base as being anterior or posterior if it is not level against the coronal plane. The term "depth of the sacral sulcus" is reserved for the difference in depth from the posterior superior iliac spine to a sacral base plane that is level against the coronal plane. The depth of the sacral sulcus then becomes a function of innominate rotation while an anterior or posterior sacral base refers to a sacroiliac diagnostic finding.

The sacral base can be evaluated in the three positions of neutral (prone on the table), forward-bent (during the seated flexion test), and backward-bent (in the sphinx position). Again one is following a motion challenge to S1 by palpating its posterior arch.

One now proceeds to evaluate the lumbar lordosis and to accomplish the spring test.

—The heel of the hand is placed over the spinous processes of the mid to lower lumbar spine.

—The examiner evaluates whether the lumbar lordosis appears to be flattened, normal, or increased.

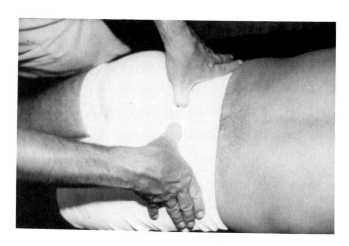

**Figure 17.18.** Palpation of sacral base, bilaterally.

—The examiner uses a short and quick push with the heel of the hand toward the examining table to evaluate the yielding of the lumbar spine.

—If the lumbar lordosis yields freely, it is recorded as a negative spring test.

—If the lumbar spine appears to be more rigid and resists the springing maneuver, it is recorded as a positive spring test.

The presence or absence of a normal lumbar lordosis, and the presence of a positive or negative spring test are confirmatory tests useful in the diagnosis of torsional dysfunction of the sacroiliac mechanism.

There are other tests that can be used to evaluate movement of the sacrum between the two innominates. These tests can be used independently or to confirm a diagnosis. One variation is

—Each thumb is placed over the sacral base and inferior lateral angle on the same side.

—Rocking is made by downward pressure with alternate thumbs (Fig. 17.19).

—This tests for nutational—counternutational movement of the sacrum across a horizontal axis.

—Place a thumb on one sacral base and the other thumb on the opposite inferior lateral angle.

—Alternating pressure with each thumb evaluates the coupled movement of sidebending and rotation around the "oblique axis" (Fig. 17.20).

An alternative method for this springing test uses the index and middle fingers overlying the sacral base and the thenar eminence over the inferior lateral angle (Fig. 17.21). By springing anteriorly and superiorly on the ILA while monitoring with the sacral base on the same side, one can test the nutation, counternutation movement. By monitoring the opposite

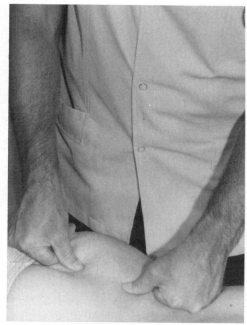

**Figure 17.19.** Sacroiliac motion tests by alternate rocking of thumbs on same side.

sacral base and pressing anteriorly and superiorly toward it with the thenar eminence on the inferior lateral angle, one can evaluate the coupled sidebending and rotational movement around the "oblique axis" (Fig. 17.22).

When the prone examination has been completed and any sacroiliac dysfunctions appropriately diagnosed and treated, the patient is now returned to the supine position. The first anatomical landmark to be evaluated is the anterior superior iliac spine. One is interested in its relationship to the three cardinal planes.

—The palm of the hand is placed over the anterior superior iliac spine to identify its location bilaterally.

—The thumb is placed on the inferior aspect of the anterior superior iliac spine and evaluation is made against the horizontal plane to see which one is inferior or superior (Fig. 17.23).

—The thumb is now placed on the most anterior aspect of the anterior supe-

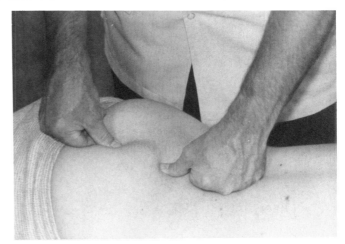

**Figure 17.20.** Sacroiliac motion tests by alternate rocking of thumbs across oblique axis.

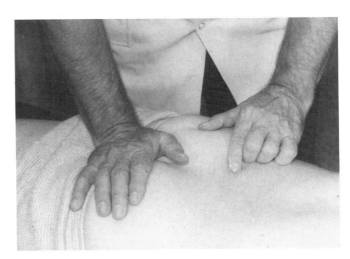

**Figure 17.21.** Sacroiliac motion tests by springing at inferior lateral angle on same side.

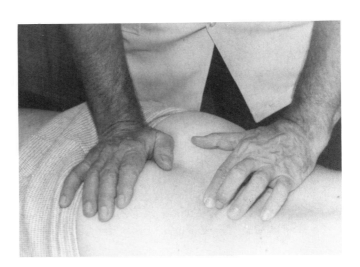

**Figure 17.22.** Sacroiliac motion tests by springing inferior lateral angle across oblique axis.

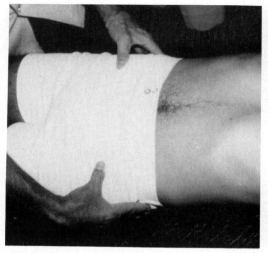

**Figure 17.23.** Palpation inferior aspect ASIS.

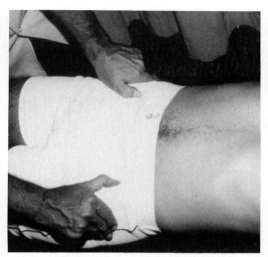

**Figure 17.25.** Palpation medial side ASIS.

rior iliac spine evaluating which is more anterior or posterior against the coronal plane (Fig. 17.24).

—The thumbs are now hooked over the medial aspect of each anterior superior iliac spine to evaluate which is more medial or lateral in relation to the midsagittal plane (Fig. 17.25).

The length of the leg in the supine position is now evaluated by

—Palpating the most inferior aspect of the medial malleolus to identify which one is longer or shorter (Fig. 17.26).

The length of the leg in the supine position, and in the absence of significant sacroiliac dysfunction, is a function of innominate rotation on one side or the other in relation to the midline sacrum.

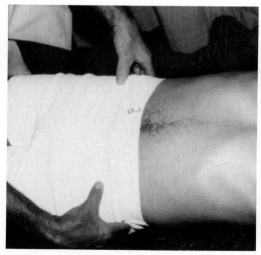

**Figure 17.24.** Palpation anterior aspect ASIS.

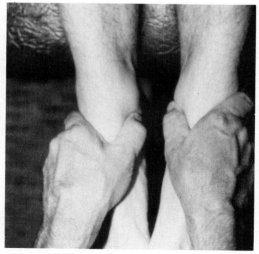

**Figure 17.26.** Supine position, palpation inferior aspect medial malleolus.

## MANAGEMENT OF PELVIC GIRDLE DYSFUNCTION

The pelvic girdle is approached with the therapeutic goal of restoring the normal mechanics of the walking cycle. In the treatment sequence, the pelvic girdle follows the lumbar spine. The rationale is that the lumbar spine is frequently used as a lever in treatment of sacral dysfunction, and lumbar dysfunction is a frequent restrictor of pelvic girdle function. The treatment sequence for the management of pelvic girdle dysfunction is:

1) Pubic symphysis;
2) Sacroiliac dysfunction;
3) Iliosacral dysfunction.

### Pubic Symphysis Dysfunction

**Table 17.1**
**Pubic Symphysis Dysfunction**

| Diagnosis | | Standing Flexion Test Positive | Pubic Tubercle Height | Tension and Tenderness of Inguinal Ligament |
|---|---|---|---|---|
| Superior | Right | Right | Right superior | Right |
| | Left | Left | Left superior | Left |
| Inferior | Right | Right | Right inferior | Right |
| | Left | Left | Left inferior | Left |

### Muscle Energy: Symphysis Pubis

Position: Symphysis superior on left

1. Patient supine on left side of table, right hand holds right side of table, left leg hanging off side of table. (Left ilium still on edge of table.)
2. Operator stands on left side of table and supports extended, freely hanging leg.
3. Operator's left hand reaches across and supports right ASIS of patient (Fig. 17.27).
4. Operator's right hand presses down on left knee to barrier limit and maintains (Fig. 17.28).
5. Patient instructed to raise left foot to ceiling while operator resists.
6. When patient completely relaxes, operator takes up slack by depressing knee.
7. Patient repeats 5.
8. Repeat 5 and 6 about three times.
9. Retest!!

Position: Symphysis inferior on right

1. Patient supine, right knee and hip flexed, adducted, and slightly internally rotated.
2. Operator on left side, places patient's flexed knee in right axilla or lateral right shoulder (Fig. 17.29).
3. Operator's left hand (or fist) placed against patient's right ischial tuberosity; pushing cephalad. Right hand holds edge of table (Fig. 17.30) or right ASIS (Fig. 17.31).
4. Patient attempts to straighten leg caudally as operator resists. Patient *relaxes*
5. Operator takes up slack as in 3 and patient repeats 4.
6. Repeat 5 approximately three times.
7. Retest!!

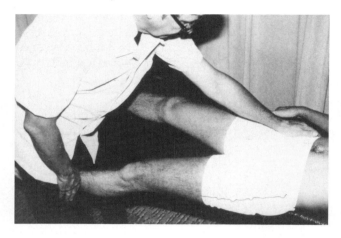

**Figure 17.27.** Supine, muscle energy technique, superior symphysis. Operator's left hand supports right ASIS.

### High Velocity Thrust: Symphysis Pubis

Position: Either superior or inferior symphysis "Shotgun" Technique

1. Patient supine on table with hips flexed, knees flexed, and feet flat on table.
2. Patient holds knees together in adducted position.
3. Operator pulls both knees apart into abduction with high velocity thrust (Fig. 17.32).
4. Retest.

### Alternative Technique: Muscle Energy "Shotgun"

1. Patient supine with hips flexed, knees flexed, and feet together.
2. Patient's knees abducted.

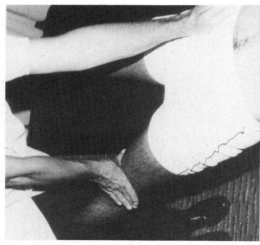

**Figure 17.28.** Supine, muscle energy technique, superior symphysis. Barrier engaged by depressing left knee while operator resists patient's effort to lift left leg.

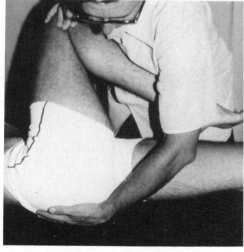

**Figure 17.29.** Supine, muscle energy technique, symphysis pubis inferior dysfunction. Operator holds patient's flexed right knee and hip in axilla or lateral shoulder.

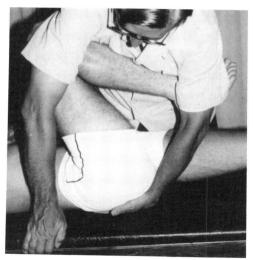

**Figure 17.30.** With operator's left hand against ischial tuberosity, right hand holds edge of table.

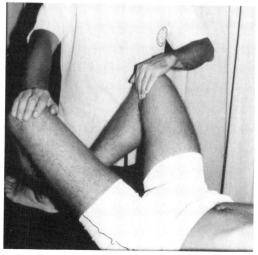

**Figure 17.32.** Supine, high-velocity thrust, symphysis pubis. Operator applies abduction thrust to patient's knees.

3. Operator places forearm between knees (Fig. 17.33).
4. Patient exerts adduction effort of both knees with a quick muscle action attempting to distract symphysis pubis.
5. Retest.

## Muscle Energy Procedures: Sacroiliac Joint

Prone Position: Unilateral sacrum flexed on left
Motion restriction: Unilateral posterior nutation on left

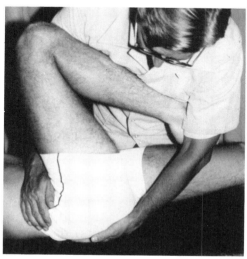

**Figure 17.31.** With operator's left hand against ischial tuberosity, alternative right hand position on right ASIS.

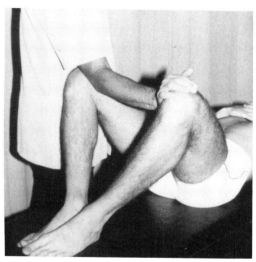

**Figure 17.33.** Supine, muscle energy technique, symphysis pubis. Operator's forearm resists patient's adduction effort of both knees.

**Table 17.2**
**Sacroiliac Dysfunctions**

| Diagnosis | Seated Flexion Test Positive | Base of Sacrum | Inferior Lateral Angle Position | Inferior Lateral Angle Motion | Lumbar Scoliosis | Lumbar Lordosis | Medial Malleolus Prone |
|---|---|---|---|---|---|---|---|
| Unilateral flexed (flexion) | Right | Anterior right | Inferior right | | Convex right | Normal to increased | Long right |
| Inferior shear | Left | Anterior left | Inferior left | | Convex left | Normal to increased | Long left |
| Unilateral extended (extension) | Right | Posterior right | Superior right | | Convex left | Decreased | Short right |
| Superior shear | Left | Posterior left | Superior left | | Convex right | Decreased | Short left |
| Anterior torsion — Left on left | Right | Anterior right | Posterior left | Left, increased on forward-bending | Convex right | Increased | Short left |
| Anterior torsion — Right on right | Left | Anterior left | Posterior right | Right, increased on forward-bending | Convex left | Increased | Short right |
| Backward torsion — Right on left | Right | Posterior right | Posterior right | Right, increased on backward-bending | Convex left | Reduced | Short right |
| Backward torsion — Left on right | Left | Posterior left | Posterior left | Left, increased on backward-bending | Convex right | Reduced | Short left |
| Bilateral flexed | Bilateral | Anterior | Posterior | | | Increased | Even |
| Bilateral extended | Bilateral | Posterior | Anterior | | | Reduced | Even |

1. Patient prone.
2. Operator stands on left side of patient.
3. Operator's left hand palpates left sacral base to monitor motion at sacroiliac joint (Fig. 17.34).
4. Abduct patient's leg (approximately 15° and internally rotate to maximum "gapping freedom" at sacral sulcus. Patient maintains this position.
5. Heel of operator's right hand, with arm straight, places pressure on patient's left inferior lateral angle in direction of maximum motion at sacral base (Fig. 17.35).
6. Patient instructed to maximally inhale and hold breath as long as possible, operator maintains pressure on ILA.
7. As patient exhales *slowly*, operator maintains pressure.

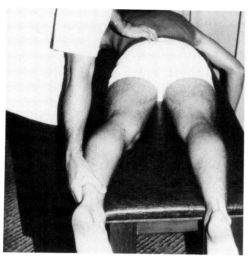

**Figure 17.34.** Prone, muscle energy technique, lateral sacrum flexed. Operator's left hand monitors left sacral base.

8. Repeat several times.
9. Retest!!

Sims Position

Position: Forward sacral torsion to left (on left axis) (Left on left sacral torsion)

Motion restriction: Right rotation, left sidebending, and posterior nutation of right sacral base

1. Patient in left lateral Sims position, close to edge of table, right arm over side of table, left arm behind and on table.
2. Operator faces patient, palpates lumbosacral junction.
3. Operator flexes patient's legs (knees and feet together) until motion felt at sacral side of LS junction (Fig. 17.36).
4. Patient's legs maintained in this position against operator's abdomen, hip, or thigh.
5. Operator's right hand now moved to patient's right shoulder. As patient exhales, instructed to reach to floor with right hand. Operator maintains pressure on right shoulder. Repeat until L5 is rotated to left. (Fig. 17.37).
6. Operator's left hand moves to patient's feet, which are placed off edge of table, and pressed downward (Fig. 17.38).
7. Patient instructed to push feet to ceiling as operator maintains pressure on patient's feet and monitors L5 junction.

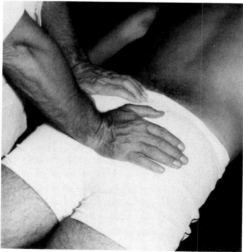

**Figure 17.35.** Prone, muscle energy technique, lateral sacrum flexed. Operator's right hand contacts left ILA.

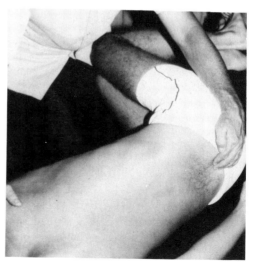

**Figure 17.36.** Sims' position, muscle energy technique, sacroiliac joint left on left torsion. Operator flexes lower extremities to sacral base.

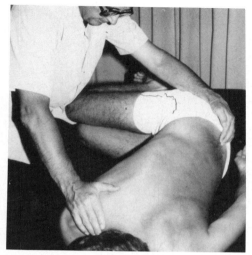

**Figure 17.37.** Sims' position, muscle energy technique, sacroiliac joint left on left torsion. Operator rotates L5 left from above.

8. When patient relaxes, slack is taken up by operator with left hand.
9. Repeat 7 two or three times. (Right sacral base should be felt to move posteriorly.)
10. Retest!!
  Note: A variation allows the operator to sit on the table with the left hand monitoring the sacral base, while the right hand resists elevation of patient's legs toward ceiling (Fig. 17.39).

Lateral Recumbent
  Position: Backward sacral torsion to right (on left axis) (Right on left sacral torsion)
  Motion restriction: Left rotation, right sidebending and anterior nutation of the right sacral base.

1. Patient lies on left side, operator facing patient, close to front of table.
2. Operator pulls left arm forward introducing right rotation down to L5.
3. Patient's lower leg fully extended, upper leg in front.
4. Operator's right hand palpates lumbosacral junction as lower leg is extended until motion palpated at sacral base (Fig. 17.40).
5. Operator's right hand now switched to patient's right shoulder. As patient exhales, upper shoulder pressed backward toward table until all right rotation to L5 has occurred. Patient grasps edge of table with right hand (Fig. 17.41).

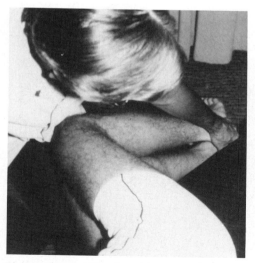

**Figure 17.38.** Sims' position, muscle energy technique, sacroiliac joint left on left torsion. With patient's feet off edge of table, operator resists lifting feet to ceiling.

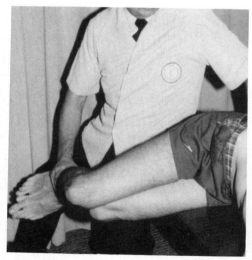

**Figure 17.39.** Sims' position, muscle energy technique, sacroiliac joint left on left torsion. Alternative operator position sitting on edge of table.

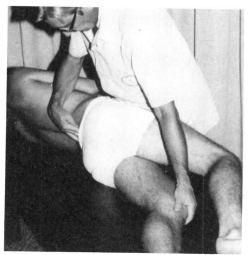

**Figure 17.40.** Lateral recumbent, muscle energy techniques, sacroiliac joint right on left torsion. Operator extends lower leg to sacral base.

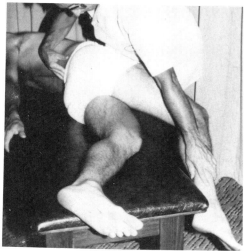

**Figure 17.42.** Lateral recumbent, muscle energy technique, sacroiliac joint right on left torsion. Operator resists patient's effort to lift right knee to ceiling.

6. Operator's left hand now drops patient's right leg off front of table and depresses right knee to barrier (Fig. 17.42).
7. Patient instructed to "raise knee toward ceiling" against resistance.
8. Repeat several times (3-4).
9. Retest!!

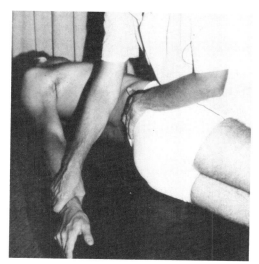

**Figure 17.41.** Lateral recumbent, muscle energy technique, sacroiliac joint right on left torsion. Operator extends upper trunk to L5 with right rotation of patient's shoulder.

Prone

Position: Unilateral right sacrum extended

Motion restriction: Unilateral anterior nutation on right (right sacral flexion)

1. Patient lies prone on table resting on elbows with hands supporting chin (sphinx position).
2. Operator stands at right side of patient and right hand monitors over cephalic end of right sacroiliac joint.
3. Operator's left hand abducts extended right leg to maximum freedom palpated at S1 joint (approximately 15°). Leave right foot externally rotated (Fig. 17.43).
4. Heel of operator's hand placed over right sacral base while opposite hand stabilizes right innominate by grasping the ASIS (Fig. 17.44).
5. Patient instructed to inhale slightly and then forcibly exhale.
6. Operator applies anterior and caudad force on right sacral base, following the motion accompanying exhalation, and holds in that position as,

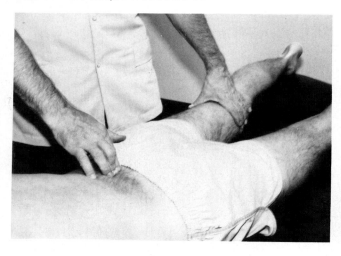

**Figure 17.43.** Prone, muscle energy technique, sacroiliac joint, unilateral extended. Operator abducts extended right leg.

7. Patient repeats step 5.
8. Repeat steps 5 and 6 several times until release is felt and motion improves.
9. Retest.

Sitting
Position: Bilateral flexed sacrum
Motion restriction: Bilateral posterior nutation

1. Patient sits on stool with feet apart and internally rotated.
2. Patient flexes trunk forward with elbows between knees (Fig. 17.45).
3. Operator places heel of left hand over apex of the sacrum.

4. Operator places right hand over the upper trunk (Fig. 17.46).
5. With operator's continued pressure over sacral apex in an anterior direction, patient is instructed to lift the shoulders toward the ceiling against resistance offered by the operator's right hand.
6. Following 3 to 5 efforts of 3 to 5 seconds of muscle contraction, posterior nutation of the base of the sacrum should occur.
7. Retest.

Sitting
Position: Bilateral extended sacrum

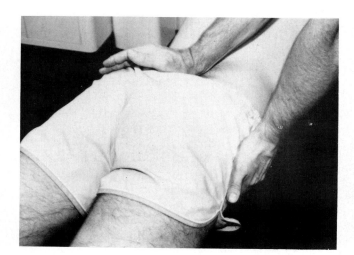

**Figure 17.44.** Prone, muscle energy technique, sacroiliac joint, unilateral extended. Operator's pisiform contacts right sacral base with left hand on right ASIS.

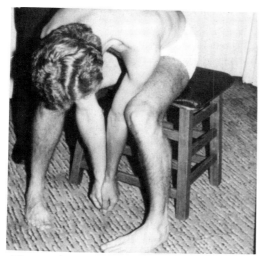

**Figure 17.45.** Sitting, muscle energy procedure, sacroiliac joint, bilateral flexed. Patient's trunk flexed.

Motion restriction: Bilateral anterior nutation

1. Patient sits on stool with feet together and knees separated.
2. Patient reaches posteriorly and holds the edge of the stool.
3. Operator places heel of the hand, or fist, against the sacral base, with an-

terior pressure maintained throughout the procedure.
4. Operator's hand applied over anterior chest wall near sternum (Fig. 17.47).
5. While maintaining forward pressure on the sacral base operator resists patient's effort to forward-bend at trunk against resistance offered by operator's left hand to the sternal area.
6. Repeat 3 to 5 times.
7. Retest.

## High-Velocity Low-Amplitude Thrust: Sacroiliac Joint

Lateral Recumbent
Diagnosis:
      Position: Unilateral left sacrum flexed (unilateral left sacral flexed shear; left sacral flexion)
      Motion restriction: Unilateral posterior nutation on left (left sacral extension)

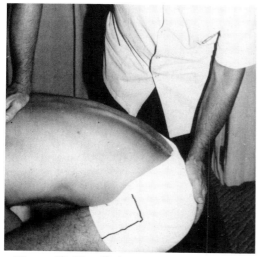

**Figure 17.46.** Sitting, muscle energy procedure, sacroiliac joint, bilateral flexed. With heel of hand on sacral apex, operator resists lifting of upper trunk.

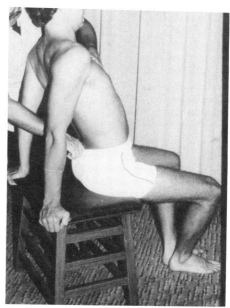

**Figure 17.47.** Sitting, muscle energy technique, sacroiliac joint, bilateral extended. With heel of hand at sacral base, operator resists patient's effort of forward-bending of trunk.

1. Patient in left lateral recumbent position with both knees flexed.
2. Operator stands in front of the patient and pulls the inferior shoulder anteriorly and inferiorly (introducing neutral movement of lumbar spine down to L5) (Fig. 17.48).
3. Operator flexes upper knee and hip and places palm contact over left inferior lateral angle of the sacrum (Fig. 17.49).
4. Operator's left forearm is parallel to the table and takes up slack in a cephalic and anterior direction.
5. Operator's right hand takes out all slack down to L5.
6. With slack taken out with the operator's left hand a direct action, high-velocity, low-amplitude thrust is directed straight cephalicly.
7. Retest.

Prone
Diagnosis

Position: Unilateral sacrum flexed (unilateral left sacral flexed shear; unilateral left sacral flexion)

Motion restriction: Unilateral posterior nutation on left. (left sacral extension)

1. Patient prone on table.
2. Operator's left hand monitors at sacral sulcus and right hand abducts left leg to loose pack position (approximately 15 to 20°). Left leg

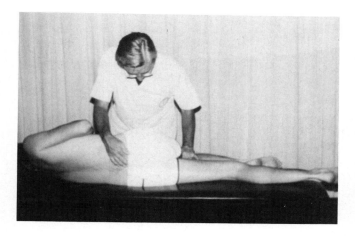

**Figure 17.48.** Lateral recumbent, high-velocity, low-amplitude thrust, sacroiliac joint, unilateral flexed. Operator introduces left sidebending, right rotation to L5 by pulling inferior shoulder anteriorly and caudally.

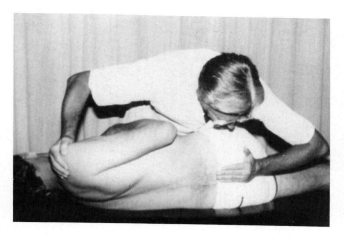

**Figure 17.49.** Lateral recumbent, high-velocity, low-amplitude thrust, sacroiliac joint, unilateral flexed. Operator's pisiform contacts left inferior lateral angle with thrust direction straight cephalic.

then internally rotated and held by patient.

3. Operator's right hand (thenar eminence) contacts left inferior lateral angle of the patient's sacrum.
4. Operator springs sacrum to point of maximum mobility of the sacrum (Fig. 17.50).
5. Patient takes a deep breath and operator takes up slack in an anterior and superior direction with the contact on the left inferior lateral angle of the sacrum.
6. A high velocity thrust is directed anteriorly and superiorly by the operator's right hand on the patient's left inferior lateral angle of the sacrum.
7. Retest.

Sitting
Diagnosis
   Position: Forward sacral torsion to left (on left axis)
   Motion restriction: Right rotation, left sidebending, and posterior nutation of the right sacral base

1. Patient sitting astride table with left hand holding right shoulder.
2. Operator stands at right side of patient with pisiform contact over the left sacral base (Fig. 17.51).

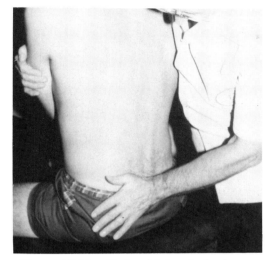

**Figure 17.51.** Sitting, high-velocity, low-amplitude thrust, sacroiliac joint, left on left torsion. Operator's pisiform contacts left sacral base.

3. Operator forward-bends patient down to and including the sacrum.
4. Right rotation and left sidebending of the trunk, including the sacrum (Fig. 17.52).
5. A direct action, high-velocity thrust is made with the operator's left forearm to the pisiform contact on the left sacral base moving anteriorly, and the operator's right arm exaggerating patient's position (Fig. 17.53).
6. Retest.

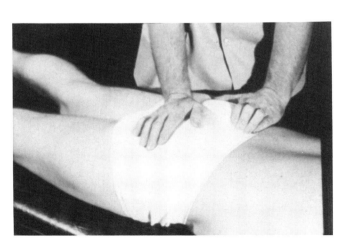

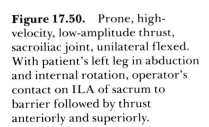

**Figure 17.50.** Prone, high-velocity, low-amplitude thrust, sacroiliac joint, unilateral flexed. With patient's left leg in abduction and internal rotation, operator's contact on ILA of sacrum to barrier followed by thrust anteriorly and superiorly.

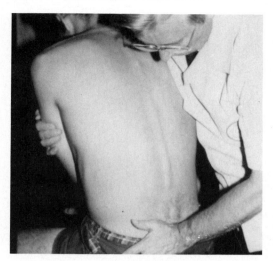

**Figure 17.52.** Sitting, high-velocity, low-amplitude thrust, sacroiliac joint, left on left torsion. Operator introduces right rotation and left sidebending to include sacrum.

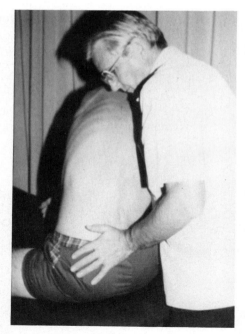

**Figure 17.53.** Sitting, high-velocity, low-amplitude thrust, sacroiliac joint, left on left torsion. A thrust is made against left sacral base while exaggerating patient's position.

### Lateral Recumbent
Diagnosis

Position: Forward sacral torsion to left (on left axis)

Motion restriction: Right rotation, left sidebending and posterior nutation of the right sacral base

1. Patient in left lateral recumbent position with both knees flexed and shoulders perpendicular to the table.
2. Operator flexes the patient's trunk down from above while maintaining patient's weight on left shoulder.
3. Right shoulder moved posteriorly locking down to L4.
4. Heel of operator's hand contacts apex of the sacrum with the pisiform overlying the left inferior lateral angle, elbow flexed.
5. Operator's right hand on superior aspect of patient's right shoulder.
6. All slack taken out with operator's right hand taking patient's right shoulder caudad (introducing right sidebending down to the lumbosacral junction) (Fig. 17.54).
7. Operator's left hand takes up slack on inferior lateral angle in the direction of the patient's right shoulder (Fig. 17.55).
8. When all slack is taken out between the operator's two hands, a high-velocity, low-amplitude thrust, with the left hand in a "scooping" motion, is directed toward the patient's right shoulder.
9. Retest.

### Patient Sitting
Diagnosis

Position: Backward sacral torsion to right (on left axis) (right posterior torsion)

Motion restriction: Left rotation, right sidebending, anterior nutation of the right base

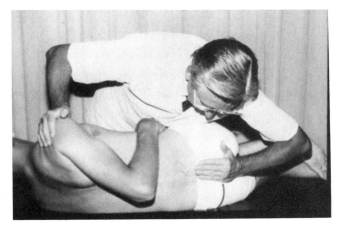

**Figure 17.54.** Lateral recumbent, high-velocity, low-amplitude thrust, sacroiliac joint, left on left torsion. Operator introduces right sidebending to lumbosacral junction by taking patient's right shoulder caudad.

1. Patient sitting astride table with the left hand holding the right shoulder.
2. Operator stands at left side of patient and grasps patient's right shoulder.
3. Operator's left anterior shoulder is against the patient's lateral left shoulder.
4. Heel of operator's hand (pisiform) overlying the right sacral base (Fig. 17.56).
5. Patient's trunk is sidebent right and rotated left with operator's right hand taking right sacral base anterior (Fig. 17.57).
6. Patient's trunk extended while right sidebent and left rotated.

7. When all slack is taken out a high-velocity, low-amplitude thrust is made by exaggerating patient's extension position and with an anterior force with the operator's right hand.
8. Retest.

Supine
Diagnosis
Position: Backward sacral torsion to right (on left axis) (right on left sacral torsion)
Motion restriction: Left rotation, right sidebending, anterior nutation of the right sacral base

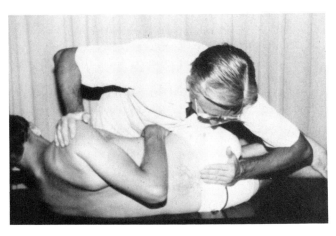

**Figure 17.55.** Lateral recumbent, high-velocity, low-amplitude thrust, sacroiliac joint, left on left torsion. Operator's pisiform on left ILA thrust in direction of patient's right shoulder with scooping motion.

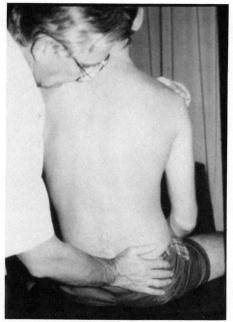

**Figure 17.56.** Sitting, high-velocity, low-amplitude thrust, sacroiliac joint, right on left torsion. Heel of operator's hand on right sacral base.

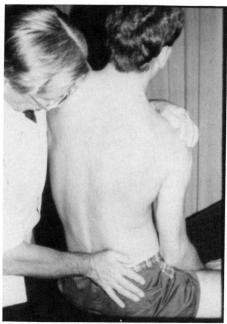

**Figure 17.57.** Sitting, high-velocity, low-amplitude thrust, sacroiliac joint, right on left torsion. Patient sidebent right and rotated left, then extended with thrust by operator's right hand and exaggeration of patient's position.

1.  Patient's position is supine on table with operator standing on patient's left side.
2.  Operator translates osseous pelvis to left introducing right sidebending of trunk.
3.  Patient clasps hands behind neck.
4.  Operator sidebends trunk to the right down to and including the sacrum (Fig. 17.58).
5.  Operator threads right hand through patient's right arm with back of operator's right hand against the sternum.
6.  Operator holds right innominate with hand over the right anterior superior iliac spine.
7.  Slack is taken out from above by left rotation of patient's trunk (Fig. 17.59).
8.  When all slack is taken out, a high-velocity thrust is made by the operator's right arm in a left rotational mode while operator's left hand holds patient's right innominate in a fixed position.
9.  Retest.

### Muscle Energy Procedures. Iliosacral Joint

Lateral Recumbent
Diagnosis
  Position: Anterior innominate dysfunction (right)
  Motion Restriction: Posterior rotation of innominate (right)

1.  Patient in left lateral recumbent position, operator facing patient.
2.  Patient's right leg flexed at hip and knee, and foot placed against operator's hip (Fig. 17.60).
3.  Operator's left hand monitors right sacroiliac joint motion (Fig. 17.61).
4.  Operator controls patient's right knee with adduction, abduction, internal and external rotation, and flexion to barrier.

**Table 17.3**
**Iliosacral Dysfunctions**

| Diagnosis | | Standing Flexion Test Positive | Anterior Superior Iliac Spine Supine | Medial Malleolus Supine | Posterior Superior Iliac Spine Prone | Sacral Sulcus Prone | Ischial Tuberosity Prone | Sacro-tuberous Ligament Prone |
|---|---|---|---|---|---|---|---|---|
| Anterior | Right | Right | Inferior right | Long right | Superior right | Shallow right | | |
| Rotated | Left | Left | Inferior left | Long left | Superior left | Shallow left | | |
| Posterior | Right | Right | Superior right | Short right | Inferior right | Deep right | | |
| Rotated | Left | Left | Superior left | Short left | Inferior left | Deep left | | |
| Outflare | Right | Right | Lateral right | | Medial right | Narrow right | | |
| | Left | Left | Lateral left | | Medial left | Narrow left | | |
| Inflare | Right | Right | Medial right | | Lateral right | Wide right | | |
| | Left | Left | Medial left | | Lateral left | Wide left | | |
| Superior shear (Upslip) | Right | Right | Superior right | Short right | Superior right | | Superior right | Lax right |
| | Left | Left | Superior left | Short left | Superior left | | Superior left | Lax left |
| Inferior shear (Downslip) | Right | Right | Inferior right | Long right | Inferior right | | Inferior right | Tight right |
| | Left | Left | Inferior left | Long left | Inferior left | | Inferior left | Tight left |

5. Patient pushes foot into operator as though to straighten leg. Operator resists.
6. After patient relaxes operator takes up slack by increased flexion.
7. Patient repeats step 5 about three times.
8. Retest!
   Note: Patient may also attempt to adduct or abduct knee against resistance as well as extend leg. This uses other muscle groups for mobilization.

Prone
Diagnosis
   Position: Anterior innominate dysfunction (right)

   Motion restriction: Posterior rotation of innominate (right)

1. Patient in the prone position with the right leg over the edge of the table.
2. Operator stands at right side of patient facing toward head and supporting the patient's right leg.
3. Operator's left hand monitors the right sacroiliac joint (Fig. 17.62).
4. The operator's right hand controls the patient's right knee with abduction, external rotation, and flexion until the barrier to posterior innominate rotation is reached.

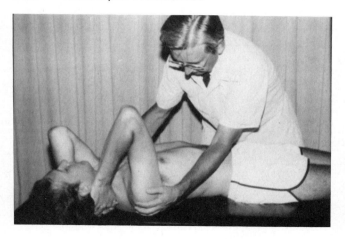

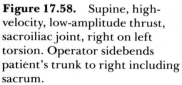

**Figure 17.58.** Supine, high-velocity, low-amplitude thrust, sacroiliac joint, right on left torsion. Operator sidebends patient's trunk to right including sacrum.

5.  Patient's right foot is placed against operator's thigh and patient is instructed to straighten the right leg while the operator's thigh resists (Fig. 17.63).
6.  Operator takes up slack by increased flexion of the knee and hip.
7.  Patient repeats step 5 about three to five times.
8.  Retest.

    Note: Occasionally it is useful for the operator's left hand to provide resistance against the posterior aspect of the sacrum so that it remains fixed during the patient's effort of extending the right leg.

Supine
Diagnosis
    Position: Anterior innominate dysfunction (right)

Motion restriction: Posterior rotation of innominate (right)

1.  Patient in the supine position with the right hip and knee flexed.
2.  Operator stands on the left side of the patient with the heel of the left hand in contact with the ischial tuberosity and the left ring and little fingers monitoring motion over the sacroiliac joint.
3.  Operator flexes, externally rotates, and abducts patient's right leg.
4.  Operator's right hand overlies the patient's right anterior superior iliac spine (Fig. 17.64).
5.  Patient instructed to extend the right leg against resistance offered by the operator's shoulder or chest wall while the operator exerts a posterior rotational counter force on

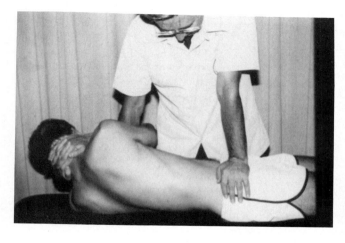

**Figure 17.59.** While operator holds right ASIS, a left rotary thrust is made by operator's right arm.

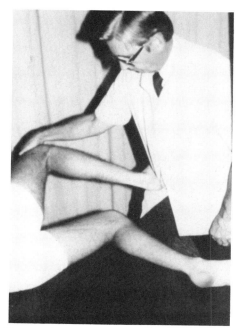

**Figure 17.60.** Lateral recumbent, muscle energy, iliosacral region, right anterior innominate. Patient's right leg flexed and foot placed against operator's hip.

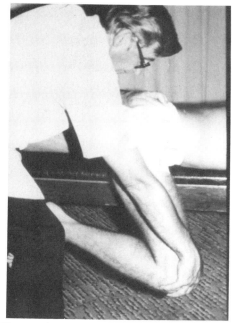

**Figure 17.62.** Prone, muscle energy technique, iliosacral region, right anterior innominate. Operator monitors right sacroiliac joint.

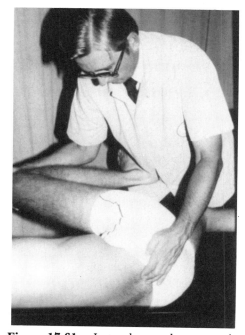

**Figure 17.61.** Lateral recumbent, muscle energy, iliosacral region, right anterior innominate. Operator's left hand monitors right sacroiliac joint and resists patient's leg extension.

the patient's right innominate maintaining the plane of the SI joint in the loose pack position.

6. Repeat 3 to 5 times.
7. Retest.
   Note: This procedure is quite similar to an inferior pubic symphysis dysfunction with the difference being the loose pack position of the sacroiliac joint and the force of the left hand on the ischial tuberosity being in the direction of innominate rotation rather than toward the symphysis pubis.

Prone
Diagnosis
> Position: Posterior innominate dysfunction (left)
> Motion restriction: Anterior rotation of innominate (left)

1. Patient lies prone on table, operator on right side of patient.
2. Operator controls patient's left leg by grasping knee in the left hand.

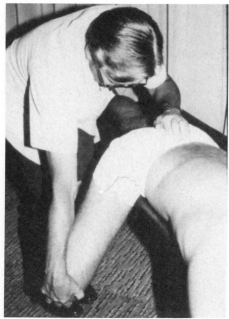

**Figure 17.63.** Prone, muscle energy technique, illiosacral region, right anterior innominate. Operator's thigh resists patient's right foot when instructed to extend leg.

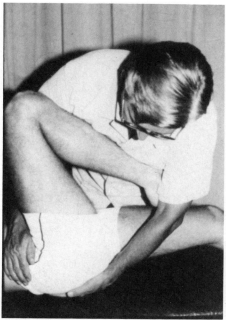

**Figure 17.64.** Supine, muscle energy technique, iliosacral region, right anterior innominate. While holding patient's right ASIS, operator's left hand contacts ischial tuberosity and operator's shoulder resist leg extension.

Leg abducted to freedom of movement at left sacroiliac joint.

3. Operator's right hand placed on left iliac crest 2-2½ in anterior to the PSIS (Fig. 17.65).
4. Operator extends patient's leg to barrier and exerts pressure along iliac crest with right hand (Fig. 17.66).
5. Patient pulls leg down to table and relaxes.
6. Slack taken out by added extension by operator after patient relaxes.
7. Patient repeats number 5 about three times.
8. Retest.

Lateral Recumbent
Diagnosis
  Position: Posterior innominate dysfunction (left)
  Motion restriction: Anterior rotation of innominate (left)

1. Patient lies in the right lateral recumbent position on table, operator behind.
2. Operator's right hand placed on iliac crest 2-2½ in anterior to the PSIS (Fig. 17.67).
3. Operator controls patient's left leg by grasping knee in the left hand and supporting the left lower leg. Leg abducted to point of freedom of movement at sacroiliac joint.
4. Operator extends patient's leg to barrier and exerts pressure along iliac crest with right hand (Fig. 17.68).
5. Patient pulls leg anteriorly against resistance offered by operator's right hand and relaxes.
6. Slack taken out by added extension of hip by operator after patient relaxes.

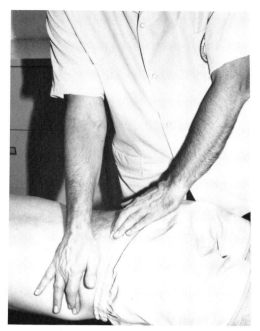

**Figure 17.65.** Prone, muscle energy technique, iliosacral region, posterior left innominate. Operator's hand contacts iliac crest anterior to PSIS.

7. Repeat numbers 5 & 6 approximately three times.
8. Retest.

Supine
Diagnosis
    Position: Posterior innominate dysfunction (left)

Motion restriction: Anterior rotation of innominate (left)

1. Patient lies supine on table, operator standing on patient's left side.
2. Operator controls patient's left leg which is brought off the edge of the table so that the innominate is free and the sacrum rests on the edge of the table.
3. Operator's left hand stabilizes the patient's right anterior superior iliac spine.
4. Operator extends patient's left leg to barrier and operator's extended right arm resists patient's effort to lift the left leg toward the ceiling (Fig. 17.69).
5. Following patients relaxation, operator takes slack out by dropping foot and leg toward floor.
6. Patient repeats step 5 about three times.
7. Retest.
   Note: This procedure is similar to that for a superior pubic symphysis dysfunction. The difference is that here the sacrum, not the posterior aspect of the innominate, is the fixed point on the edge of the table.

Supine
Diagnosis
    Position: Superior innominate shear dysfunction (right)

**Figure 17.66.** Prone, muscle energy technique, iliosacral region, posterior left innominate. Operator extends patient's leg to barrier and resists patient's effort to pull leg to table.

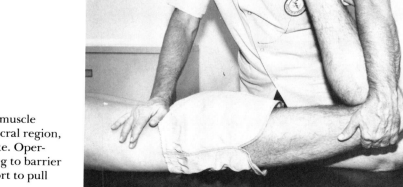

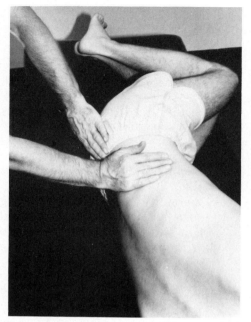

**Figure 17.67.** Lateral recumbent, muscle energy technique, iliosacral region, posterior left innominate. Operator's right hand on iliac crest anterior to PSIS.

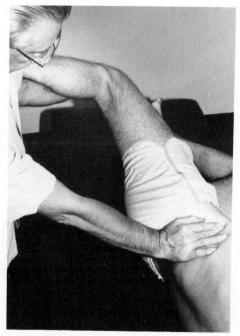

**Figure 17.68.** Lateral recumbent, muscle energy technique, iliosacral region, posterior left innominate. Operator extends patient's leg to barrier and resists patient's hip flexion.

1. Patient supine on table with feet off end of table.
2. Operator stands at end of table and places one thigh against left foot. (An assistant to do this task is useful.)
3. Operator grasps distal right tibia and fibula above ankle.
4. Operator internally rotates extended right leg to close pack the right hip joint (Fig. 17.70).
5. Operator abducts extended right leg to "point of maximum ease" (loose packed position) for the right sacroiliac joint.
6. Long axis extension is maintained on abducted and internally rotated right leg while the patient breathes deeply in and out approximately 3-4 times.
7. At end of last exhalation effort patient is instructed to cough and simultaneously the operator "tugs" caudally on right leg.
8. Retest.
   Note: Same procedure can be done in the prone position.

Left Lateral Recumbent
Diagnosis
  Postion: Inferior innominate shear dysfunction (right)

1. Patient lies in the left lateral recumbent position.
2. Operator stands at back of patient with right arm and shoulder supporting the patient's right lower extremity.
3. Operator's left hand grasps the posterior aspect of the right innominate bone from the ischial tuberosity to the posterior superior iliac spine and the right hand grasps the patient's right innominate from the ischial tuberosity to the inferior pubic ramus (Fig. 17.71).
4. Operator's combined hand effort distracts the patient's right innominate by lifting toward the ceiling.

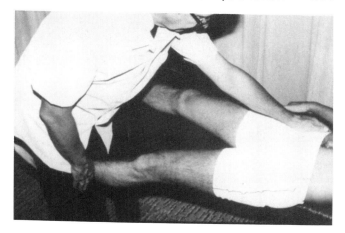

**Figure 17.69.** Supine, muscle energy technique, iliosacral region, posterior left innominate. With patient's innominate off edge of table and operator's left hand stabilizing right ASIS, operator resists patient's hip-flexion effort.

5. Operator's two hands then exert effort on the right innominate in a cephalic direction (Fig. 17.72).
6. Patient is instructed to breathe deeply, in and out, while the operator maintains distraction and cephalic compression on the right innominate.

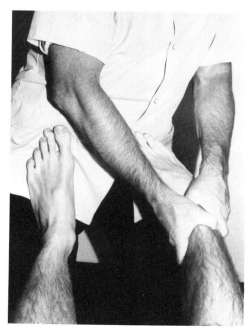

**Figure 17.70.** Supine, muscle energy technique, iliosacral region, right superior innominate shear. Operator holds distal leg in abducted and internally rotated position, and provides long-axis extension.

7. Repeat respiratory effort until release is felt.
8. Retest.

Supine
Diagnosis
    Position: Inflare (internally rotated) innominate (right)

1. Patient supine on table with operator standing to right side.
2. Patient flexes hip and knee and places right foot on the left side of the left knee (Fig. 17.73).
3. Operator's left hand is placed on the patient's left anterior superior iliac spine.
4. Operator's right hand is placed on the medial side of the patient's right knee and the hip is externally rotated until barrier is felt (Fig. 17.74).
5. Patient attempts to internally rotate right hip against resistance.
6. Operator takes up slack and patient repeats internal rotation effort approximately three times.
7. Retest.

Supine
Diagnosis
    Position: Outflare (externally rotated) innominate (right)

1. Patient supine on table with operator standing to right side

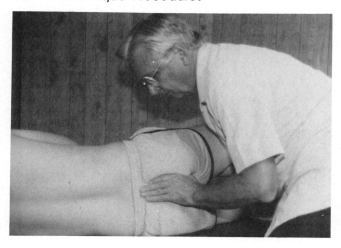

**Figure 17.71.** Lateral recumbent, muscle energy technique, iliosacral region, right inferior innominate shear. Operator's two hands grasp right innominate and distract laterally.

2. Operator flexes patient's hip and knee to approximately 90°.
3. Operator's left hand is placed under the patient's right innominate bone with the fingertips grasping the medial side of the right posterior superior iliac spine.

4. Operator adducts patient's flexed knee and pulls laterally on the posterior superior iliac spine (Fig. 17.75).
5. Patient attempts to push right knee to the right (abduction) against resistance.

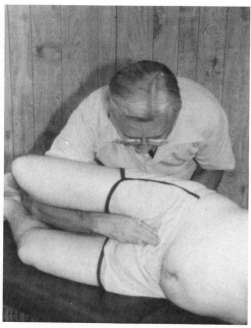

**Figure 17.72.** Lateral recumbent, muscle energy technique, iliosacral region, right inferior innominate shear. Operator directs right innominate in cephalic direction.

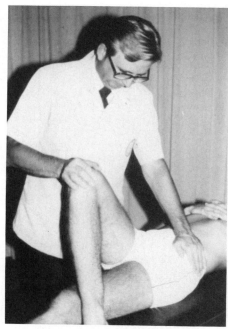

**Figure 17.73.** Supine, muscle energy technique, iliosacral region, right innominate internally rotated. Patient's hip and knee flexed and right foot on left side of left knee.

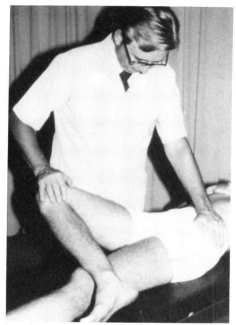

**Figure 17.74.** Supine, muscle energy technique, iliosacral region, right innominate internally rotated. Operator externally rotates right innominate to barrier and resists effort of internal rotation.

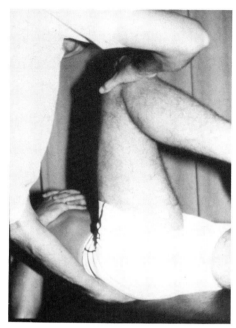

**Figure 17.75.** Supine, muscle energy technique, iliosacral region, right innominate externally rotated. Operator pulls laterally on PSIS with patient's flexed knee adducted.

6. Operator increases adduction and lateral traction of PSIS to new barrier (Fig. 17.76).
7. Patient repeats abduction effort approximately three times.
8. Retest.

### High Velocity Thrust: Iliosacral Joint

Lateral Recumbent
Diagnosis
    Position: Posterior innominate right
    Motion restriction: Innominate anterior rotation right

1. Patient in left lateral recumbent position with knees flexed. Operator stands in front of patient.
2. Operator extends bottom leg of patient and allows top leg to lie on table in front of bottom leg.
3. Operator pulls patient's left arm forward and caudad down to the sacrum with sacrum remaining perpendicular to the table (Fig. 17.77).
4. Operator places pisiform contact on the patient's right posterior superior iliac spine with left elbow flexed and forearm pointed in direction of iliac crest (Fig. 17.78). (Alternative arm position is operator's left forearm along posterior aspect of the patient's right iliac crest) (Fig. 17.79).
5. With all slack taken out (sacrum locked) a high-velocity, low-amplitude thrust occurs through the operator's left forearm in an anterior rotary direction.
6. Retest.

Lateral Recumbent
Diagnosis
    Position: Anterior innominate right
    Motion restriction: Right innominate posterior rotation

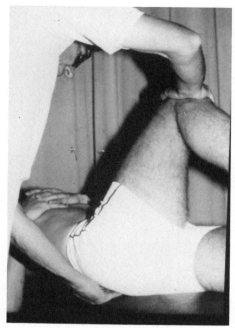

**Figure 17.76.** Supine, muscle energy technique, iliosacral region, right innominate externally rotated. While maintaining lateral traction of PSIS, operator resists abduction effort.

1.  With patient in left lateral recumbent position and knees flexed. Operator stands in front of patient.
2.  All slack taken down from above through vertebral axis to the sacrum by pulling patient's left arm anterior and caudad.

3.  Operator flexes patient's right leg, hip, and knee.
4.  With sacrum perpendicular to table, operator's two hands make contact with the right innominate bone, with the right on the patient's right ASIS and the left on the ischial tuberosity. All slack is taken out in a posterior rotary movement and a high-velocity, low-amplitude thrust exaggerates the posterior rotation (Fig. 17.80).
5.  Alternative hand position has operator's left forearm on the patient's right ischial tuberosity. The sacrum is fixed from above downward by the operator's right hand on the patient's right shoulder, and posterior rotation of the innominate is accomplished by the operator's left forearm moving anterior and superior with a high-velocity, low-amplitude thrust (Fig. 17.81).
6.  Retest.

Supine
Diagnosis
> Position: Superior innominate shear dysfunction (right)

1.  Patient supine on table with feet off end of table.
2.  Operator stands at end of table and grasps patient's distal right tibia and fibula above ankle (Fig. 17.82).

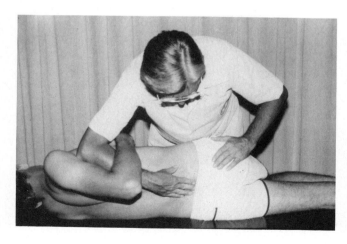

**Figure 17.77.** Lateral recumbent, high-velocity, low-amplitude thrust, iliosacral region, right posterior innominate. Localization to sacrum by introducing neutral mechanics by pulling left arm forward and caudad.

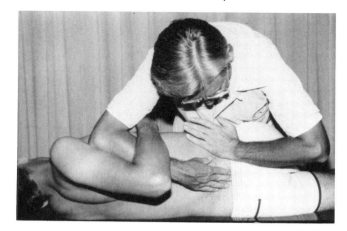

**Figure 17.78.** Lateral recumbent, high-velocity, low-amplitude thrust, iliosacral region, right posterior innominate. Pisiform contact on PSIS with forearm pointed in direction of crest.

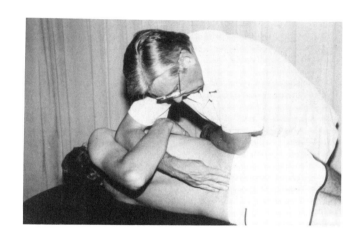

**Figure 17.79.** Lateral recumbent, high-velocity, low-amplitude thrust, iliosacral region, right posterior innominate. Alternate position with left forearm along posterior aspect iliac crest.

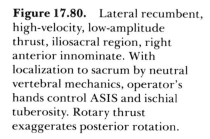

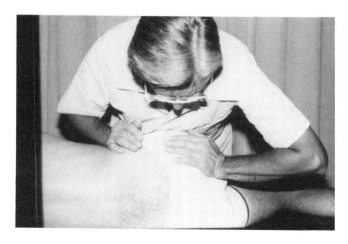

**Figure 17.80.** Lateral recumbent, high-velocity, low-amplitude thrust, iliosacral region, right anterior innominate. With localization to sacrum by neutral vertebral mechanics, operator's hands control ASIS and ischial tuberosity. Rotary thrust exaggerates posterior rotation.

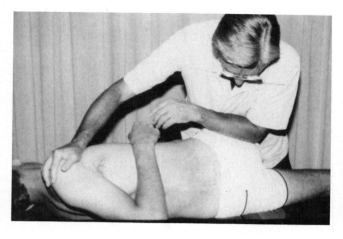

**Figure 17.81.** Lateral recumbent, high-veloicty, low-amplitude thrust, iliosacral region, right anterior innominate. Alternate left forearm contact on ischial tuberosity with thrust moving anterior and superior.

3. Operator abducts right leg to point of maximum ease (loose pack position) for the right sacroiliac joint.
4. Operator flexes and extends patient's right hip and knee several times while patient completely relaxes (Fig. 17.83).
5. Following a series of flexions and extensions in a caudad direction, the operator puts a long axis extension tug on the right leg with a high-velocity force (Fig. 17.84).
6. Retest.
   Note: The patient's knee and hip should be in the loose packed position and the high-velocity tug must be in the plane of the loose packed position of the sacroiliac joint. This procedure should not be used in the presence of organic hip or knee disease.

Lateral Recumbent
Diagnosis: Inferior innominate shear dysfunction (right)

1. Patient on left side.
2. Operator stands in front of patient.
3. Operator pulls patient's left arm anteriorly and caudally, introducing movement down to and including the sacrum.
4. Operator's right arm stabilizes patient's trunk and sacrum.
5. Operator's left forearm contacts patient's ischial tuberosity (Fig. 17.85).

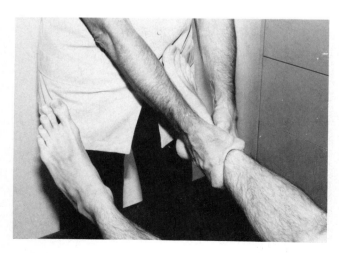

**Figure 17.82.** Supine, high-velocity, low-amplitude thrust, iliosacral region, right superior innominate shear. Operator grasps distal leg above ankle.

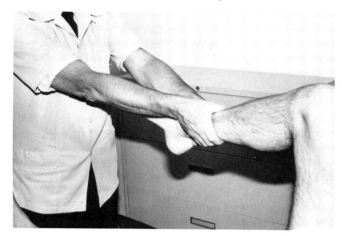

**Figure 17.83.** Supine, high-velocity, low-amplitude thrust, iliosacral region, right superior innominate shear. Operator flexes patient's right hip and knee.

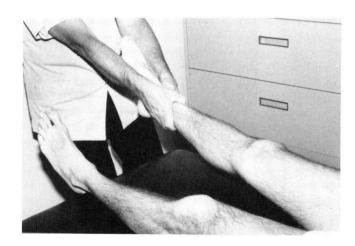

**Figure 17.84.** Supine, high-velocity, low-amplitude thrust, iliosacral region, right superior innominate shear. A long-axis extension tug that completes leg extension.

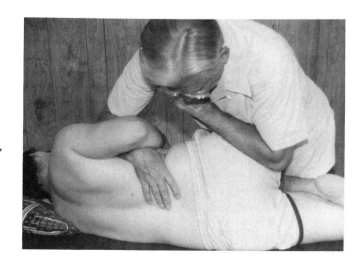

**Figure 17.85.** Lateral recumbent, high-velocity, low-amplitude thrust, iliosacral region, right inferior innominate shear. With localization to sacrum, operator's left forearm contacts ischial tuberosity for thrust in cephalic direction.

6. A high-velocity, low-amplitude thrust is made by the operator's forearm in a cephalic direction.
7. Retest.

### Dysfunction of the Pelvic Diaphragm

In dysfunctions of the pelvic girdle it is frequently observed that there is bilateral alteration of the pelvic diaphragm tone. This is particularly true with long-standing dysfunction at the public symphysis and with innominate shear dysfunctions. Dysfunctions of the pelvic diaphragm can have widespread effect, causing symptoms in the lower urinary tract, the male and female genitalia, and the rectum. Alteration in the tone of the pelvic diaphragm should be suspected when there is inequality in the tone of the sacrotuberous ligaments during palpation in the prone position. The therapeutic goal is to restore symmetry of tone to the pelvic diaphragm and symmetry to its excursion during the inhalation—exhalation respiratory cycle. The usual palpable dysfunction is unilateral tension with concurrent reduction in the inhalation—exhalation respiratory excursion. A combined muscle energy and respiratory technique for the pelvic diaphragm is as follows:

Diagnosis: Dysfunction of the pelvic diaphragm (Fig. 7.32)
Lateral Recumbent

1. Patient lies in the left lateral recumbent position with the hips and knees flexed.
2. Operator stands behind with the left hand supporting the pelvis to prevent rotation and the right hand palpating just medial to the ischial tuberosity.
3. The operator's fingers move along the lateral wall of the osseous pelvis in a cephalic direction until tension is felt.
4. The patient is instructed to take a deep inhalation and then a forced exhalation.
5. The operator's right hand follows the diaphragm in a cephalic direction through the exhalation phase and holds it in that position.
6. With the patient's next inhalation effort the operator resists the descent of the pelvic diaphragm.
7. During the exhalation phase additional cephalic compression is made by the operator's fingerpads.
8. Repeat 3 to 4 times.
9. Retest.

This procedure can be accomplished on both sides until symmetry of tone and excursion is achieved.

### CONCLUSION

Dysfunctions of the pelvic girdle are frequently complex and not easily understood. It is not uncommon to find several dysfunctions present within the same pelvic girdle. Each needs to be individually diagnosed and appropriately treated. The diagnostic and therapeutic system described here allows the operator to deal with any combination of physical findings present within the pelvic girdle. It is again emphasized that the restoration of pelvic girdle function within the walking cycle is a major therapeutic goal from the biomechanical, postural—structural point of view.

# 18 UPPER EXTREMITY TECHNIQUE

Highly developed hand dexterity is one of man's distinguishing characteristics. The upper extremity functions to place the hand in positions which allow it to perform its unique intricate movements. The upper extremity is attached to the trunk primarily through muscular attachments; the only articulation of the upper extremity with the trunk is the sternoclavicular joint. The arrangement of the muscular attachments allow the extremity a wide range of movement in relation to the trunk. The multiple muscle relationships of the upper extremity account for its strong interrelationship with the cervical spine, thoracic spine, and thoracic cage.

In approaching dysfunctions within the upper extremity, the operator should first examine and treat any dysfunctions within the cervical spine, thoracic spine, and thoracic cage. This is particularly true for the cervicothoracic junction, one of the major transitional regions of the body, because of the relationship of T1 to the first rib, and, subsequently, the relationship of the first rib to the sternoclavicular joint. Dysfunctions of T1 strongly influence the first rib and lead to dysfunctions there. Dysfunctions of the first rib influence the manubrium of the sternum and the sternoclavicular joint. Evaluation of symptoms in the upper extremity should proceed from proximal to distal because of the influence of the cervical spine and thoracic inlet on circulatory and neural functions. Therefore, whether the therapist is using a circulatory or a neurologic model evaluation of the cervical and thoracic spine is appropriate before looking distally in the upper extremity.

One of the common mistakes in upper extremity complaints is for the operator to evaluate only at the joint where the symptom is present and proximal thereto. From a structural diagnostic perspective, a patient with pain in the upper extremity under the general rubric of "brachialgia", has five potential entrapment sites for elements of the brachial plexus.

1. The cervical roots are at risk at the intervertebral foramen as they exit from the vertebral canal. Productive change of the uncovertebral joint of Luschka anteriorly may reduce the space available for the roots. Alteration in function of the apophyseal joints posteriorly, or disease process within these joints, can likewise negatively affect the foraminal size and shape. Not only are the osseous changes of significance, but swelling and congestion from acute or chronic inflammation can also cause entrapment.

2. The roots are transported through the muscles between the transverse processes of the cervical vertebra.

Hypertonicity of these short, fourth layer, spinal muscles, with accompanying chronic passive congestion, may also be a site of potential entrapment.

3. The roots forming the brachial plexus pass through the scalene muscles. Hypertonicity and passive congestion of these muscles, commonly found in cervical and upper rib cage dysfunction, can also be a negative influence upon the brachial plexus.

4. As the plexus traverses laterally, it passes through the costoclavicular canal. This triangular-shaped region is bounded by the lateral portion of the second rib and the posterior aspect of the clavicle. Dysfunctions of the second rib, particularly those where the second rib is held in a position of inhalation in the lateral bucket-handle range of motion, and dysfunction of the sternoclavicular and acromioclavicular articulations, can result in potential entrapment at the costoclavicular canal. Remember, a great deal of soft tissue occupies space within this region; if congested, the costoclavicular canal can narrow.

5. More laterally, the neurovascular bundle passes under the tendon of the pectoralis minor muscle as it attaches to the coronoid process of the scapula. Hypertonicity, shortening, and thickening of the pectoralis muscle and its tendon can compress the nerves as they pass distally.

In addition to the neural structures, the vascular and lymphatic channels are also at risk at the scalenes, the first rib, the costoclavicular canal underlying the pectoralis minor tendon. The examiner must thoroughly evaluate the cervical, upper thoracic, and upper rib cage before proceeding with the evaluation and management of the distal region of the upper extremity.

The screening examination (see Chapter 2) for the upper extremities involves the patient actively abducting the upper extremities with the elbows extended and attempting to bring the backs of the hands together over the head. Inability to accomplish this maneuver symmetrically demands further diagnostic evaluation. The upper extremities should be evaluated by traditional orthopedic and neurological testing. There are many systems for the structural diagnosis and manual medicine therapies of the extremities. This author has found many of the procedures found in Mennell's *Joint Pain*[1] to be of considerable therapeutic value. These procedures will not be repeated here and the reader is encouraged to study Mennell's text.

The shoulder, elbow, and wrist are not single joints; each of the regions contains several articulations. For that reason we will approach the upper extremity on a regional basis and evaluate the specific articulations individually.

## SHOULDER REGION

The shoulder region consists of the sternoclavicular, acromioclavicular, and glenohumeral articulations. The scapulocostal junction is not a true articulation, but the ability of the concave costal surface of the scapula to move smoothly over the thoracic cage is of major importance in the function of the upper extremity, particularly the shoulder region. The direct restrictors of scapulocostal motion are the muscles and fascia which hold the scapula to the trunk. These myofascial elements are best approached by soft tissue and myofascial release techniques. Particular attention must be given to the trapezius, levator scapulae, rhomboids, and latissimus dorsi muscles and their fascias. This should precede evaluation and treatment of the other articulations in the shoulder region.

### Sternoclavicular Joint

The medial end of the clavicle articulates with the manubrium of the sternum. Within this joint is found a meniscus. The medial

---

[1] Mennell, J McM: *Joint Pain*. Boston, Little, Brown & Co., 1964.

end of the clavicle is intimately related to the anterior aspect of the first rib. The joint is polyaxial in its movement with the primary motions being abduction, horizontal flexion, and rotation. As the clavicle is abducted, it externally (posteriorly) rotates, and as it returns to neutral, it internally (anteriorly) rotates. Rotation then becomes a coupled movement with abduction.

## Tests for Restricted Abduction

1. Patient supine on table with arms resting easily at the side.
2. Operator stands at side or head of table with paired fingers over the superior aspect of the medial end of the clavicle (Fig. 18.1).
3. The patient is asked to actively "shrug the shoulders" by attempting to bring the shoulder tip to the ear bilaterally (Fig. 18.2).

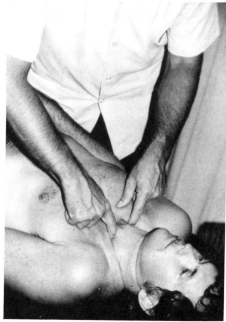

**Figure 18.2.** Test for abduction, sternoclavicular joint. Patient shrugs shoulders toward ear.

4. The operator's palpating fingers follow the movement at the medial end of the clavicle.
5. The normal finding is equal movement of the medial end of both clavicles in a caudad direction.
6. A positive finding is the failure of one clavicle to move caudad when compared to the opposite. It appears to be held in the original starting position.

   Note: This test can also be done with patient sitting.

## Treatment for Restricted Abduction - Articulatory Procedure

1. Patient sits on the examining table or stool.
2. Operator stands behind patient with the thenar eminence of one hand over the superior aspect of the medial end of the dysfunctional clavicle, the other hand grasps the patient's forearm (Fig. 18.3).

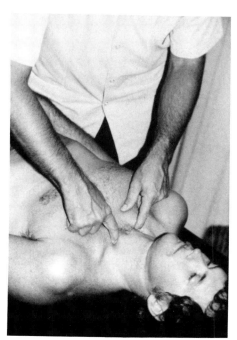

**Figure 18.1.** Test for abduction, sternoclavicular joint. Operator palpates superior aspect, medial end of clavicle.

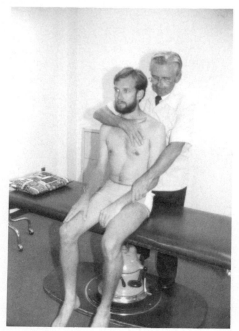

**Figure 18.3.** Sitting, articulatory technique for restricted abduction, sternoclavicular joint. Thenar eminence over superior aspect, medial end of clavicle, with other hand grasping forearm.

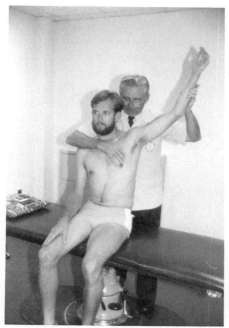

**Figure 18.4.** Sitting, articulatory technique for restricted abduction, sternoclavicular joint. Operator abducts extended extremity to barrier.

3. The operator abducts the extended upper extremity to the resistant barrier (Fig. 18.4) and sweeps it across the patient's torso in the direction of the opposite knee while constant caudad pressure is maintained by the thenar eminence on the medial end of the clavicle (Fig. 18.5).
4. Several repetitions are done increasing the abduction movement of the patient's extended arm. (A high-velocity thrust by the thenar eminence may be used)
5. Retest.

*Muscle Energy Procedure* (1)

1. Patient supine on table with the dysfunctional upper extremity at the edge of the table.
2. Operator stands on the side of dysfunction facing cephalward (Fig. 18.6).

3. The operator places one hand over the medial end of the dysfunctional clavicle while the other grasps the patient's forearm just above the wrist (Fig. 18.7).
4. The operator internally rotates the dysfunctional upper extremity and takes it off the edge of the table into extension to the resistant barrier while the monitoring with the opposite hand at the sternoclavicular region.
5. The patient is instructed to raise the extended arm toward the ceiling for 3 to 5 seconds against resistance offered by the operator.
6. Following relaxation, the operator increases the extension of the upper extremity to a new resistant barrier and patient again repeats the effort of lifting the arm toward the ceiling.

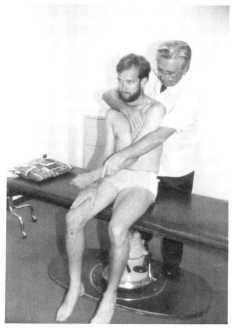

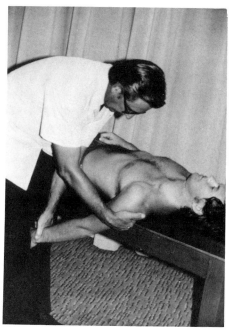

**Figure 18.5.** Sitting, articulatory technique for restricted abduction, sternoclavicular joint. Arm swept across trunk while maintaining constant caudad pressure on clavicle.

**Figure 18.6.** Supine, muscle energy procedure, restricted abduction, sternoclavicular joint. Operator stands on side of dysfunction, facing cephalward.

7. Three to five repetitions are made.
8. Retest.
   Note: This procedure also increases internal (anterior) rotation at the sternoclavicular joint.

*Muscle Energy Procedure* (2)

1. Patient sitting on table or stool.
2. Operator standing behind patient with the thenar eminence of one hand in contact with the superior aspect of the medial end of the dysfunctional clavicle, and the other hand controlling the dysfunctional upper extremity at the elbow (Fig. 18.8).
3. With the elbow at 90°, the upper extremity is externally rotated and abducted to approximately 90° with additional abduction until the resistant barrier is engaged (Fig. 18.9).

4. With a counterforce on the medial end of the clavicle, the patient is requested to adduct the upper extremity for 3 to 5 seconds against resistance offered by the operator at the elbow.
5. Additional slack is taken out in the abducted position and the patient is instructed to repeat the muscle energy effort.
6. Three to five repetitions are done.
7. Retest.
   Note: This procedure also enhances the external (posterior) rotation at the sternoclavicular joint.

### Test for Restricted Horizontal Flexion

1. Patient supine on table.
2. Operator stands at the side or head of the table with symmetrical fingers placed on the anterior aspect of the

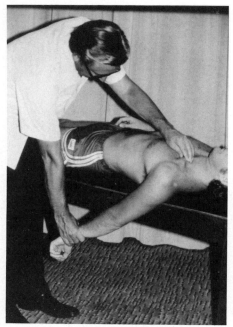

**Figure 18.7.** Supine, muscle energy procedure, restricted abduction, sternoclavicular joint. Operator holds medial end of dysfunctional clavicle, other hand grasps forearm to resist elevation of dysfunctional upper extremity.

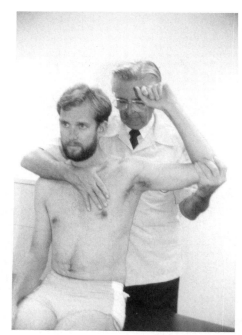

**Figure 18.8.** Sitting, muscle energy procedure, restricted abduction, sternoclavicular joint. Thenar eminence contacts superior aspect, medial end of clavicle, with other hand controlling elbow.

medial end of each clavicle (Fig.18.10).

3. The patient is asked to extend the upper extremities in front of the body toward the ceiling.

4. The operator evaluates movement of the medial end of each clavicle (Fig. 18.11).

5. The normal finding is for each clavicle to move symmetrically in a posterior direction as the lateral end of the clavicle moves anteriorly.

6. A positive finding is for one clavicle not to move in a posterior direction during the reaching effort.
   Note: This test can also be done with the patient sitting.

## Treatment of Restricted Horizontal Flexion Articulatory Procedure

1. Patient sitting on table.

2. Operator standing behind with one hand on the anterior aspect of the medial end of the dysfunctional clavicle and the lateral hand grasping the forearm (Fig. 18.12).

3. The upper extremity is taken into horizontal extension (Fig. 18.13) and then swept forward in horizontal flexion (Fig. 18.14) with slightly increasing arcs of movement, while the thenar eminence of the opposite hand maintains a posterior compressive force on the medial end of the dysfunctional clavicle. (A high-velocity thrust by the thenar eminence may be substituted.)

4. Retest.

*Muscle Energy Procedure*

1. Patient supine on table.

2. Operator stands on side of table opposite to the dysfunctional sternoclavicular joint.

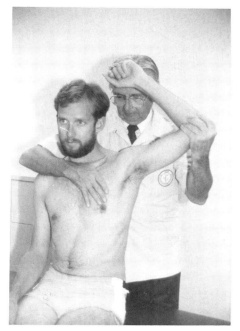

**Figure 18.9.** Sitting, muscle energy procedure, restricted abduction, sternoclavicular joint. With elbow flexed and upper extremity externally rotated, the operator resists patient's adduction of upper extremity.

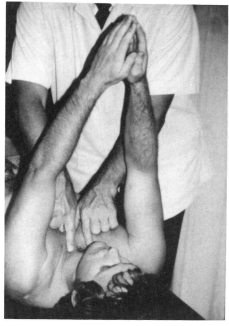

**Figure 18.10.** Test for restricted horizontal flexion, sternoclavicular joint. Operator palpates anterior aspect, medial end of each clavicle.

3. Operator places cephalic hand over the medial end of the dysfunctional clavicle (Fig. 18.15).
4. Operator's caudal hand grasps the patient's shoulder girdle over the posterior aspect of the scapula (Fig 18.16).
5. Patient grasps the back of the operator's neck.
6. With the patient's arm fully extended and continuing to grasp the back of the neck, the operator takes up all of the slack by standing more erectly and lifting the dysfunctional scapula.
7. The patient is instructed to pull down upon the operator's neck against equal and opposite resistance while the operator maintains posterior compression on the anterior portion of the medial extremity of the dysfunctional clavicle.

8. Following relaxation, additional slack is taken up in a horizontal flexion direction.
9. Patient repeats the effort three to five times.
10. Retest.

*Articulatory Procedure*

1. Patient supine, operator stands on opposite side of dysfunction.
2. Operator places caudad forearm on table between chest and humerus.
3. Patient's opposite hand grasps wrist of dysfunctional extremity. A pull places traction on the clavicle (Fig. 18.17).
4. Operator's cephalic hand applies pressure on medial end of clavicle.
5. Treatment combines distraction by the patient pull on wrist and operator springing of medial end of clavicle.

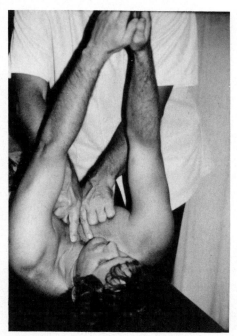

**Figure 18.11.** Test for restricted horizontal flexion, sternoclavicular joint. Operator evaluates movement as patient reaches to ceiling.

## Acromioclavicular Joint

The acromioclavicular joint contributes only a small amount of motion to the shoulder region. However, clinical experience has shown that loss of acromioclavicular joint function is highly significant, particularly the loss of abduction. This joint depends, in large measure, on ligaments for its integrity, and frequently separates during trauma. Productive change at this joint is not uncommon. The primary movements of this articulation are abduction, and internal and external rotation. In testing for motion, it is important to remember that this joint is angled at approximately 30° laterally from before backward.

### Testing for Restricted Motion

1. Patient sitting with operator standing behind.
2. Operator's medial hand palpates over superior aspect of acromioclavicular joint (Fig. 18.18).

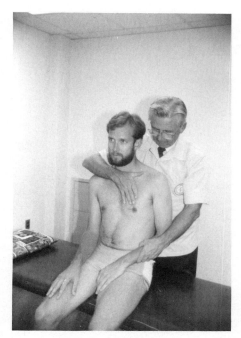

**Figure 18.12.** Sitting, articulatory procedure for restricted horizontal flexion, sternoclavicular joint. Operator's hand on anterior aspect, medial end of clavicle, other hand grasping forearm.

3. Operator's lateral hand controls patient's arm by grasping proximal forearm. Adduction and external rotation are introduced (Fig. 18.19).
4. A gapping movement is felt at the A-C joint in the absence of restriction.
5. Comparison is made with the normal joint on the opposite side.

### Testing for Restricted Abduction

1. Patient sitting on table or stool.
2. Operator standing behind patient.
3. Operator's medial hand palpates the superior aspect of the acromioclavicular joint (Fig. 18.20).
4. The operator's lateral hand controls the patient's upper extremity.
5. Operator horizontally flexes the upper extremity to approximately

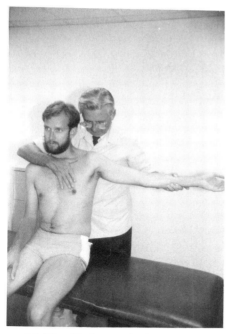

**Figure 18.13.** Sitting, articulatory procedure for restricted horizontal flexion, sternoclavicular joint. Upper extremity taken to horizontal extension.

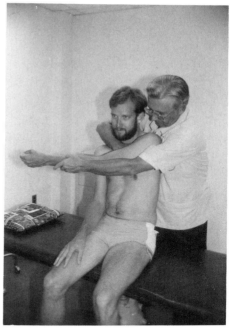

**Figure 18.14.** Sitting, articulatory procedure for restricted horizontal flexion, sternoclavicular joint. Operator sweeps arm forward while pressure maintained on medial end of clavicle.

30° and then introduces abduction (Fig. 18.21).

6. Operator's hand over acromioclavicular joint monitors for movement.
7. The opposite side is tested in similar fashion and comparison is made for restriction of abduction movement at the acromioclavicular joint.

## Treatment of Restricted Abduction

1. Patient sitting on table or stool.
2. Operator stands at side.
3. Operator places one hand on the lateral end of the clavicle just medial to the acromioclavicular joint (Fig. 18.22).
4. The operator's opposite hand takes the patient's upper extremity into horizontal flexion of approximately 30°.
5. Operator introduces abduction movement to the barrier (Fig. 18.23).

6. Patient is instructed to pull the elbow to the side of the body against equal and opposite resistance, while the operator maintains fixation of the lateral end of the clavicle.
7. Following relaxation, additional abduction is taken to the next barrier.
8. Three to five repetitions are made.
9. Retest.

## Testing for Restricted Internal and External Rotation

1. The patient sitting on table or stool.
2. Operator standing behind.
3. Operator's medial hand palpates over the acromioclavicular joint (Fig. 18.24).
4. Operator's lateral hand controls the patient's upper extremity.

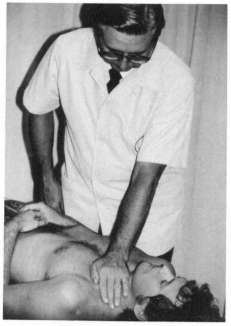

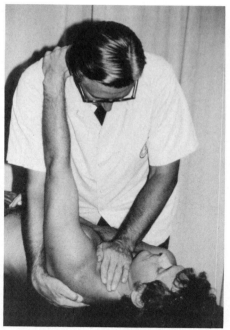

**Figure 18.15.** Supine, muscle energy procedure, restricted horizontal flexion, sternoclavicular joint. Operator contacts medial end of dysfunctional clavicle.

**Figure 18.16.** Supine, muscle energy procedure, restricted horizontal flexion, sternoclavicular joint. Operator grasps shoulder girdle while patient grasps back of operator's neck.

5. Operator takes the upper extremity into horizontal flexion to 30° and abduction to the first barrier.

6. Internal (Fig. 18.25) and external rotation (Fig. 18.26) of the upper

extremity are accomplished while the operator monitors mobility at the acromioclavicular joint sensing for restriction of internal or external rotation

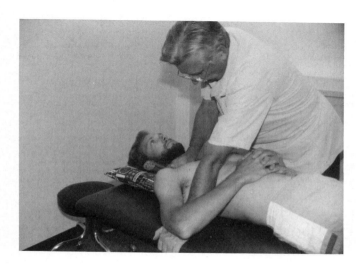

**Figure 18.17.** Supine, articulatory procedure, restricted horizontal flexions, sternoclavicular joint. With operator's forearm between chest and humerus, lateral traction applied to clavicle, operator's other hand maintains pressure on medial end of clavicle.

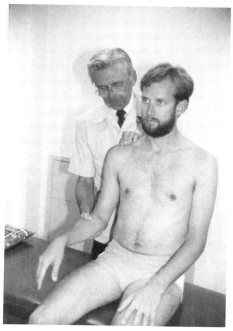

**Figure 18.18.** Test for restricted adduction motion, acromioclavicular joint. Operator's hand palpates acromioclavicular joint.

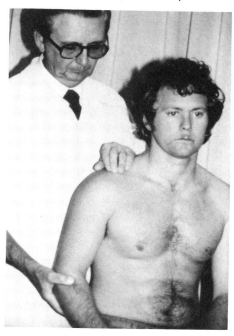

**Figure 18.20.** Test for restricted abduction, acromioclavicular joint. Operator palpates superior aspect of acromioclavicular joint.

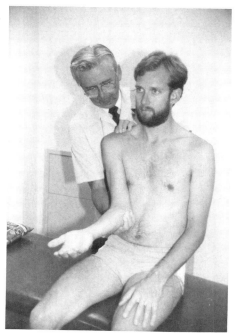

**Figure 18.19.** Test for restricted adduction motion, acromioclavicular joint. Operator's lateral hand introduces adduction and external rotation.

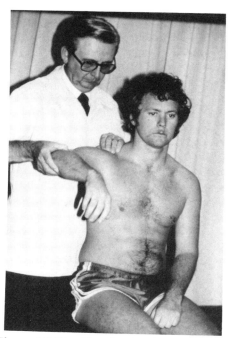

**Figure 18.21.** Test for restricted abduction, acromioclavicular joint. Operator introduces abduction at 30° of horizontal flexion.

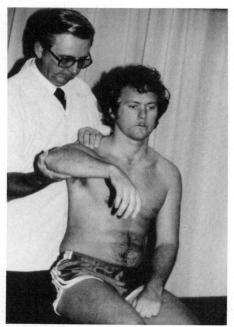

**Figure 18.22.** Sitting, muscle energy technique, restricted acromioclavicular abduction. Operator holds clavicle medial to acromioclavicular joint.

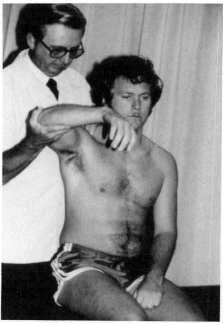

**Figure 18.23.** Sitting, muscle energy technique, restricted acromioclavicular abduction. At abduction barrier, operator resists patient's adduction effort.

7. The opposite side is tested in a similar manner and comparison is made.

## Treatment for Restricted Internal and External Rotation Muscle Energy

1. Patient sitting on table or stool.
2. Operator standing behind.
3. Operator's medial hand stabilizes the lateral aspect of the clavicle and monitors at the acromioclavicular joint (Fig. 18.27).
4. The patient's humerus is taken into 30° horizontal flexion.
5. For internal rotation restriction the operator threads his hand under the elbow and over the patient's wrist and introduces internal rotation to the first barrier (Fig. 18.28).

6. Patient attempts to externally rotate the humerus against equal and opposite resistance.
7. Increased internal rotation is taken to the barrier and the patient's effort is repeated.
8. Three to five repetitions are made.
9. For external rotation restriction the operator's forearm is on the posterior aspect of the elbow, grasping the anterior portion of the wrist, introducing external rotation of the humerus to the first barrier, and the same procedure is accomplished (Fig. 18.29).
10. Retest.
    Note: Remember to maintain the arm in 30° horizontal flexion and 90° of abduction throughout the treatment procedure.

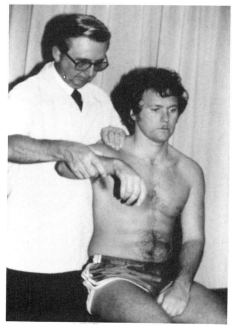

**Figure 18.24.** Test for restricted internal-external rotation, acromioclavicular joint. Operator palpates acromioclavicular joint.

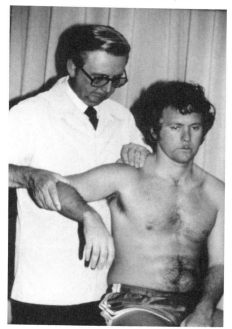

**Figure 18.25.** Test for restricted internal-external rotation, acromioclavicular joint. Operator introduces horizontal flexion and abduction, tests internal rotation.

### Glenohumeral Joint

The glenohumeral joint has one of the widest ranges of movement of any joint within the body. The articular surface of the head of the humerus is considerably larger than the small, pearshaped, articular surface of the glenoid of the scapula. The glenoid is slightly increased in depth by the cartilagenous glenoidal labrum. The articular capsule is normally quite redundant and loose, providing the wide range of movement. Joint integrity is maintained primarily by the intimate attachment of the rotator cuff muscles (supraspinatus, infraspinatus, teres minor, and subscapularis) to the articular capsule.

The extensive movements of this joint are described in relation to the vertical and horizontal planes. In the vertical or neutral plane, the humerus is at the side of the body. Movement then occurs in flexion, extension, internal rotation, and external rotation. In the horizontal plane, with the humerus at 90° to the trunk, it is also possible to have flexion, extension, internal rotation, and external rotation. Adduction moves the humerus toward the body and in front of the chest, and abduction moves the arm away from the body with full range extending so that the elbow can touch the ear. All of these motions must be tested and comparisons made to the opposite side. The primary movement loss in the glenohumeral joint affecting its function involves external rotation and abduction. Remember also that the humeral head must move from the cephalic to caudal end of the glenoid during abduction. Loss of this ability to track from superior to inferior during abduction results in major restriction at the glenohumeral joint.

Since the vast majority of dysfunctions within the glenohumeral joint are muscular in origin, muscle energy diagnostic and therapeutic procedures are most effective at

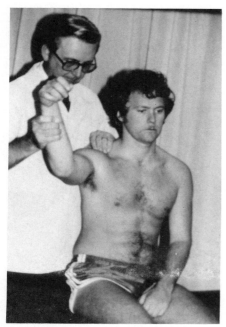

**Figure 18.26.** Test for restricted internal-external rotation, acromioclavicular joint. Operator introduces horizontal flexion, abduction, and external rotation.

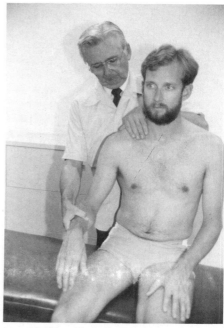

**Figure 18.27.** Sitting, muscle energy technique for restricted internal-external rotation, acromioclavicular joint. Operator stabilizes clavicle medial to the acromioclavicular joint.

this joint. The principles of diagnosis and treatment are (*a*) to evaluate range of motion in all of the motion directions described above; (*b*) to evaluate the strengths of each of the muscle groups; (*c*) to treat restricted range of movement by isometric technique at the restrictive barrier; and (*d*) if weakness is identified, to treat by means of a series of concentric isotonic contractions. Each motion should be compared with that available on the opposite side.

## Muscle Energy Procedure

1. Patient sits on table or stool.
2. Operator stands behind.
3. Operator's medial hand grasps the scapula with the index finger on the corocoid process, the web of the thumb over the acromioclavicular joint engaging the acromion, and the thumb posterior and inferior to the spine of the scapula. This stabilizes the scapula.

4. The operator controls the patient's arm at the elbow (Fig. 18.30).
5. The operator introduces movements of neutral flexion, neutral extension (Fig. 18.31), neutral internal rotation (Fig. 18.32), neutral external rotation (Fig. 18.33), horizontal flexion (Fig. 18.34), horizontal extension (Fig. 18.35), horizontal internal rotation (Fig. 18.36), horizontal external rotation (Fig. 18.37), abduction (Fig. 18.38), and adduction (Fig. 18.39).
6. Range of motion is tested for restriction and if present a series of three to five isometric contractions against operator resistance is performed.
7. Strength testing is done and if a muscle group is found to be weaker than the opposite, a series of three to five concentric isotonic contractions through total range of movement

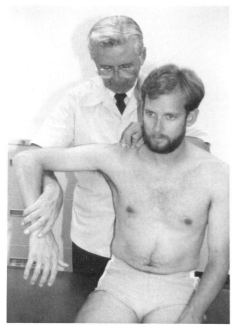

**Figure 18.28.** Sitting, muscle energy technique for restricted internal-external rotation, acromioclavicular joint. With humerus at 30° horizontal flexion, internal rotation to barrier, operator resists external rotation.

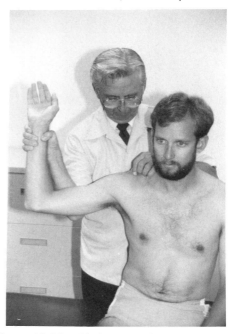

**Figure 18.29.** Sitting, muscle energy technique for restricted internal-external rotation, acromioclavicular joint. Operator resists external rotation for internal rotation restriction.

possible, against progressively increasing resistance by the operator is performed.

8. Retest.

Another technique at the glenohumeral joint that has been found to be effective is described as Green's glenoid or glenoid labrum technique. The goal of this technique is to enhance the capacity of the humeral head to move within the glenoid and particularly at the extremes of the glenoid, the glenoid labrum. In principle, it attempts to restore the normal tracking mechanism of the humeral head on the glenoid. The procedure is as follows:

1. The patient is prone on the table with the involved arm dropped off over the edge of the table (Fig. 18.40).

2. The operator sits at the side of the table facing patient's dysfunctional shoulder.

3. Operator places both hands on the distal humeral shaft at the superior epicondylar ridges, and applies caudad and anterior traction followed by internal and external rotation to barrier sense. This is repeated two or three times (Fig. 18.41).

4. Following step 3, the operator's two hands grasp the patient's humeral neck with the thumbs on the greater tuberosity, the index and middle fingers at the attachment of the rotator cuff and the ring and little fingers surrounding the proximal shaft to control the humeral shaft against the thenar eminences (Fig. 18.42).

5. Alternate movements using the fingers and the thumbs are then accomplished in and anterior-

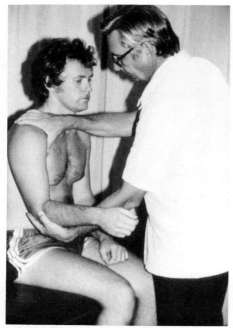

**Figure 18.30.** Sitting, muscle energy technique for glenohumeral joint. Operator grasps patient's arm at elbow.

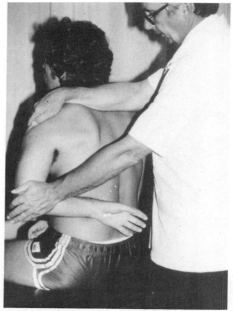

**Figure 18.32.** Sitting, muscle energy technique for glenohumeral joint. Neutral internal rotation.

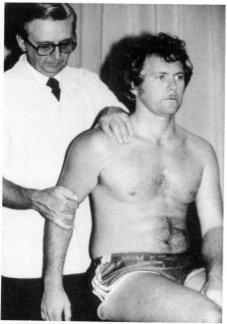

**Figure 18.31.** Sitting, muscle energy technique for glenohumeral joint. Neutral extension.

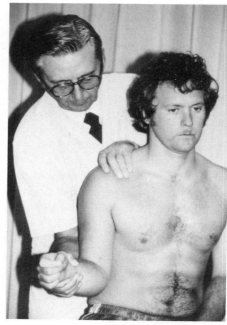

**Figure 18.33.** Sitting, muscle energy technique for glenohumeral joint. Neutral external rotation.

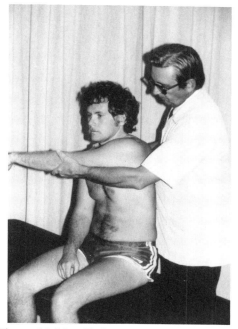

**Figure 18.34.** Sitting, muscle energy technique for glenohumeral joint. Horizontal flexion.

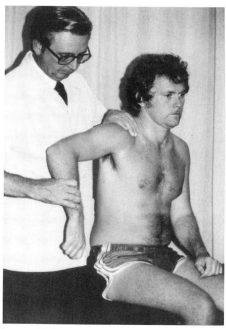

**Figure 18.36.** Sitting, muscle energy technique for glenohumeral joint. Horizontal internal rotation.

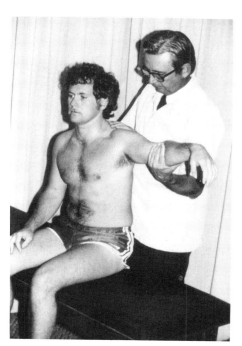

**Figure 18.35.** Sitting, muscle energy technique for glenohumeral joint. Horizontal extension.

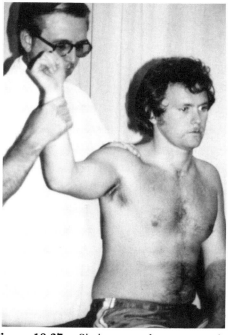

**Figure 18.37.** Sitting, muscle energy technique for glenohumeral joint. Horizontal external rotation.

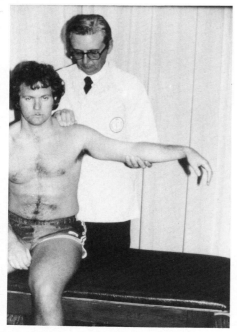

**Figure 18.38.** Sitting, muscle energy technique for glenohumeral joint. Abduction.

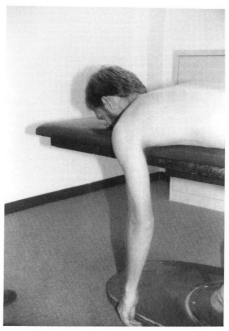

**Figure 18.40.** Prone, articulatory glenoid labrum technique. Dysfunctional arm off edge of table.

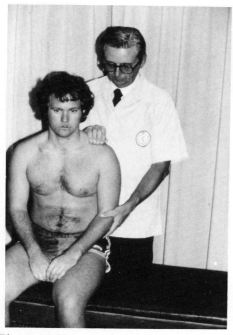

**Figure 18.39.** Sitting, muscle energy technique for glenohumeral joint. Adduction.

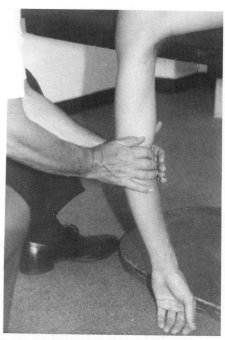

**Figure 18.41.** Prone, articulatory glenoid labrum technique. Operator grasps distal humerus and introduces internal/external rotation.

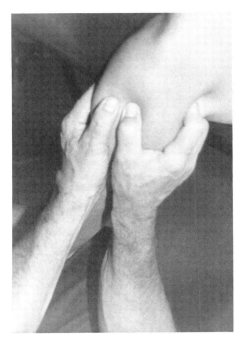

**Figure 18.42.** Prone, articulatory glenoid labrum technique. Operator grasps humeral neck with both hands and introduces movement in multiple directions.

2. Operator stands and faces patient.
3. One of operator's hands stabilizes the clavicle and the scapula, which hand varies from step to step.
4. (Step one) Gently flex (Fig. 18.43) and extend arm (Fig. 18.44) in the sagittal plane with the elbow flexed. Repetitive engagements of the restrictive barrier are made in an articulatory fashion within the limits of pain provocation.
5. (Step two) Flex arm in the sagittal plane with the elbow extended with rhythmic swinging movement. The goal is increasing range of movement so that patient's arm covers the ear (Fig. 18.45).
6. (Step three) Circumduct the abducted humerus with the elbow acutely flexed in both clockwise and counterclockwise concentric circles while stabilizing the scapula. Gradually increase the range of circular movement within the

posterior direction, cephalic-caudad direction, and in a lateral traction and medial distraction direction.
6. Circular and figure-eight motion are introduced with the combined action of both hands enhancing range of motion in all directions.
7. Of major importance is increasing the caudad translatory movement of the humeral head on the glenoid.
8. Retest.

Another procedure that has been clinically successful in glenohumeral dysfunction is the seven-step technique of Spencer. The principle is that of direct action, articulatory procedure against resistance to movement in sequential fashion.

1. Patient in lateral recumbent position with affected shoulder uppermost, head supported, knees flexed.

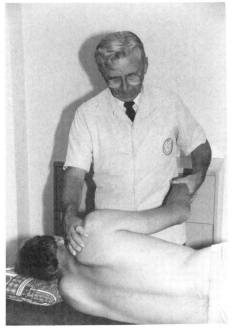

**Figure 18.43.** Lateral recumbent, Spencer articulatory technique, glenohumeral joint. While stabilizing clavicle and scapula, operator's other hand introduces flexion.

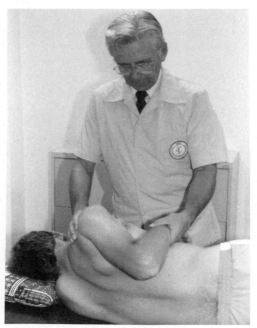

**Figure 18.44.**   Lateral recumbent, Spencer articulatory technique, glenohumeral joint. Operator introduces extension, elbow flexed.

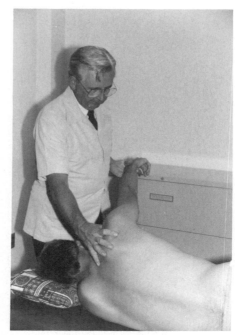

**Figure 18.45.**   Lateral recumbent, Spencer articulatory technique, glenohumeral joint. Operator increases swinging movement, elbow extended.

limits permitted by pain (Fig. 18.46).

7.  (Step four) Circumduct the humerus around the stabilized scapula with the elbow extended in clockwise and counterclockwise circles, gradually increasing the range permitted by pain (Fig. 18.47).

8.  (Step five) Abduct the arm against the stabilized shoulder girdle with the elbow flexed (Fig. 18.48).

9.  (Step six) Place the patient's hand behind the lower ribs and gently pull the elbow forward and slightly inferior increasing the internal rotation of the humerus at the glenoid. Springing repetitions are made to increase range of motion but limited by the introduction of pain (Fig. 18.49).

10.  (Step seven) Operator grasps the proximal humerus with both hands and applies lateral and

caudad traction in an alternate pumping fashion (Fig. 18.50).

11.  Retest.

## ELBOW REGION

There are three joints at the elbow region, the ulnohumeral joint, the radiohumeral joint, and the proximal radioulnar joint. The primary movements are flexion and extension, pronation and supination, and small amount of abduction-adduction. While all of the joints participate in elbow function, flexion-extension is primarily an ulnohumeral movement, and pronation—supination is a combined radiohumeral and proximal radioulnar joint movement. The abduction-adduction movement is primarily a play movement of the ulnohumeral joint, and, when dysfunctional, appears to reduce the flexion—extension range.

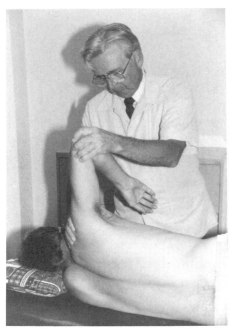

**Figure 18.46.** Lateral recumbent, Spencer articulatory technique, glenohumeral joint. Operator introduces clockwise and counterclockwise circumduction.

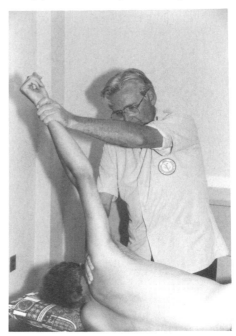

**Figure 18.47.** Lateral recumbent, Spencer articulatory technique, glenohumeral joint. Operator introduces clockwise and counterclockwise circumduction, elbow extended.

### Test for Abduction-Adduction

1. Patient sitting on table.
2. Operator standing in front.
3. Operator's two hands circumferentially grasp the proximal radio-ulnar region.
4. The operator supports the patient's hand and wrist between the lateral elbow and trunk (Fig. 18.51).
5. The operator's hands introduce translatory movement medially and laterally through an arc of flexion and extension, testing for resistance.
6. Comparison is made with the opposite side.

### Treatment of Restricted Abduction-Adduction

(*Direct action articulatory technique* may be carried through to high-velocity, low-amplitude thrust)

1. Patient sitting on table.
2. Operator controls patient's proximal ulna and radius and patient's resting hand as described in the diagnostic procedure above.
3. Caudad traction is introduced upon the ulna which is flexed at approximately 90° (Fig. 18.52).
4. The forearm is extended and either the adduction or abduction barrier is engaged (Fig. 18.53).
5. A general articulatory movement against the resistant barrier is accomplished in an oscillatory fashion.
6. Increasing extension of the forearm at the elbow region is made while the articulatory force is maintained.
7. At the final barrier, a low-amplitude, high-velocity thrust may be instituted.
8. Retest.
   Note: Adduction restriction is much

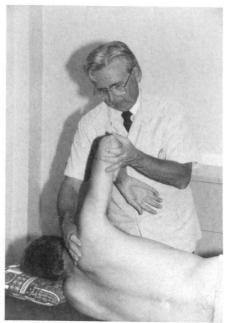

**Figure 18.48.** Lateral recumbent, Spencer articulatory technique, glenohumeral joint. Operator introduces abduction.

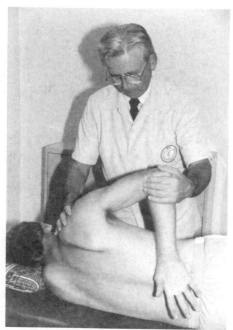

**Figure 18.49.** Lateral recumbent, Spencer articulatory technique, glenohumeral joint. Operator introduces internal rotation.

more common than abduction restriction.

## Tests for Restriction of Pronation-Supination

1. Patient sitting on table.
2. Operator standing in front of patient.
3. One hand of the operator holds the distal humerus at the patient's side (Fig. 18.54).
4. The operator's other hand grasps the distal radius and ulna and maintains the elbow at 90° of flexion.
5. The operator introduces pronation (Fig. 18.55) and supination (Fig. 18.56), testing for range of motion and restriction.
6. Strength test of pronation and supination can be made at the two extremes of movement.
7. Comparison is made with the opposite side.

## Treatment of Restricted Pronation and Supination (Muscle Energy Technique)

1. The patient and operator positions are the same as for the diagnostic procedure.
2. In the presence of restricted supination (Fig. 18.57) (or pronation) (Fig. 18.58) the restrictive barrier is engaged and the patient instructed to pronate (or supinate) against equal and opposite resistance.
3. Three to five isometric procedures are accomplished against each succeeding resistant barrier.
4. Retest.
5. If there is weakness of pronator (or supinator) muscle groups, a series of concentric isotonic contractions is made against progressively increasing resistance by the operator through the total range of pronation (or supination).
6. Retest.

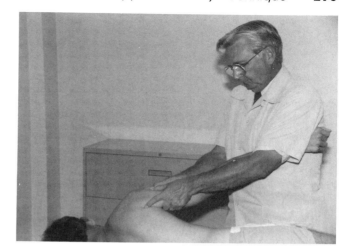

**Figure 18.50.** Lateral recumbent, Spencer articulatory technique, glenohumeral joint. Operator introduces lateral and caudad traction in pumping fashion.

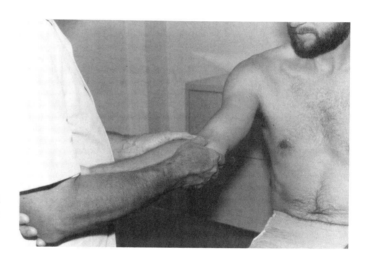

**Figure 18.51.** Restricted abduction-adduction, ulna-humeral joint, with wrist stabilized against trunk, operator introduces translatory medial and lateral movement.

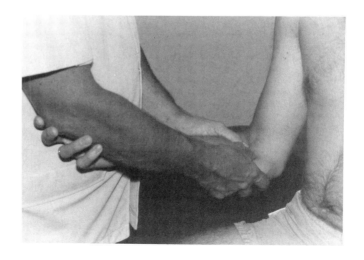

**Figure 18.52.** Sitting, articulatory technique, restricted abduction-adduction, ulna-humeral joint. Caudad traction applied with elbow flexed.

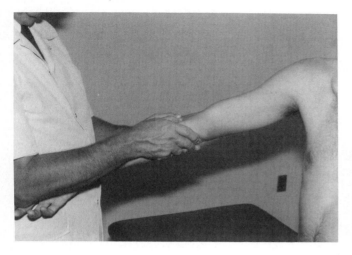

**Figure 18.53.** Sitting, articulatory technique, restricted abduction-adduction, ulna-humeral joint. As forearm is extended, adduction or abduction barrier is engaged and articulatory movement introduced.

Pronation and supination of the forearm is a combined action of the radiohumeral, proximal radioulnar, and distal radioulnar articulations. The previously described muscle energy technique deals with all three of these joints and the supinator and pronator muscles. The most common restriction in this author's experience is supination restriction at the radiohumeral and proximal radioulnar joint. It behaves as though the head of the radius does not pivot symmetrically around the capitulum. These dysfunctions are described as dysfunctions of the radial head and are classified as pos-

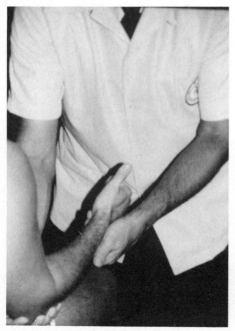

**Figure 18.54.** Test for restricted pronation-supination, elbow region. Operator stabilizes distal humerus.

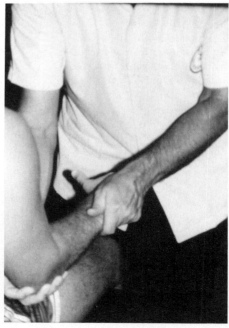

**Figure 18.55.** Test for restricted pronation-supination, elbow region. With elbow at 90° pronation is introduced.

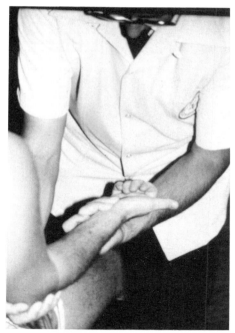

**Figure 18.56.** Test for restricted pronation-supination, elbow region. With elbow at 90°, supination is introduced.

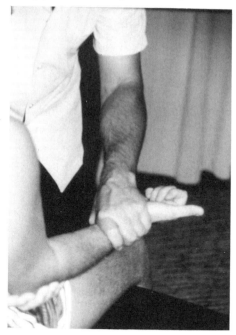

**Figure 18.57.** Sitting, muscle energy technique for restricted pronation-supination, elbow region. Operator stabilizes humerous and engages supination barrier.

terior or anterior radial head dysfunctions. Posterior radial head dysfunction appears to be the more frequent.

## Diagnosis of Radial Head Dysfunction

### Test one: Palpation for asymmetry

1. Patient sits on table with elbows flexed at 90°, forearms supinated and supported in the lap.
2. Operator stands in front of the patient and palpates both elbows with the index finger on the radial head posteriorly and with the thumb in the soft tissues anterior to the radial head (Fig. 18.59).
3. The symmetrical relationship of the radial head to the capitulum of the humerus is ascertained.
4. On the dysfunctional side there is usually tenderness and some tension of the periarticular tissues.

### Test two: Motion of the radial head

1. Patient sitting with elbow at the side, and flexed at 90°.
2. Operator stands in front with the lateral hand palpating the radial head at the radiohumeral articulation (as in the diagnostic procedure above).
3. Operator's medial hand grasps the distal radius and ulna and introduces pronation (Fig. 18.60) and supination (Fig. 18.61).
4. Comparison is made on both sides of symmetrical turning of the radial head during the pronation and supination movement. In the presence of dysfunction, asymmetry of the relationship of the radial head to the capitulum appears during this movement.

### Test three: Motion test

1. Patient sits on table.

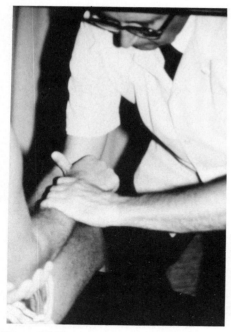

**Figure 18.58.** Sitting, muscle energy technique for restricted pronation-supination, elbow region. Operator engages pronation barrier.

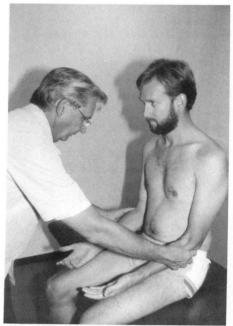

**Figure 18.59.** Test for asymmetry, radial head. With elbows flexed at 90° and forearms supinated, operator palpates posterior radial head bilaterally.

2. Patient's hands and forearms are supinated.
3. With the elbows flexed, the patient brings the elbows together in front of the chest with the medial margins of the forearm and hand approximated (Fig. 18.62).
4. The patient attempts to extend the elbows while maintaining contact of the forearms (Fig. 18.63).
5. In dysfunction at the radial head, the forearm on that side will tend to pronate from its supinated position during extension of the forearms at the elbow.

## Treatment for Radial Head Dysfunction

Diagnosis: Posterior radial head
Muscle energy procedure

1. Patient sitting on table, arm at the side, and elbow flexed at 90°.

2. Operator stands in front with the lateral hand supporting the proximal forearm and the index finger placed over the posterior aspect of the radial head.
3. Operator's medial hand grasps the distal forearm and introduces supination to the barrier (Fig. 18.64).
4. Patient is instructed to pronate the hand against equal and opposite resistance by the operator at the distal forearm, while the operator maintains anterior force on the posterior aspect of the radial head.
5. Three to five repetitions are made against succeeding supination barriers.
6. During the last muscle energy attempt, isometric contraction in an attempt to flex the elbow may be used in addition to pronation.
7. Retest.

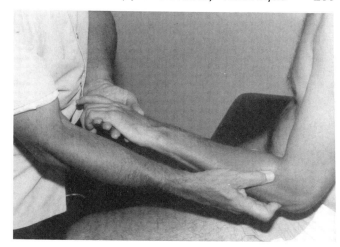

**Figure 18.60.** Motion test for radial head. While palpating radial head, operator introduces pronation.

Diagnosis: Posterior radial head
High-velocity, low-amplitude, direct action technique

1. Patient sitting on the table.
2. Operator stands in front with the medial hand grasping the proximal forearm surrounding the ulna, and the lateral hand grasping the proximal radius with the index finger overlying the posterior aspect of the radial head (Fig. 18.65).
3. The operator controls the patient's hand and wrist between the operator's elbow and chest wall.

4. The operator takes the elbow into extension, supination, and slight adduction (Fig. 18.66).
5. When all barriers are engaged in a direct action, high-velocity, low-amplitude thrust is made in a lateral and anterior direction.
6. Retest.

### Treatment for Anterior Radial Head

Diagnosis: Anterior radial head
Procedure: Direct action, high-velocity, low-amplitude thrust

1. Patient standing.

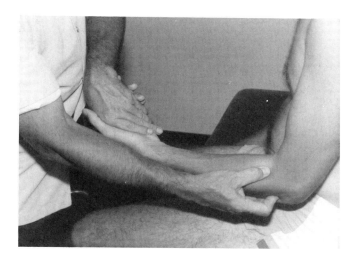

**Figure 18.61.** Motion test for radial head. While palpating radial head, operator introduces supination.

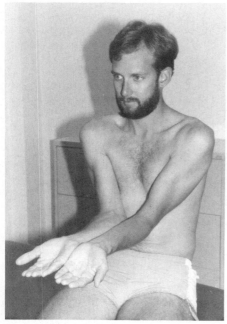

**Figure 18.62.**   Motion test, radial head, elbows flexed and forearms in front of chest.

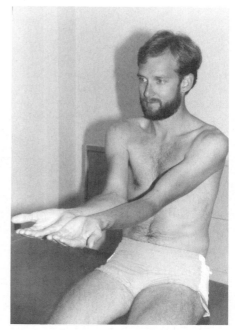

**Figure 18.63.**   Motion test, radial head, elbows flexed and forearms in front of chest. Patient attempts to extend elbows maintaining forearm contact.

2.  Operator stands at side of patient with proximal hand grasping the proximal forearm, and the thumb anterior to the radial head.
3.  Operator's caudal hand grasps the distal forearm (Fig. 18.67).
4.  The patient's forearm is pronated and flexed while the operator's thumb holds the radial head posteriorly (Fig. 18.68).
5.  When all the slack is taken out in pronation and flexion, a high-velocity thrust is made to increased flexion.
6.  Retest.

Diagnosis: Restricted flexion or extension at the elbow

1.  Patient sitting on edge of table with operator standing in front.
2.  Operator grasps upper arm above elbow, while other hand grasps forearm just above wrist.
3.  With the patient's forearm supinated, the operator introduces flex-

ion (Fig. 18.69) and extension (Fig. 18.70) at the elbow, testing for restriction.
4.  Comparison is made with the opposite side.

### Treatment of Restricted Flexion or Extension at the Elbow

Muscle energy technique

1.  With the patient and operator in the same position used for testing, the operator engages the first resistant barrier (to either flexion (Fig. 18.71) or extension) (Fig. 18.72)).
2.  The patient exerts an isometric muscle contraction against equal and opposite operator effort for 3–5 seconds.
3.  Following patient relaxation, the operator engages the next resistant barrier.
4.  Patient repeats step 2 approximately 3 times.
5.  Retest.

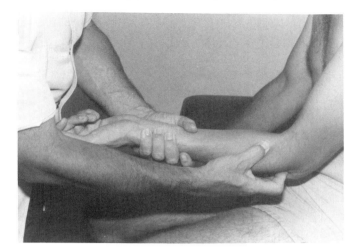

**Figure 18.64.** Sitting, muscle energy technique, radial head dysfunction. While maintaining contact over posterior aspect radial head, operator introduces supination and resists pronation and flexion.

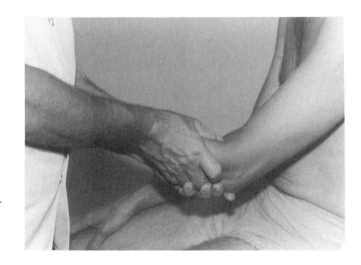

**Figure 18.65.** Sitting, highvelocity, low-amplitude thrust technique, radial head. Operator controls forearm and contacts posterior aspect radial head.

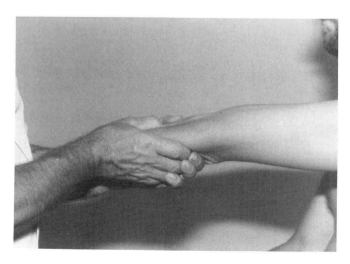

**Figure 18.66.** Sitting, highvelocity, low-amplitude thrust technique, radial head. With elbow taken to extension, supination, and slight adduction, thrust made in lateral and anterior direction.

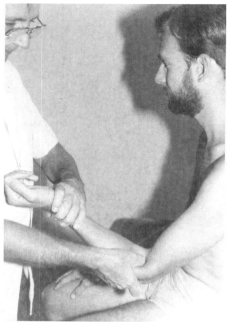

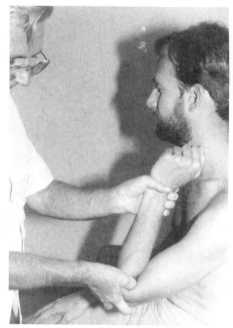

**Figure 18.67.** Standing, high-velocity, low-amplitude thrust, anterior radial head dysfunction. Operator controls distal forearm with opposite thumb anterior to radial head.

**Figure 18.68.** Standing, high-velocity, low amplitude thrust, anterior radial head dysfunction. Patients's forearm pronated and flexed while operator pulls radial head posteriorly and thrust made into flexion.

## WRIST AND HAND REGION

The articulations in this region are the radiocarpal joint (with the distal radius articulating with the carpal navicular and lunate), the ulna-meniscal-triquetral articulation, the distal radial ulnar joint, the intercarpal joints, and the carpometacarpal joints. The primary movements are pronation and supination, occurring primarily at the distal radioulnar joint, and related to the pronation—supination movement of the elbow region. Other movements at the wrist region are dorsiflexion, palmar flexion, adduction (ulnar deviation) and abduction (radial deviation).

## Tests for Restriction of Movement at the Wrist Region

1. Patient sitting on the table
2. Operator standing in front.
3. With patient's arms at the side and elbows at 90°, the operator introduces passive palmar flexion (Fig. 18.73), dorsiflexion (Fig. 18.74), radial deviation (Fig. 18.75), and ulnar deviation (Fig. 18.76) on each side, testing for restricted range of movement.
4. Muscle strength testing can be accomplished in each of these directions to test for muscle weakness as usual.

## Muscle Energy Treatment for Restriction at the Wrist Region

1. Patient sitting on table.
2. Operator standing in front.
3. Operator grasps distal forearm with proximal hand and engages resistant barrier with the distal hand.
4. Barriers of dorsiflexion (Fig. 18.77), palmar flexion (Figure 18.78), ulnar deviation (Fig. 18.79),

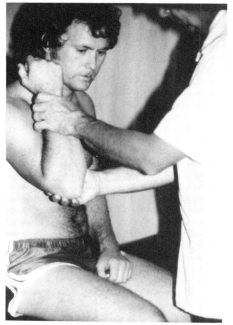

**Figure 18.69.** Test for restricted flexion-extension at elbow. With forearm supinated, operator introduces flexion.

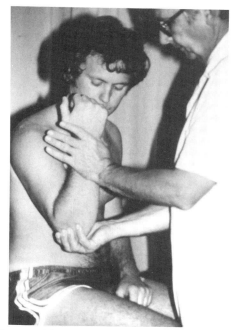

**Figure 18.71.** Sitting, muscle energy technique, restricted flexion-extension at elbow. Operator engages flexion barrier and resists extension effort.

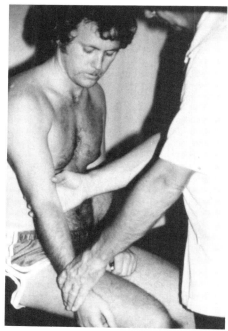

**Figure 18.70.** Test for restricted flexion-extension at elbow. With patient's forearm supinated, operator introduces extension.

or radial deviation (Fig. 18.80) are engaged.

5. Patient instructed to use isometric contraction in the opposite direction against equal and opposite resistance.
6. Three to five repetitions are made against succeeding resistant barriers.
7. Retest.

### Direct Action High Velocity Techniques for the Wrist Region

Diagnosis: Restriction of dorsiflexion
High-velocity, low-amplitude technique

1. Patient sitting on table or standing.
2. Operator stands facing patient.
3. Operator's thumbs contact the dorsal aspect of the navicular and lunate bones (Fig. 18.81), with the pads of the index fingers grasping the volar aspect of the navicular and lunate

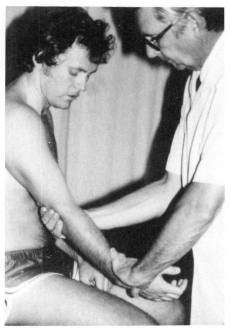

**Figure 18.72.** Sitting, muscle energy technique, restricted flexion-extension at elbow. Operator engages extension barrier and resists flexion effort.

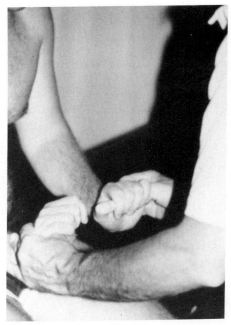

**Figure 18.74.** Test for restriction at wrist region. Operator introduces dorsiflexion.

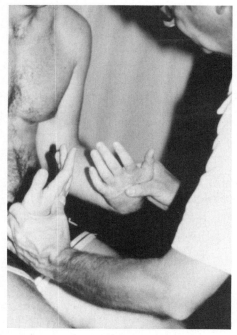

**Figure 18.73.** Test for restriction at wrist region. Operator introduces palmar flexion.

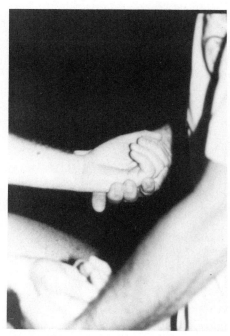

**Figure 18.75.** Test for restriction at wrist region. Operator introduces radial deviation.

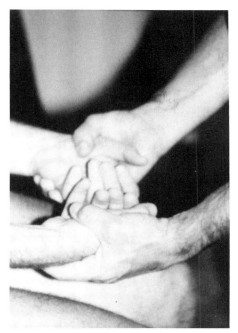

**Figure 18.76.** Test for restriction at wrist region. Operator introduces ulnar deviation.

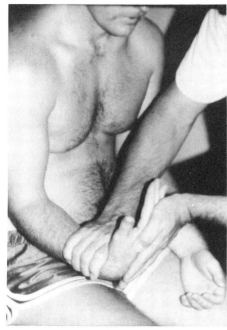

**Figure 18.78.** Sitting, muscle energy technique for restriction at wrist region. Operator stabilizes forearm and introduces palmar flexion.

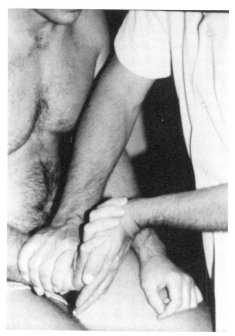

**Figure 18.77.** Sitting, muscle energy technique for restriction at wrist region. Operator stabilizes forearm and engages dorsiflexion barrier.

bones (Fig. 18.82), and the palms of the hands controlling the remainder of the hand.

4. The operator introduces a small amount of palmar flexion, then traction.
5. The hand is taken into dorsiflexion to the barrier (Fig. 18.83).
6. High-velocity, low-amplitude thrust is made by taking the hand into dorsi-flexion with the thumbs carrying the proximal carpal bones anteriorly.
7. Retest.

Diagnosis: Restriction of palmar flexion

1. Patient sitting or standing.
2. Operator standing in front of patient.
3. Operator's two hands grasp the patient's hand, with the operator's thumbs on the dorsal aspect of the

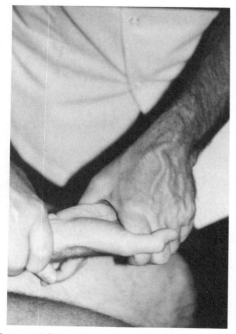

**Figure 18.79.** Sitting, muscle energy technique for restriction at wrist region. Operator stabilizes forearm and introduces ulnar deviation.

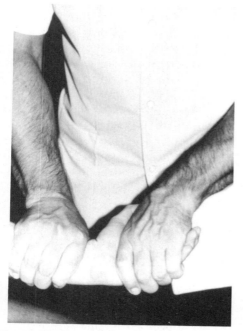

**Figure 18.80.** Sitting, muscle energy technique for restriction at wrist region. Operator introduces radial deviation.

navicular and lunate, and the index fingers on the volar aspect of the navicular and lunate.

4. The operator's hands control the rest of the patient's hand and wrist.
5. A small amount of dorsiflexion is introduced and then traction applied.
6. The palmar flexion barrier is now engaged.
7. A high-velocity, low-amplitude thrust is made with the index fingers being carried posteriorly, and the patient's hand being carried into palmar flexion (Fig. 18.84.).
8. Retest.

Diagnosis: Restriction of ulnar deviation
High-velocity, low-amplitude technique

1. Operator grasps distal radius and ulna with the proximal hand, and the carpals and hand in the distal hand, with the two thumbs adjacent to each other on the ulnar side.
2. The barrier to ulnar deviation is engaged, and a high-velocity thrust is made in the direction of ulnar deviation (Fig. 18.85).
3. Retest.

Diagnosis: Restriction of radial deviation
High-velocity, low-amplitude technique

1. This procedure is exactly the same as the preceding except that the operator's hand positions are reversed, with the thumbs on the radial side.
2. The thrust is in the direction of radial deviation (Fig. 18.86).

The intercarpal joints can be treated individually by articulatory methods, holding one carpal bone and moving the adjacent one upon it. The intercarpal articulations function in an integrated fashion within the dorsal carpal arch. Restriction within the dorsal carpal arch can be treated with the

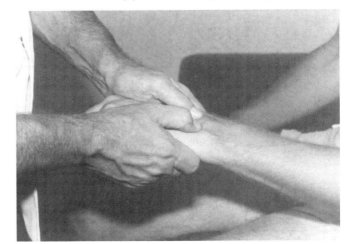

**Figure 18.81.** Sitting, high-velocity, low-amplitude technique, restriction of dorsiflexion, wrist region. Operator's thumbs contact dorsum navicular and lunate.

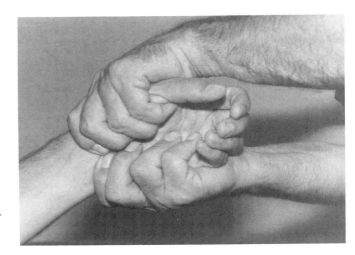

**Figure 18.82.** Sitting, high-velocity, low-amplitude technique, restriction of dorsiflexion, wrist region. Index fingers grasp volar aspect navicular and lunate.

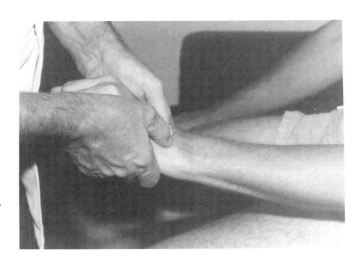

**Figure 18.83.** Sitting, high-velocity, low-amplitude technique, restriction of dorsiflexion, wrist region. Dorsiflexion barrier is engaged and low-amplitude thrust applied.

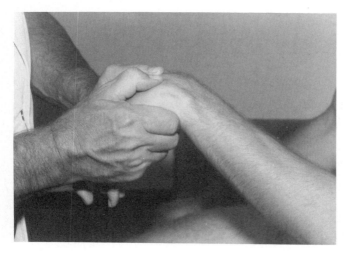

**Figure 18.84.** Sitting, high-velocity, low-amplitude technique, restriction of dorsiflexion, wrist region. With same finger contact, palmar flexion barrier is engaged and thrust into palmer flexion.

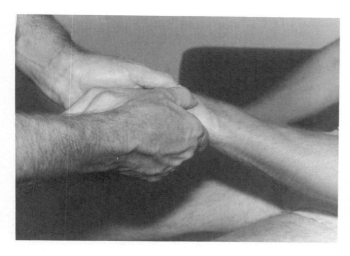

**Figure 18.85.** High-velocity, low-amplitude technique, restriction ulnar deviation at wrist. Operator stabilizes radius and ulna with one hand and carpal bones with other and engages barrier to ulnar deviation.

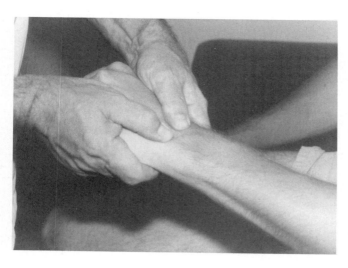

**Figure 18.86.** High-velocity, low-amplitude thrust technique, restriction radial deviation, wrist region. Operator stabilizes distal radius and ulna with one hand and grasps bones with the other, radial deviation barrier engaged.

following direct action, combined compressive technique and muscle energy assist.

1. Patient sits on table.
2. Operator stands in front.
3. Operator's thenar eminences are placed on the dorsal and volar surfaces of the carpal arch with the fingers interdigitating.
4. The operator puts a compressive force from volar to dorsal with the heels of both hands.
5. Patient is instructed to forcefully make a fist and then extend the fingers while the operator maintains progressive increasing compression on the costal arch.
6. Retest.

## SUMMARY

The upper extremity is the site for frequent complaints such as bursitis, tendonitis, epicondylitis, tennis elbow, golfer's elbow, carpal tunnel syndrome, and many others. Most, if not all, of these conditions, will be found to have dysfunciton at the symptomatic joint, as well as dysfunctions at other joints both proximal and distal. The ability to identify and appropriately treat dysfunctions within the entire extremity is very helpful in the management of patients with problems in the area.

# 19
## *LOWER EXTREMITY TECHNIQUE*

The primary function of the lower extremities is ambulation. The complex interactions of the foot, ankle, knee, and hip regions provide both a stable base for the trunk in standing, and a mobile base for walking and running. Alterations in function of the lower extremities can alter function of the rest of the body, particularly the pelvic girdle. In the screening examination (Chapter 2) we evaluated the lower extremities while standing, during walking, performing the squat test, the straight leg raising test (for hamstring length), and during the standing flexion test (for influence on the pelvic girdle and trunk flexion). If significant alteration in function is present in the lower extremities, the examiner proceeds to further evaluate the hip, knee, foot and ankle.

As with the upper extremities, evaluation should be made from proximal to distal for several reasons. First, consider the respiratory circulatory model in proceeding from proximal to distal to enhance venous and lymphatic return. If edema and inflammation are part of the restrictive process, this sequence assists fluid movement. Secondly, by proceeding from proximal to distal, the examiner sequentially develops points of reference for evaluating one bone in relation to the other at an articulation. The ultimate goal of evaluation and treatment of the lower extremities is to return

the walking cycle to the maximum possible symmetry. Shortening of one of the components of a lower extremity can result in a pelvic tilt syndrome which appears to have clinical significance in somatic dysfunction of the vertebral column and pelvic girdle. Alterations in foot mechanics which result in a pronated and flattened medial arch can likewise alter function within the vertebral axis and pelvic girdle.

As with the upper extremity, study of the diagnostic and therapeutic joint play movements advocated by Mennell for the joints within the lower extremity is recommended.

## HIP JOINT

The hip joint is a ball-and-socket articulation which provides for movement in six directions: flexion—extension, abduction—adduction, internal rotation—external rotation. The musculature surrounding the hip joint can be divided into six groups, each being responsible for one of the movement directions. The primary dysfunctions of the hip joint are imbalance of length and strength of these muscles. The principles for structural diagnosis and manual medicine treatment are as follows:

1. The operator passively carries the hip joint through a range of motion, evaluating total range, quality of

movement during the range, and quality of the end point.

2. Comparison is made on the opposite side for the similar range.

3. In the presence of asymmetry, there may be shortening of a muscle group on the restricted side, or weakness of the contralateral muscle group on the side with increased range.

4. Comparison of strength is made by asking the patient to maximally contract the muscle against equal and opposite resistance, testing for comparable strength on each side.

5. With restricted range of movement due to shortened and tightened muscle, a series of three to five isometric contractions by the patient against the operator's equal and opposite resistance are accomplished against succeeding resistant barriers to lengthen the shortened muscle through postisometric relaxation.

6. With extended range on one side, due to functional weakness of the muscle group on that side, a series of three to five concentric isotonic contractions are made throughout the range of movement against a yielding counterforce offered by the operator.

7. Retest is made both for length and strength of comparable muscles.

The following positions are used to evaluate and treat (with muscle energy principles) the six major muscle groups of the hip region.

Motion tested: Abduction
Muscles tested: Adductors (adductor magnus, adductor brevus, adductor longus)

1. Patient supine on table.
2. Operator standing at end of table grasping each lower extremity at the heel.
3. Operator takes each extended lower extremity in turn through abduc-

tion movement to end point, evaluating total range and quality of movement (Fig. 19.1).

4. For strength testing, Operator offers resistance against the abducted leg and the patient is instructed to maximally adduct the extended leg. (Note: The knee should be fully extended, with the operator offering resistance to the patient's adduction movement above the knee joint to protect the medial collateral ligaments) (Fig. 19.2).

5. Treat either shortness or weakness as appropriate.

6. Retest.

Motion tested: Adduction
Muscles tested: Abductors (gluteus medius, gluteus minimus)

1. Patient supine on table.
2. Operator standing at end of table.
3. Operator adducts the extended leg across the front of the opposite leg testing for range and quality of movement (Fig. 19.3).

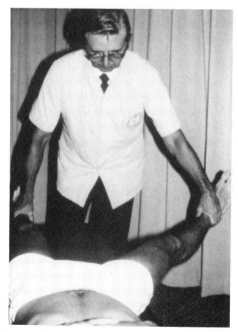

**Figure 19.1.** Test for abduction motion, hip joint.

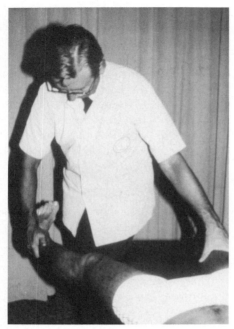

**Figure 19.2.** Muscle energy technique for restricted abduction of hip joint.

4. Opposite leg is tested in similar fashion.
5. Strength is tested by asking the patient to maximally abduct the leg against resistance offered by the operator holding the leg in the adducted position (Fig. 19.4).
6. Treatment for shortness or weakness is accomplished as appropriate.
7. Retest.
   Note: An alternate method is to lift the leg not being tested and adduct the extended leg (being tested) beneath it. Testing in this position also evaluates the tensor fasciae latae muscle.

Motion tested: External rotation (hip flexed to 90°)
Muscles tested: Internal rotators (gluteus medius, gluteus minimus)

1. Patient supine on table.
2. Operator stands at side of table next to extremity being tested.

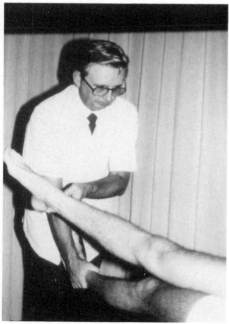

**Figure 19.3.** Test for adduction movement, hip joint.

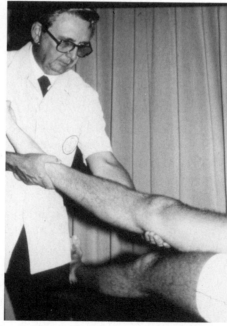

**Figure 19.4.** Muscle energy technique for restricted adduction of hip joint.

3. Operator holds lower extremity with 90° flexion at both the hip and knee.
4. Operator externally rotates the femur by carrying the foot and ankle medially, evaluating range and quality of movement (Fig. 19.5).
5. Strength test is made with patient attempting to internally rotate the femur against equal and opposite resistance offered by operator (Fig. 19.6).
6. Shortness or weakness are treated as appropriate.
7. Retest.

Motion tested: Internal rotation (hip flexed to 90°)
Muscles tested: External rotators (primarily piriformis)

1. Patient supine on table.
2. Operator standing on side of leg to be tested.

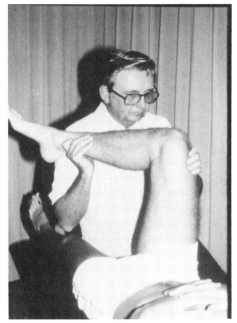

**Figure 19.6.** Muscle energy technique for restricted external rotation, hip joint, flexed to 90°.

3. Operator holds the knee flexed at 90° with the hip also flexed at 90°.
4. Operator introduces internal rotation, testing range and quality of movement (Fig. 19.7).
5. Strength is tested by asking the patient to attempt to externally rotate against resistance offered by the operator holding leg in the internal rotated position (Fig. 19.8).
6. Shortness and weakness treated as appropriate.
7. Retest.

Motion tested: Partial hip flexion (straight leg raising)
Muscles tested: Hip extensors primarily hamstring muscles (semitendinosis, semimembranosus, biceps femoris) (Note: gluteus maximus and adductor magnus become hip extensor when thigh is flexed.)

1. Patient supine on table.
2. Operator stands at side of table.

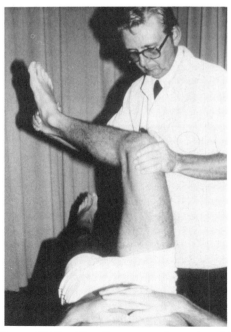

**Figure 19.5.** Test for external rotation, hip joint, with hip flexed 90°.

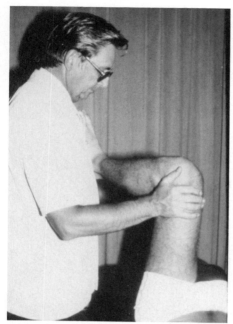

**Figure 19.7.** Test for internal rotation, hip joint, flexed to 90°.

3. Operator monitors anterior superior iliac spine on side opposite to leg being tested.

4. Operator lifts extended leg introducing hip flexion testing for range and quality of movement (Fig. 19.9).

5. Shortness and tightness are treated by a series of isometric contractions against resistance, the direction of effort is the patient pulling the heel toward the buttocks (Fig. 19.10).

6. To test for strength, the patient is prone on the table and operator resists attempts at knee flexion bilaterally.

7. To treat for weakness, the patient exerts a series of concentric isotonic contractions throughout the full range of knee flexion against operator resistance.

8. Retest.

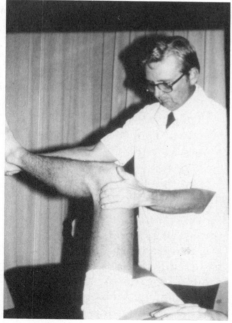

**Figure 19.8.** Muscle energy technique for restricted internal rotation, hip joint at 90°.

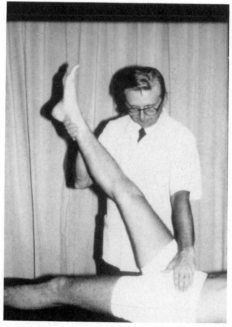

**Figure 19.9.** Test for hip flexion (hamstring length).

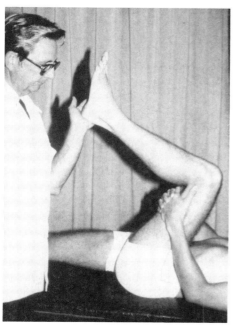

**Figure 19.10.** Muscle energy technique for shortness and tightness, hamstrings.

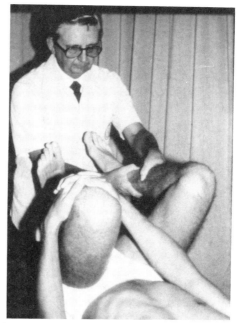

**Figure 19.11.** Test for hip extension. Patient holds leg opposite the one being tested.

Motion tested: Hip extension
Muscle tested: Iliopsoas

1. Patient supine with pelvis close to the end of the table so that lower extremity below the knee is free of the table.
2. Operator stands at end of table facing patient.
3. Both hips and knees are flexed.
4. Patient holds leg opposite that being tested in the flexed position (Fig. 19.11).
5. Operator passively extends the leg being tested, ascertaining if the back of the thigh is able to strike the table, with the knee fully flexed at the endpoint (Fig. 19.12).
6. The opposite side is tested in similar manner.
7. Strength test is done by having the patient attempt to lift the knee to the ceiling against operator resistance at the distal femur.

8. Shortness is treated by isometric contraction against operator resistance. In addition to resisting hip flexion at the distal femur, the operator also resists attempts at external rotation of the hip (iliopsoas function) by offering a resistance with the leg against the medial side of the patient's foot and ankle (Fig. 19.13).
9. Weakness is treated by a series of concentric isotonic contractions of hip flexion and external rotation.
10. Retest.
   Note: Before testing for length and strength of the iliopsoas, the lumbar spine should have been evaluated and treated appropriately. The test for iliopsoas function put stress on the lumbar spine, particularly the lumbosacral junction.

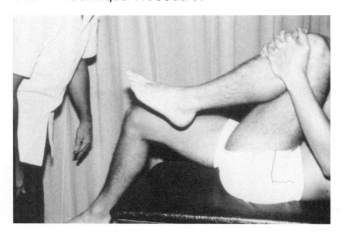

**Figure 19.12.** Test for hip extension. Operator extends leg to test iliopsoas length.

Motion tested: Internal rotation with hips at neutral
Muscles tested: External rotators (obturator internis, obturator externis, gemellus superior, gemellus inferior, quadratus femoris, and piriformis)

1. Patient prone on table.
2. Operator stands at foot of table facing patient.

3. Operator flexes the knees to 90° and internally rotates both hips by letting the feet drop laterally, testing for range and quality of movement (Fig. 19.14).

4. Strength is tested bilaterally by asking the patient to pull the feet together from the endpoint of the position in step 3.

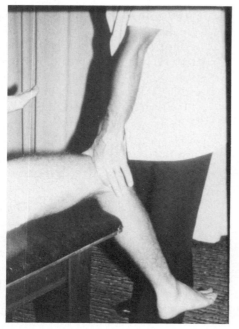

**Figure 19.13.** Muscle energy treatment for shortness and tightness, iliopsoas.

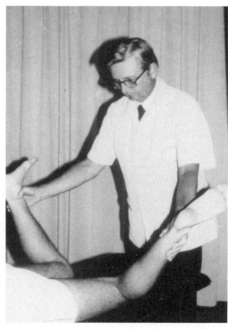

**Figure 19.14.** Test for internal rotation of hips, in neutral.

5. Treatment for shortening is accomplished by the operator holding the opposite leg with knee flexed and hip internally rotated while the operator resists patient attempts at external rotation of the hip with the knee in the 90° flexed position against the internal rotation barrier (Fig. 19.15).
6. Weakness is treated by a series of concentric isotonic contractions throughout a range of external rotation with the knee at 90°.
7. Retest.

Motion tested: External rotation with the hips at neutral
Muscles tested: Internal rotators (gluteus medius, gluteus minimus)

1. Patient prone on the table.
2. Operator standing at foot of table facing patient.
3. Operator fixes leg opposite one being tested with slight knee flexion and hip external rotation.

4. Leg being tested is flexed to 90° and externally rotated, testing for range and quality of movement (Fig. 19.16).
5. Steps 3 and 4 are performed on the opposite side.
6. Strength is tested by asking the patient to internally rotate against resistance.
7. Shortness and weakness are treated as appropriate (Fig. 19.17).
8. Retest.

Motion tested: Knee flexion
Muscles tested: Quadriceps muscles (rectus femoris, vastus lateralis, vastus intermedius, vastus medialis)

1. Patient prone on table.
2. Operator stands at foot of table facing patient.
3. Operator flexes both knees while holding at the patient's ankles (Fig. 19.18).
4. Test is made for range and quality of movement.

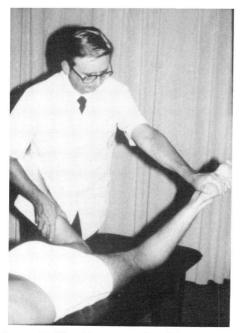

**Figure 19.15.** Treatment for tightness, external rotator muscles.

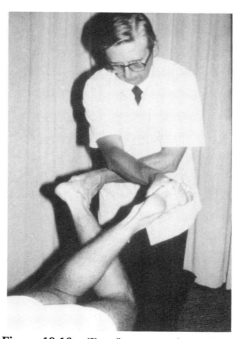

**Figure 19.16.** Test for external rotation of hips, in neutral.

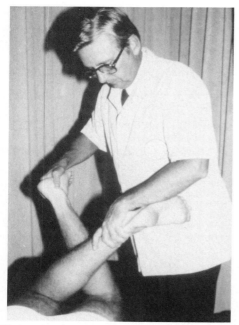

**Figure 19.17.** Muscle energy technique for tightness, internal rotation muscles.

5. With the knee fully flexed, strength is tested by asking the patient to extend the knee against resistance offered by operator. (Both sides tested simultaneously.)
6. Shortness is treated by a series of isometric tractions against resistance (Fig. 19.19).
7. Weakness is treated by a series of concentric isotonic contractions against resistance.
8. Retest.

Although there are some differences of opinion on treatment sequence, this author has found it most effective to treat the shortness and tightness before treating for weakness. It is common to find shortness of a muscle group reflexly inhibit its antagonist, resulting in apparent weakness of that antagonist muscle. However, once the shortness and tightness of the agonist is removed, the apparent weakness of the antagonist is no longer present. Once shortness and

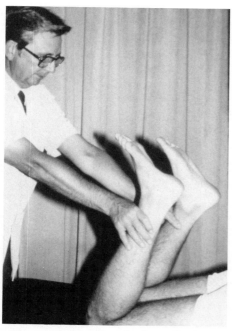

**Figure 19.18.** Test for knee flexion.

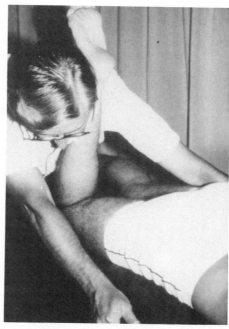

**Figure 19.19.** Muscle energy treatment for tightness, quadriceps muscle.

tightness have been removed, then muscles that still appear to be functionally weak should be treated for weakness using the techniques described.

It has also been observed that there are certain patterns of muscle imbalance in the six muscle groups. For example, when the right adductors are tight, the left adductors appear weak, and the left abductors appear to be tight. Similar relationships of tightness to weakness are found from agonist to antagonist and between comparable muscle groups on opposite sides. These observations are clearly consistent with those found in the tight—loose concept of myofascial release technique.

In addition to the muscle energy procedures found above, the hip joint can be treated with particular reference to the relationship of the femoral head to the acetabulum by the following articulatory technique:

Hip joint: Acetabular technique
Articulatory procedure

1. Patient supine on table.
2. Operator stands at side of table of dysfunctional hip joint.
3. Operator's caudal hand controls the patient's lower extremity which is flexed to 90° at the hip joint and knee. This arm will control internal—external rotation and adduction—abduction, while exerting an articulatory force in an anteroposterior translation movement.
4. Operator's cephalic hand overlies the lateral hip with the thenar eminence against the lateral aspect of the greater trochanter. The heel of the hand exerts impaction in an anteromedial direction which alternates with the posterior translatory movement of the patient's thigh by the operator's opposite hand (Fig. 19.20).
5. Articulatory efforts are made in internal—external rotation, adduc-

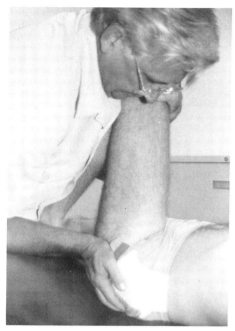

**Figure 19.20.** Supine articulatory technique for hip joint. Operator's hand contacts greater trochanter and exerts medial impaction, alternating with posterior translation from operator's opposite hand.

tion—abduction, anterior—posterior translation, and impaction—distraction to enhance total range of movement.

### KNEE JOINT

The primary movement at the knee joint is the flexion and extension of the tibia under the femur. Because of the difference in the length of the medial and lateral femoral condyles, there is an internal—external rotational component to the flexion—extension arc of movement. During extension the tibia rotates externally, and during flexion, the tibia rotates internally. When this minor internal—external rotation is lost, there is interference with the normal flexion—extension movement. Both the flexion—extension and the internal—external rotation depend upon a small amount of anteroposterior glide and medial to lateral gapping of the opposing surfaces of the femur and tibia. These minor play movements are present with ligamentous stability and are increased with ligamentous damage to the knee joint. The primary dysfunctions of the knee joint are at the medial meniscus and internal—external rotation of the tibia on the femur.

### Diagnosis: Medial Meniscus "Lock" Technique: Direct Action Operator Guiding

Procedure #1

1. Patient supine on table.
2. Operator stands at side of table near dysfunctional knee.
3. Operator's caudal arm grasps distal leg between upper arm and chest with hand surrounding proximal tibia and thumb overlying anteromedial aspect of knee joint (Fig. 19.21).

4. Operator's cephalic hand placed over distal femur with heel of hand on lateral side exerting a force medially.
5. Operator gaps medial side of knee joint by holding distal leg laterally, with medial pressure on distal femur.
6. Operator maintains posterolateral compressive force on medial meniscus as leg is carried into extension at the knee (Fig. 19.22).
7. Several repetitions of this movement may be necessary to release restriction of the medial meniscus.
8. Retest.

Procedure #2

1. Patient supine on table.
2. Operator stands at caudal end of the table facing patient.
3. Patient's dysfunctional leg is carried over the edge of the table and distal

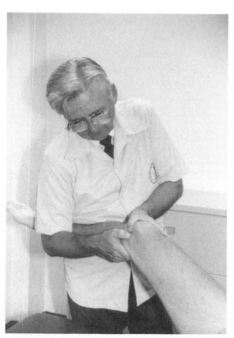

**Figure 19.21.**  Supine, operator guiding technique for medial meniscus. Operator controls distal leg and thumb overlays medial meniscus.

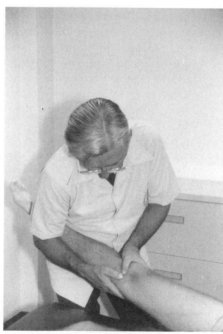

**Figure 19.22.**  Supine, operator guiding technique for medial meniscus. Operator maintains posterolateral force on medial meniscus as leg is carried into extension.

leg is supported between the operator's thighs.

4. Operator's two hands grasp proximal tibia with both thumbs over anteromedial aspect of knee joint (Fig. 19.23).
5. A circumduction movement carrying first into medial translation and then extension at the knee is accomplished, attempting to result in full extension (Fig. 19.24).
6. Several repetitions may be necessary.
7. Retest

Note: This technique may also be used for restriction of the lateral meniscus, but with the thumbs overlying the anterolateral aspect of the knee and the circumduction movement being a lateral translation rather than medial. Dysfunction of the lateral meniscus is more uncommon than that of the medial meniscus.

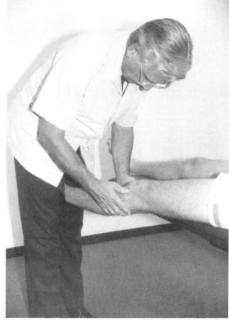

**Figure 19.24.** Supine, operator guiding technique for medial meniscus. Operator introduces medial translation, then extension.

Muscle energy procedures for the treatment of rotational restriction of the tibia on the femur are as follows:

## Diagnosis of Internal-External Rotation:

1. Patient sits on edge of table with lower legs dangling off the edge.
2. Operator sits in front of patient.
3. Operator grasps foot and dorsiflexes ankle to barrier.
4. Operator introduces external rotation (Fig. 19.25) and internal rotation (Fig. 19.26) by medial and lateral movement of the distal foot, testing for range, quality of range, and endfeel.
5. Both sides tested for comparison.
6. Strength is tested in both directions with both lower extremities in usual manner.

Note: The same principles apply to this procedure with the patient prone and the knee flexed to 90°.

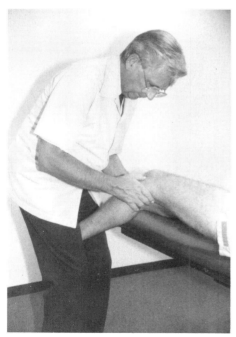

**Figure 19.23.** Supine, operator guiding technique for medial meniscus. Operator's hands grasp proximal tibial with thumbs over medial meniscus.

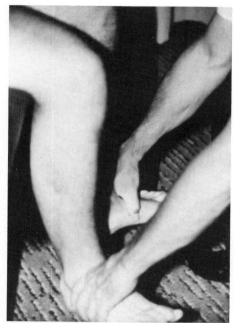

**Figure 19.25.** Diagnosis of internal-external rotation of tibia. Operator introduces external rotation.

## Technique: Direct Action Muscle Energy

Diagnosis
Position: Tibia internally rotated
Motion restriction: External rotation of tibia

1. Patient sits on edge of table with lower legs dangling.
2. Operator sits in front of patient.
3. Operator grasps heel of foot in one hand and forefoot in the other.
4. Operator dorsiflexes foot at ankle and introduces external rotation to barrier (Fig. 19.27).
5. Patient internally rotates forefoot against operator resistance for 3-5 seconds.
6. Following patient relaxation, operator externally rotates foot to new barrier.
7. Patient repeats step 5 approximately 3 times.
8. Retest.

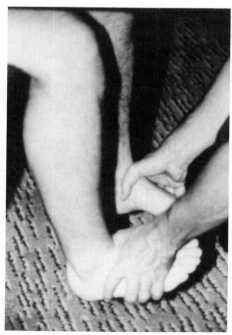

**Figure 19.26.** Diagnosis of internal-external rotation of tibia. Operator introduces internal rotation.

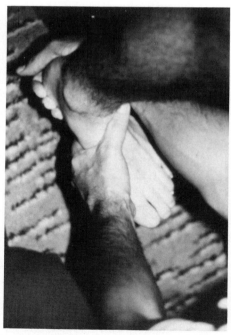

**Figure 19.27.** Sitting, muscle energy technique, internally rotated tibia. Operator dorsiflexes ankle and introduces external rotation to barrier and resists internal rotation.

Diagnosis:
Position: Tibia externally rotated
Motion restriction: Internal rotation of tibia

Steps 1-3 as above.
4. Operator dorsiflexes foot and introduces internal rotation to barrier (Fig. 19.28).
5. Steps 5-8 as above except patient effort is to external rotation against resistance.
   Note: The same principles can be used with the patient prone on the table with the knee at 90° (Figs. 19.29, 19.30).

With internal or external rotators, a series of three to five concentric isotonic contractions are made throughout the range of movement against yielding resistance by the operator.

The restoration of normal internal— external rotational movement of the tibia

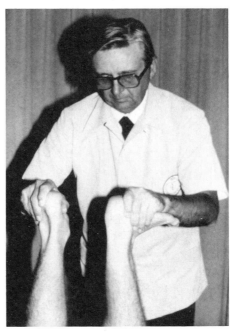

**Figure 19.29.** Prone, muscle energy technique, internally rotated tibia. Operator dorsiflexes foot, externally rotates tibia, and resists internal rotation.

on the femur is made before addressing the proximal tibiofibular joint.

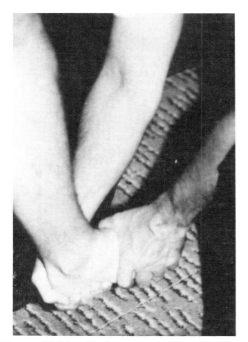

**Figure 19.28.** Sitting, muscle energy technique, tibia externally rotated. Operator dorsiflexes ankle, introduces internal rotation to barrier, and resists external rotation.

### PROXIMAL TIBIOFIBULAR JOINT

This articulation, while being intimately related to the knee joint, is equally important in its relationship to the ankle. The proximal tibiofibula joint normally has an anteroposterior glide, and is influenced by the action of the biceps femoris muscle inserting on the fibular head. The proximal tibiofibular joint will be restricted either anteriorly or posteriorly. Restoration of the normal AP glide and its normal relationship to the tibia, are the goals of treatment.

Testing for anteroposterior movement of the proximal tibiofibular joint can be accomplished with the patient either supine or sitting on the edge of the table. Remember that the plane of the joint is approximately 30° from lateral to medial and from before backward. The test is performed as follows:

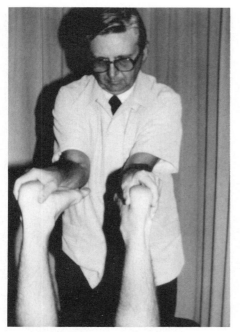

**Figure 19.30.** Prone, muscle energy technique, externally rotated tibia. Operator dorsiflexes ankle, introduces internal rotation, and resists external rotation.

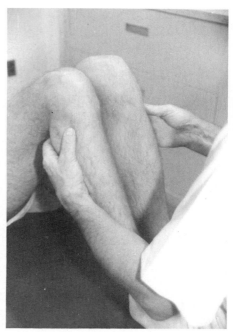

**Figure 19.31.** Supine, test for anteroposterior movement, proximal tibiofibular joint.

1. Patient supine on table with both feet flat on table for fixation purposes (Fig. 19.31) or patient sits on edge of table with the operator sitting in front and holding the medial sides of both feet together (Fig. 19.32).
2. The operator grasps the proximal fibula between the thumb and the fingers of each hand. (Note: be careful of the perineal nerve behind the fibular head.)
3. The operator translates the fibular head anteriorly and posteriorly within the plane of the joint, testing for comparability of range from side to side, quality of movement, and endfeel.

Muscle energy treatment for the proximal tibiofibular joint is as follows:

Position: Fibular head posterior
Motion restriction: Anterior glide of the fibular head

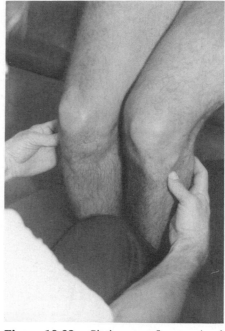

**Figure 19.32.** Sitting, test for proximal tibiofibular joint.

1. Patient sits on edge of table with the dysfunctional leg dangling.
2. Operator sits in front with the medial hand grasping the patient's forefoot.
3. The operator inverts and internally rotates the patient's foot (Fig. 19.33).
4. Fingers of the operator's lateral hand reach behind the fibular head and exert an anterolateral force.
5. The patient is instructed to evert and dorsiflex the foot against resistance offered by the operator's medial hand (Fig. 19.34).
6. Three or four repetitions of this effort are applied.
7. Retest.

Position: Fibular head anterior
Motion restriction: Posterior glide of fibular head

1. Patient sits on edge of table with dysfunctional foot dangling.

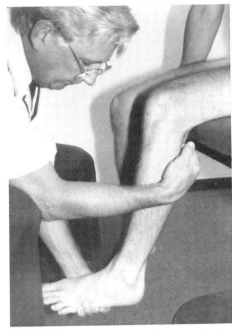

**Figure 19.34.** Sitting, muscle energy technique for posterior fibular head. Operator resists patient's eversion and dorsiflexion of foot.

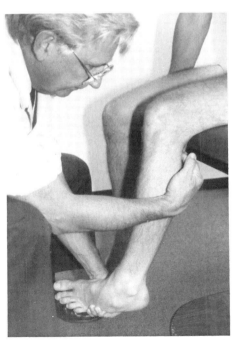

**Figure 19.33.** Sitting, muscle energy technique for posterior fibular head. Operator inverts and internally rotates patient's foot.

2. Operator sits in front of the patient.
3. Operator's medial hand grasps the patient's forefoot and inverts and externally rotates the foot (Fig. 19.35).
4. The thumb of the operator's lateral hand is anterior to the fibular head and exerts a force posteromedially.
5. The patient is instructed to evert and plantar flex the foot against resistance offered by the operator's medial hand (Fig. 19.36).
6. Three to five repetitions are performed.
7. Retest.

Direct action, high-velocity, low-amplitude thrusting procedures for the proximal tibiofibular joint are as follows:

Position: Posterior fibular head
Motion restriction: Anterior glide of fibular head

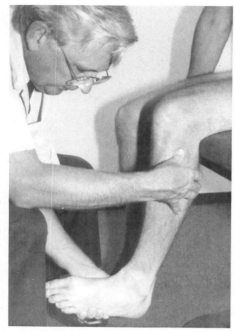

**Figure 19.35.** Sitting, muscle energy technique for anterior fibular head. Operator inverts and externally rotates foot.

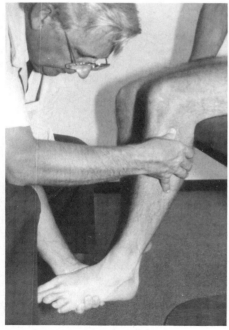

**Figure 19.36.** Sitting, muscle energy technique for anterior fibular head. Operator resists patient's eversion and plantar flexion of foot.

*Alternative #1*

1. Patient supine on table.
2. Operator stands at side of dysfunction with caudal hand controlling lower leg above ankle.
3. Operator's cephalic hand supports the flexed knee with the metacarpophalangeal joint of the index finger just posterior to the fibular head (Fig. 19.37).
4. The hip and knee are flexed, pinching the metacarpophalangeal joint between the distal femur and the fibular head.
5. The operator's distal hand takes the flexed knee into external rotation to the barrier.
6. A high-velocity, low-amplitude thrust is made by an exaggeration of knee flexion, bringing the fibular head anterior (Fig. 19.38).
7. Retest.

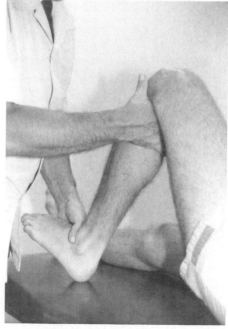

**Figure 19.37.** Supine, high-velocity, low-amplitude thrust for posterior fibular head. Operator's metatarsal phalangeal joint posterior to fibular head.

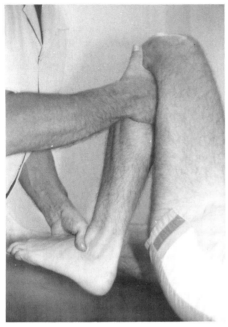

**Figure 19.38.** Supine, high-velocity, low-amplitude thrust for posterior fibular head. Thrust applied by exaggeration of knee flexion.

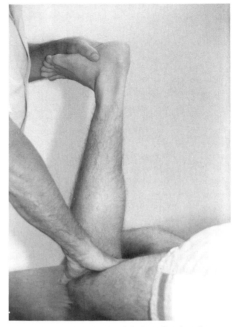

**Figure 19.39.** Prone, high-velocity, low-amplitude thrust for posterior fibular head. Operator's metacarpophalangeal joint posterior to fibular head.

*Alternative #2*

1. Patient prone on table.
2. Operator stands on side of dysfunction.
3. Operator's distal hand controls the ankle and foot.
4. Operator's proximal hand laid over the popliteal space with a metacarpophalangeal joint of the index finger posterior to the fibular head (Fig. 19.39).
5. The knee is flexed, pinching the metacarpophalangeal joint between the fibular head and the femur.
6. With a slight amount of external rotation of the leg, all slack is taken out, and a high-velocity, low-amplitude thrust is made by exaggerating the flexion (Fig. 19.40).
7. Retest.

Position: Fibular head anterior
Motion restriction: Posterior glide fibular head

1. Patient supine on table.
2. Operator standing on the side of dysfunction.
3. Operator's distal hand controls the lower leg and holds the leg in knee extension.
4. Operator internally rotates distal leg to approximately 30°.
5. The thenar eminence of the operator's proximal hand is placed anterior to the proximal fibula (Fig. 19.41).
6. The operator takes up all of the anteroposterior slack at the fibular head by downward compression with the arm extended.
7. When all slack is taken up a direct action high-velocity thrust is per-

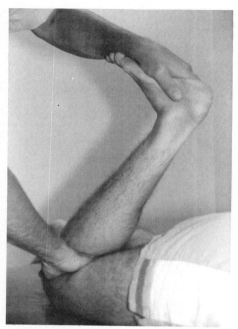

**Figure 19.40.** Prone, high-velocity, low-amplitude thrust for posterior fibular head. High-velocity thrust by exaggerating knee flexion.

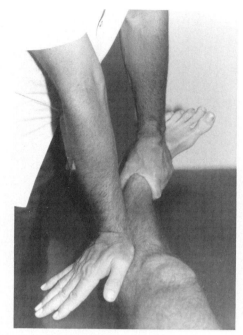

**Figure 19.41.** Supine, high-velocity, low-amplitude thrust for anterior fibular head. With patient's leg internally rotated 30°, operator's thenar eminence thrusts posteriorly on anterior aspect proximal fibula.

formed by dropping the weight of the operator's body through the extended arm to the anterior aspect of the fibular head.

## ANKLE REGION

The ankle region consists of the distal tibiofibular articulation, the articulation of the superior aspect of the talus to the tibiofibular joint mortice, and, for functional purposes, the talocalcaneal articulation. Although the talocalcaneal joint is frequently classified as being in the foot, the key to ankle function is movement on the talus. If the talus is restricted, from either above or below, ankle movement is restricted. The talus is an interesting bone with no muscular attachments. Its movement is determined by muscle action influencing bones above and below it. Alteration of function of the talus at the tibiofibular joint mortice is one of the more common dysfunctions in the lower extremity. An-

other functionally important anatomical feature of the talus is that its superior surface is wedge-shaped, with the posterior aspect being narrower than the anterior as it articulates with the tibiofibular joint mortice. Therefore, the ankle is more stable when dorsiflexed than when plantar flexed, and the most common dysfunction present at this joint is restricted dorsiflexion.

The distal tibiofibular joint is basically quite stable and is infrequently dysfunctional. This articulation is strongly influenced by the function of the proximal tibiofibular articulation, and frequently dysfunctions at the distal tibiofibular articulation are removed by appropriate treatment at the proximal one.

Diagnostic evaluation of the distal tibiofibular articulation is as follows:

1. Patient supine on table.
2. Operator standing at foot of table.

3. Operator's medial hand grasps the posterior and medial aspects of the patient's ankle and heel.
4. The operators lateral hand grasps the lateral malleous between the thumb and index finger (Fig. 19.42).
5. The operator's lateral hand moves the lateral malleous anterior and posterior against the fixed foot and ankle held by the operator's medial hand.
6. A posterior distal tibiofibular joint has anterior movement restriction and an anterior distal tibiofibular joint has posterior motion restriction.

Direct action, high-velocity, low-amplitude thrusting procedures for the distal tibiofibular joint are as follows:

Position: Anterior distal tibiofibular joint
Motion restriction: Posterior movement of the lateral malleous

1. Patient supine on table.
2. Operator standing at foot of table.
3. Operator's medial hand grasps the patient's heel and maintains the ankle at 90° flexion. The thumb is placed over the anterior aspect of the patient's lateral malleous (Fig. 19.43).
4. The thenar eminence of the operator's lateral hand is superimposed on the opposite thumb and the fingers are curled around the posterior aspect of the ankle (Fig. 19.44).
5. All of the slack is taken out in a posterior direction and a high-velocity thrust is made posteriorly against the anterior aspect of the lateral malleous by combined effort of the thenar eminence of the lateral hand and the thumb of the medial hand.
6. Retest.

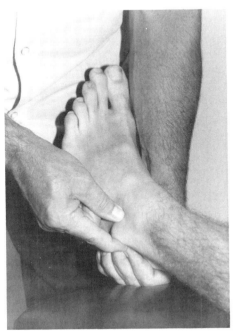

**Figure 19.42.** Test for distal tibiofibular articulation.

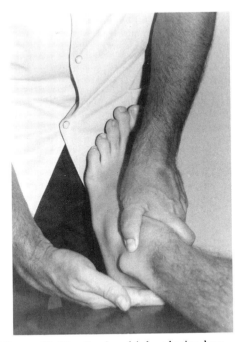

**Figure 19.43.** Supine, high-velocity, low-amplitude thrust for anterior distal tibiofibular joint. Operator maintains ankle at 90° flexion with thumb over anterior aspect lateral malleolus.

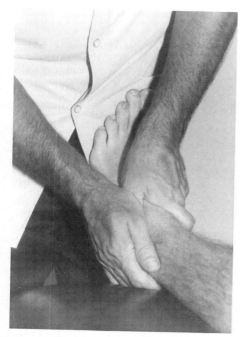

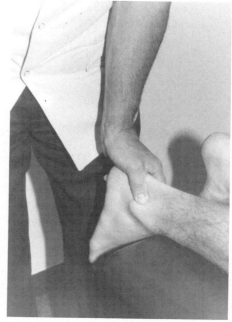

**Figure 19.44.** Supine, high-velocity, low-amplitude thrust for anterior distal tibiofibular joint. Operator's thenar eminence over thumb thrusts distal malleolus in posterior direction.

**Figure 19.45.** Prone, high-velocity, low-amplitude thrust for posterior distal tibiofibular joint. Operator maintains dorsiflexion of ankle and thumb over posterior aspect lateral malleolus.

Position: Posterior distal tibiofibular joint

Motion restriction: Anterior movement of the lateral malleous

1. Patient prone with feet over edge of table.
2. Operator stands at foot of table facing cephalad.
3. Operator's medial hand grasps the calcaneous and maintains dorsiflexion at the ankle. The thumb is placed over the posterior aspect of the later malleous (Fig. 19.45).
4. The operator's lateral hand is placed with the thenar eminence overlying the opposite thumb (Fig. 19.46).
5. All of the slack is taken out in an anterior direction and a direct action, high-velocity thrust by the reinforced thumb is made carrying the lateral malleous toward the floor.
6. Retest.

The talotibial joint is evaluated for its capacity to plantar flex and dorsiflex, with particular attention to possible restriction of dorsiflexion. To test for this movement the following procedure is performed:

1. Patient sitting on table with legs dangling.
2. Operator sits in front of patient.
3. To test for plantar flexion, the operator grasps the forefoot and plantar flexes to the barrier, evaluating each side for restriction of movement.
4. To test for dorsiflexion, each thumb is placed on the anterior surface of the neck of the talus with the fingers underlying the forefoot and the legs are passively swung back toward the table resulting in dorsiflexion of the talotibial joint. Restriction of dorsiflexion on one side is evaluated. Frequently the neck of the talus on the dysfunctional side will be tender during this procedure (Fig. 19.47).

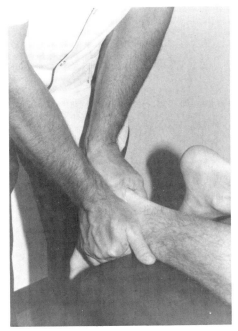

**Figure 19.46.** Prone, high-velocity, low-amplitude thrust for posterior distal tibiofibular joint. Thenar eminence over thumb thrusts lateral malleolus anteriorly.

5. Restricted dorsiflexion of the talotibial joint is frequently related to shortening and tightening of the gastrocnemius-soleus mechanism in the calf.

A muscle energy procedure for restricted dorsiflexion of the talotibial joint, which lengthens the gastocnemius-soleus mechanism, is as follows:

Position: Talus plantar flexed
Motion restriction: Dorsiflexion of the talus

1. Patient sitting on the table with both legs dangling freely.
2. Operator sits in front of the dysfunctional talus.
3. Operator puts lateral hand under the plantar surface of the forefoot.
4. Operator crosses lower legs underneath patient's forefoot.
5. The web of the operator's medial hand is placed overlying the neck of the talus (Fig. 19.48).

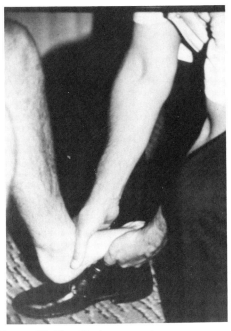

**Figure 19.48.** Sitting, muscle energy procedure for restricted dorsiflexion tibiofibular joint. Operator's hand over neck of talus resists plantar flexion with other hand.

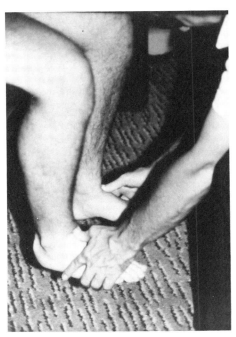

**Figure 19.47.** Sitting, test for talotibial joint.

6. Dorsiflexion to the barrier is taken, with combined action of a caudad and posterior force on the talar neck and a dorsiflexion movement of the sole of the foot.
7. The patient is instructed to plantar flex the forefoot against equal and opposite resistance.
8. Several repetitions are accomplished against progressive dorsilexion barrier.
9. Retest.

Direct action high-velocity thrusting procedures for the talotibial joint are as follows:

Position: Talus plantar flexed
Motion restriction: Dorsiflexion of the talus

1. Patient supine on table with operator standing at foot.
2. Operator's two hands encircle patient's foot, both middle fingers overlapping on top of talar neck and thumbs on sole of foot (Fig. 19.49).
3. Operator takes up slack into dorsiflexion and long-axis extension.
4. A high-velocity long-axis extension thrust is made.
5. Retest.

Position: Dorsiflexed or plantar flexed talus
Motion restriction: Dorsiflexion or plantar flexion of talus

1. Patient supine on table.
2. Operator sits on edge of table on dysfunctional side facing caudad.
3. Patient's hip is flexed to 90° and externally rotated. The knee is flexed to 90° with the thigh against the operator's posterior trunk.
4. Webs of the thumb and index finger of operator's two hands are placed on the neck of the talus anteriorly and the tubercle of the talus posteriorly (through the Achilles tendon) (Fig. 19.50).

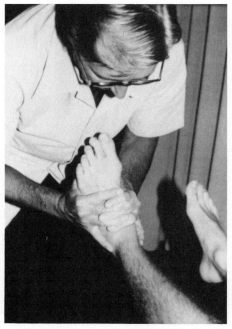

**Figure 19.49.** Supine, high-velocity, low-amplitude thrust for plantar flexed talus. Operator's two hands encircle foot with middle fingers over talar neck and long-axis extension thrust made.

5. The talus is dorsiflexed or plantar flexed against the resistant barrier as appropriate.
6. All of the slack is taken up by the operator's hands moving caudad.
7. When all slack is taken up, a direct action high-velocity, low-amplitude thrust in a long-axis distraction mode is accomplished.
8. Retest.

The talocalcaneal joint consists of two small articular surfaces, and the motion is primarily an anteromedial to posterolateral glide. The test for motion restriction is as follows:

1. Patient supine on table.
2. Operator stands at side of table facing dysfunctional ankle.
3. Operator's proximal hand grasps the ankle joint with the web of the

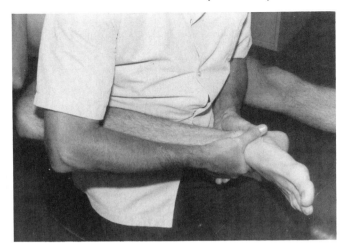

**Figure 19.50.** Supine, high-velocity, low-amplitude thrust for talotibial joint.

thumb and index finger over the neck of the talus, the fingers grasping the medial malleous, and the thumb grasping the lateral malleous, stabilizing the talus.

4. The operator's distal hand grasps the calcaneous, and maintaining the foot and ankle at 90°, the caudal hand translates the calcaneous anteromedially and posterolaterally under the talus, sensing for restricted movement (Fig. 19.51).

5. The opposite side is tested for comparison in a similar manner.

Direct action, high-velocity, low-amplitude thrusting procedure for talocalcaneal dysfunction is as follows:

1. Patient supine on table.
2. Operator sits on table facing caudally.
3. Patient's hip is flexed to 90° and externally rotated while the knee is flexed to 90° resulting in the posterior thigh being against the posterior trunk of the operator.
4. Operator's medial hand grasps the superior aspect of the calcaneous.
5. The operator's lateral hand grasps the anterior and lateral aspect of the calcaneous incorporating the cuboid within the web of the thumb

and index finger, with thumb on the tarsal navicular.

6. In the presence of an anteromedial talus (calcaneous posterolateral), the calcaneous is medially rotated (inverted) to the barrier (Fig. 19.52).

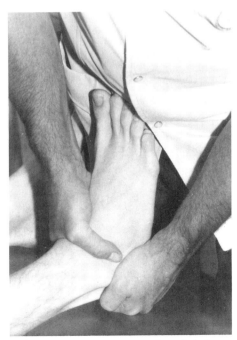

**Figure 19.51.** Motion test for talocalcaneal joint.

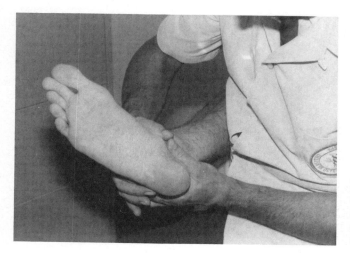

**Figure 19.52.** Supine, direct action high-velocity, low-amplitude thrust for talocalcaneal joint. For anteromedial talus, calcaneus medial rotated to barrier.

7. In the presence of a posterolateral talus (calcaneous anteromedial), the slack is taken up with lateral rotation of the calcaneous (inverted) (Fig. 19.53).
8. All of the slack is taken out in a caudad direction and a high-velocity, low-amplitude thrust is made in a long-axis distraction direction.
9. Retest.

## FOOT

The foot is a complex structure incorporating the tarsals, metatarsals, and the phalanges. There are four arches identified in the foot. The lateral arch is referred to as the weight-bearing arch and runs from the calcaneous, through the cuboid, to the fourth and fifth metatarsal bones, and to the fourth and fifth toes. The key to the lateral, weight-bearing arch, is the cuboid which rotates medially and laterally around the anterior articulation of the calcaneous. The medial, spring arch, includes the talus, the navicular, the medial cuneiform, the first metatarsal, and the great toe. The function of the navicular, which medially and laterally rotates around the head of the talus, largely determines the function of the medial, spring arch. The transverse arch con-

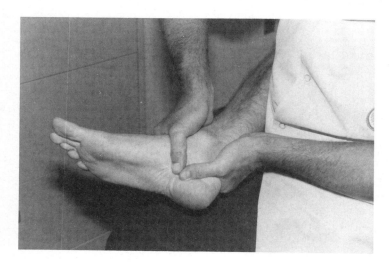

**Figure 19.53.** Supine, direct action high-velocity, low-amplitude thrust for talocalcaneal joint. For posterolateral talus, calcaneus laterally rotated.

sists of the cuboid laterally and the navicular medially, with the accompanying relationship to the cuneiforms.

The major restrictors of the transverse arch are dysfunction at the cuboid laterally and the navicular medially. Most common in the transverse arch is cuboid dysfunction, with the cuboid being rotated laterally (pronated). The so-called metatarsal arch is not a true arch at all but refers to the relationship of the heads of the five metatarsals. With normal foot mechanics there is free mobility and springing of the metatarsal heads during normal walking. Restrictions of the metatarsal arch are usually secondary to alteration in the other arches of the foot, and are accompanied by restriction of the soft tissues of the forefoot, primarily the plantar fascia.

The primary goals of manual medicine management of the foot are to restore function of the cuboid laterally and the navicular medially, followed by mobilization of the remaining intertarsal, tarsometatarsal joints, metatarsal heads, and metatarsophalangeal and interphalangeal joints.

### The Calcaneocuboid Joint

Dysfunction of the cuboid occurs with it rotating medially into a position of eversion, with the medial margin being depressed.

To test for cuboid dysfunction, one looks for asymmetry in relationship with the cuboid of the opposite side; alteration in tissue texture, primarily tenderness over the plantar surface of the cuboid; and motion restriction, primarily external rotation (supination).

1. Patient supine on table.
2. Operator stands at end of table.
3. Operator palpates plantar surface of each cuboid looking for prominence of the tuberosity of the cuboid on the dysfunctional side.
4. Operator palpates plantar surface of both cuboids for tenderness and tension.
5. Operator motion tests cuboid on each side by having the medial hand

grasp the heel of the foot and holding the foot in 90° at the ankle. The lateral hand grasps the lateral side of the forefoot encircling the cuboid and internally and externally rotates the forefoot monitoring for movement at the cuboidcalcaneal joint (Fig. 19.54).

A high-velocity, low-amplitude thrusting procedure for a cuboidcalcaneal dysfunction is as follows:

Position: Right cuboid depressed (pronated, internally rotated)
Motion restriction: Cuboid supination (external rotation)

1. Patient prone on table with the dysfunctional leg off edge of table.
2. Operator stands at side of table on dysfunctional side facing cephalad.
3. Operator's two hands grasp the forefoot.
4. The thumb of the lateral hand is placed over the medial side of the plantar surface of the cuboid, rein-

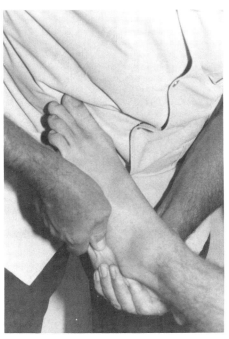

**Figure 19.54.** Motion test for calcaneocuboid joint.

forced with the thumb of the medial hand (Fig. 19.55).

5. The operator swings the foot in a series of oscillating movements with the heel of the foot toward the operator and with the forefoot plantar flexed.

6. On the final efforts the foot is "thrown" toward the floor with acute plantar flexion of the forefoot, with reinforced thumbs carrying the cuboid dorsally and into external rotation (Fig. 19.56).

A muscle energy procedure for cuboid dysfunction is as follows:

Position: Cuboid depressed (internally rotated, pronated)
Motion restriction: Cuboid external rotation and inversion

1. Patient supine on table.
2. Operator standing at foot of table facing dysfunctional foot.

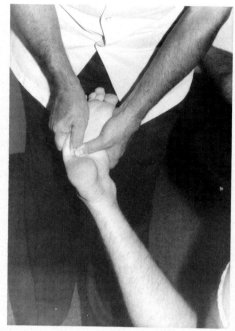

**Figure 19.56.** Prone, high-velocity, low-amplitude thrust for pronated cuboid. Thrust made by foot toward floor with acute plantar flexion forefoot.

3. Medial hand grasps the heel and maintains the foot in 90° flexion.

4. Operator's left hand grasps the lateral side of the foot with the middle and ring fingers overlying the plantar surface of the cuboid, and the hypothenar eminence overlying the dorsal aspect of the fourth and fifth metatarsal shafts (Fig. 19.57).

5. Resistant barrier is engaged by lifting with the middle finger and depressing with the hypothenar eminence on the metatarsals.

6. The patient is instructed to lift (dorsiflex) the little toe against resistance.

7. Three to four repetitions are made.

8. Retest.

Note: The same position can be utilized with a high-velocity, low-amplitude thrust procedure. With all of the slack taken out, an acute

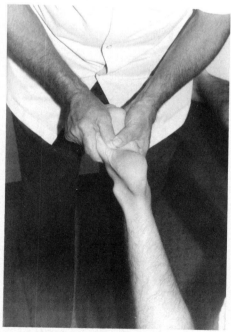

**Figure 19.55.** Prone, high-velocity, low-amplitude thrust for pronated cuboid. Operator's hands grasp forefoot with thumbs on plantar surface cuboid.

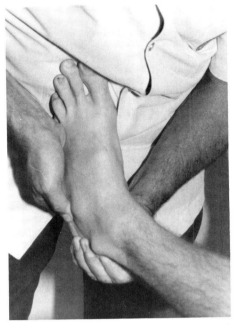

**Figure 19.57.** Supine, muscle energy technique, pronated cuboid.

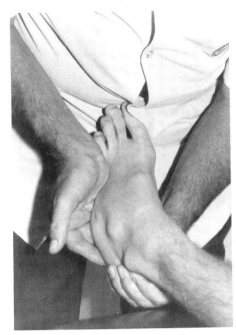

**Figure 19.58.** Supine, high-velocity, low-amplitude thrust for pronated cuboid.

thrust is made by lifting with the reinforced middle finger and depressing the fourth and fifth metatarsal shafts (Fig. 19.58).

## *Talonavicular Joint*

The navicular will be dysfunctional either having been internally or externally rotated. The usual dysfunction which accompanies a depressed cuboid is for the navicular to rotate externally with elevation of its medial tubercle. The navicular will also become dysfunctional if rotated medially (internally) and with depression of the medial tubercle. While this dysfunction is less common, it still does occur.

To test for dysfunction of the talonavicular joint one looks for asymmetry, tissue texture abnormality, and motion restriction.

1. Patient supine on table.
2. Operator stands and faces cephalad.
3. Operator palpates the medial tubercle of each navicular for symmetry.

4. Operator palpates for tenderness and tissue texture abnormality overlying the medial—plantar surface of the navicular.
5. The operator tests for movement of each navicular by having the medial hand grasp the proximal foot with the web of the thumb and index finger surrounding the head of the talus, and the web of the thumb and index finger of the lateral hand surrounding the tarsal navicular. Internal and external rotation is tested by movement of the operator's lateral hand throughout a "wringing" movement.

A muscle energy procedure for talonavicular dysfunction is as follows:

1. Patient supine on table.
2. Operator stands at foot of table facing cephalad.
3. Operator's medial hand grasps the ankle and proximal foot with the web of the thumb and index fingers circling the head of the talus and

holding the foot in 90° at the ankle.

4. Operator's lateral hand encircles the navicular with the web of the thumb and index finger controlling rotation of the navicular.

5. In the presence of external rotation, the operator's lateral hand internally rotates the navicular against the barrier and the patient is instructed to invert the foot against resistance. This is repeated 3-5 times (fig. 19.59).

6. In the presence of internal rotation of the navicular, the lateral hand externally rotates the navicular to the resistant barrier and the patient is instructed to evert the foot against resistance. Three to five repetitions are made (Fig. 19.60).

7. Retest.

Note: A direct action high-velocity, low-amplitude thrust can be substituted for the muscle energy activating force in exactly the same manner of localization as described above.

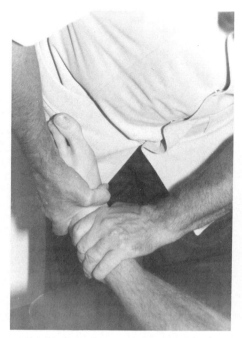

**Figure 19.60.** Supine, muscle energy technique for talonavicular joint with navicular internal rotation.

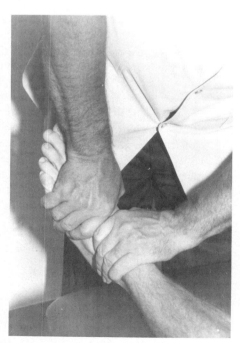

**Figure 19.59.** Supine, muscle energy technique for talonavicular joint with navicular external rotation.

## The Cuneiform Bones (Intertarsal Joints)

The cuneiforms function in response to normal motion, or dysfunction, of the navicular and cuboid. The first cuneiform can rotate internally and externally on the navicular. The remaining cuneiforms have a gliding movement on each other and their usual dysfunction is depression in which the transverse arch is flattened.

The first cuneiform—navicular articulation is tested and treated in exactly the same fashion as the talonavicular articulation with the exception of the grasp of the two hands. At this joint level, the medial hand grasps the navicular and the lateral hand grasps the first cuneiform.

To test for intercuneiform movement, the following procedure is used.

1. Patient supine on table.
2. Operator standing at foot of table facing cephalad.
3. The forefoot is grasped by both hands with the thumbs overlying the dorsal aspect of the three cuneiforms (Fig. 19.61).
4. The thumbs are used to direct a plantar force against the dorsum of the cuneiforms ascertaining the presence or absence of a springing-type movement.
5. Both sides are tested for comparison.
6. Individual gliding movement is tested by the medial hand grasping one cuneiform between the thumb on the dorsal aspect and the index finger on the plantar aspect, and the lateral hand on the adjacent cuneiform in similar fashion. A dorsal to plantar gliding movement is performed by holding one cuneiform and moving the other on it.

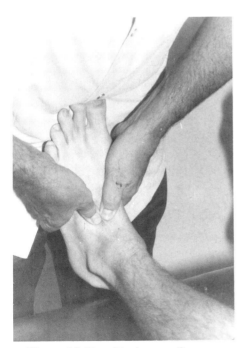

**Figure 19.61.** Motion test for cuneiform movement.

A muscle energy procedure for depression of the cuneiforms is as follows:

1. Patient supine on table.
2. Operator standing at foot of table facing cephalad.
3. Operator's hands grasp each side of the patient's foot with the hypothenar eminence over the dorsal aspect of the metatarsal shafts.
4. The middle fingers are placed against the dysfunctional cuneiform bone (first, second, or third) and exerts a dorsal force (Fig. 19.62).
5. The forefoot is plantar flexed and the patient is instructed to lift the toes cephalward against equal and opposite resistance (Fig. 19.63).
6. Three to five repetitions are made.
7. Retest.

A high-velocity, low-amplitude thrust procedure for depressed cuneiforms is similar to that for the depressed cuboid with the patient in the prone position. In this instance the reinforced thumb is on the dysfunctional cuneiform and the counterforce of the thumbs is in the plane of the intertarsal joint. Again the high-velocity thrust is accomplished by acute plantar flexion of the forefoot against the counterforce with the thumbs in a "J stroke" manner.

### The Tarsometatarsal Joints

The first tarsometatarsal joint has movement very similar to that of the navicular on the talus and the first cuneiform on the navicular. It is diagnosed and treated for dysfunction in a similar manner but with localization at the tarso-first metatarsal articulation. The remaining tarsometatarsal joints have primarily a dorsal to plantar glide function which responds to the transverse tarsal arch. This motion is evaluated by grasping the base of one metatarsal between the thumb and index finger of one hand and moving the adjacent metatarsal, similarly grasped between the thumb and index finger (Fig. 19.64), in a dorsal to plantar glide fashion. If restriction is noted, an

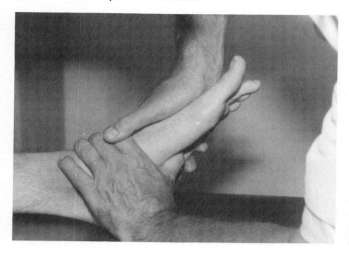

**Figure 19.62.** Supine, muscle energy technique for depression of cuneiforms. Fingers applied against dysfunction of cuneiforms exerting dorsal force.

articulatory to-and-fro movement is used to enhance the gliding movement between the bases of the metatarsal bones and the tarsometatarsal articulations.

### The Metatarsal Heads

The metatarsal heads form the "pseudo-" metatarsal arch. They do not have individual articulations with each other, but they must have mobility between each other.

To test for mobility, grasp the distal shafts of two adjacent metatarsals just proximal to the heads and move one on the other in a dorsal an plantar direction (Fig. 19.65).

The second metatarsal appears to be the axis of the forefoot and so the first metatarsal is moved on the second; the third on the second; the fourth on the third; and, the fifth on the fourth. The most common restriction appears to be between the third and second. In the presence of restriction of metatarsal head mobility, there is frequently identified tension and tenderness of the interosseous muscles.

### The Metatarsal-Phalangeal Joints and the Interphalangeal Joints

These movements are primarily those of dorsiflexion and plantar flexion. Restric-

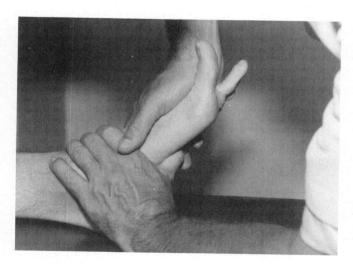

**Figure 19.63.** Supine, muscle energy technique for depression of cuneiforms. Operator resists patient's lifting of toes.

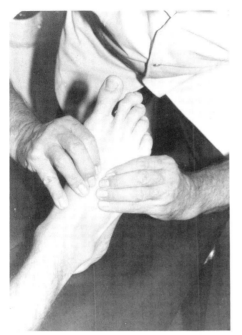

**Figure 19.64.** Motion test of tarsometatarsal joints.

tion is identified by grasping the head of the proximal bone between the thumb and index finger of one hand and the base of the distal bone between the thumb and index finger of the other (Fig. 19.66) and introducing dorsi- and plantar flexion. If found restricted, a high-velocity, low-amplitude thrust is made on the distal bone against the resistant barrier with the thrust direction being long-axis distraction thrust.

Identification and appropriate treatment for dysfunctions within the lower extremities can be most useful in treating pain problems in this area, particularly those resulting from injury. Treatment for dysfunctions has a positive influence on the effect of the lower extremities on the trunk during the walking cycle. The effort to master lower extremity technique is well worthwhile.

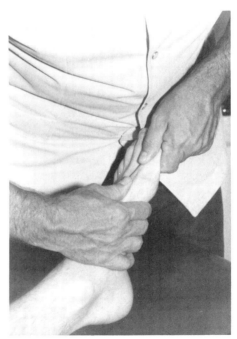

**Figure 19.66.** Motion test of metatarsophalangeal and interphalangeal joints.

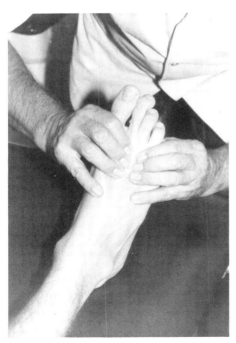

**Figure 19.65.** Motion test of metatarsal heads.

# Recommended Reading

Beal MC: Motion sense. *Osteopath Assoc* 53:151–153, 1953.

Beal MC: *Spinal Motion.* Yearbook of the Academy of Applied Osteopathy Carmel, CA, 1970, pp 11–16.

Bourdillon JF: *Spinal Manipulation*, ed 3. East Norwalk, CT, Appleton-Century-Crofts, 1982.

Bowles CH: Functional technique: a modern perspective. *J Am Osteopath Assoc* 80: 326–331, 1981.

Buerger AA, Greenman PE (eds), *Empirical Approaches to the Validation of Spinal Manipulation.* Springfield, IL, Charles C Thomas, 1985.

Buerger AA, Tobis JS: *Approaches to the Validation of Manipulation Therapy.* Springfield, IL, Charles C Thomas, 1977.

Cyriax J: *Textbook of Orthopedic Medicine*, ed 7., East Sussex, England, Baillière-Tindall. vol. I, 1978.

Dvorak V, Dvorak V, Schneider W (eds): *Manual Medicine 1984.* Heidelberg, Springer-Verlag, 1985.

Farfan HF: The scientific basis of manipulative procedures. *Clin Rheum Dis* 6(1):159, 1980.

Fisk JW: *The Painful Neck and Back.* Springfield, IL, Charles C Thomas, 1977.

Fryette HH: *Principles of Osteopathic Technic.* Carmel, CA, American Academy of Osteopathy, 1954.

Gevitz N: *The D.O.'s - Osteopathic Medicine in America.* Baltimore, Johns Hopkins University Press, 1982.

Good AB: Spinal joint blocking. *J. Manipulative Physio Therapy* 8 (1): 1–8, 1985.

Greenman, PE: The osteopathic concept in the second century: is it still germane to specialty practice. *J Am Osteopath Assoc* 75: 589–595, 1976.

Greenman PE: Layer palpation. *Mich Osteopath J*, 47 (9): 936–937, 1982.

Greenman PE, (ed): *Concepts and Mechanisms of Neuromuscular Functions.* Berlin, Springer-Verlag, 1984.

Greenman PE: Models and Mechanisms of Osteopathic Manipulative Medicine. *Osteopathic Medical News*, 4 (5): 1-20, 1987.

Grieve GP: *Common Vertebral Joint Problems.* Edinburgh, Churchill Livingstone, 1981.

Haldeman S: *Modern Developments in the Principles and Practice of Chiropractic.* East Norwalk, CT, Appleton-Century-Crofts, 1980.

Hoag JM, Cole WV, Bradford SG: *Osteopathic Medicine.* New York, McGraw-Hill, 1969.

Hoover HW: *Functional Technique.* Yearbook of the Academy of Applied Osteopathy, Carmel, CA, 1958, pp 47–51.

Johnston WL, Robertson JA, Stiles EG: *Finding a common denominator for the variety of manipulative techniques.* Yearbook of the Academy of Applied Osteopathy, Carmel, CA, 1969, pp 5–15.

Jones LH: *Strain and Counterstrain.* American Academy of Osteopathy. Colorado Springs, CO, 1981.

Kimberly PE: Formulating a prescription for osteopathic manipulative treatment. *J Am Osteopath Assoc* 75:486–499, 1976.

Kimberly PE (ed): *Outline of Osteopathic Manipulative Procedures,* ed 2. Kirksville College of Osteopathic Medicine, Kirksville, MO, 1980.

Kirkaldy-Willis WH: *Managing Low Back Pain.* Edinburgh, Churchill Livingstone, 1983.

Korr IM (ed): *The Neurologic Mechanisms in Manipulative Therapy.* New York, Plenum, 1978.

Lamax E: Manipulative therapy: a historical perspective from ancient times to the modern era. In Goldstein M (ed): *The Research Status of Spinal Manipulative Therapy.* National Institute of Neurological and Communicative Disorders and Stroke Monograph No. 15., pp 11–17, 1975.

Lewit K: *Manipulative Therapy in Rehabilitation of the Motor System.* Stoneham, MA, Butterworth, 1985.

Magoun HI: *Osteopathy in the Cranial Field,* ed 2, Kirksville, MO, Journal Printing Co., 1966.

Maigne R: *Orthopedic Medicine.* Springfield, IL, Charles C Thomas, 1972.

Maitland GD: *Vertebral Manipulation,* ed 4, Stoneham, MA, Butterworths, 1980.

Mennell J McM: *Back Pain.* Boston, Little, Brown & Co, 1960.

Mennell J McM: *Joint Pain.* Boston, Little, Brown & Co, 1964.

Mitchell FL Sr: *Motion Discordance.* Yearbook of the Academy of Applied Osteopathy, Carmel, CA, 1967, pp 1–5.

Mitchell FL Jr, Moran PS, Pruzzo NA: *An Evaluation and Treatment Manual of Osteopathic Muscle Energy Procedures.* Valley Park, MO, Mitchell, Moran, and Pruzzo Associates, 1979.

Nicholas NS: *Atlas of Osteopathic Techniques.* Philadelphia, Philadelphia College of Osteopathic Medicine, 1974.

Northup G: *Osteopathic Medicine. An American Reformation.* ed 2. Chicago, American Osteopathic Association, 1979.

Northup GW, Korr IM, Buzzell KA, Hix EL: *The Physiological Basis of Osteopathic Medicine.* New York, Postgraduate Institute of Osteopathic Medicine and Surgery, 1970.

Northup GW (ed): *Osteopathic Research: Growth and Development.* Chicago, American Osteopathic Association, 1987.

Page LE: *The Principles of Osteopathy.* Kansas City, MO, American Academy of Osteopathy, 1952.

Retzlaff EW, Mitchell FL Jr: *The Cranium and Its Sutures.* Berlin, Springer-Verlag, 1987.

Sandoz R: Some physical mechanisms and effects of spinal adjustments. *Ann Swiss Chiro Assoc* 6:91–141, 1976.

Schiotz EH: Manipulation treatment of the spinal column from the medical-historical viewpoint. *Tidsskr Nor Laegeforn* 78:359–372, 429–438, 946–950, 1003, 1958. (NIH Library Translation NIH-75-22C, 23C, 24C, 25C).

Schiotz EH, Cyriax J: *Manipulation Past and Present.* London, William Heinemann Medical Books, 1975.

Stiles EG: Manipulative techniques: four approaches. *Osteopath Med,* 1. (6): 27–30, 1976.

Stoddard A: *Manual of Osteopathic Technique.* London, Hutchinson Medical Publications, 1959.

Stoddard A: *Manual of Osteopathic Practice.* New York, Harper & Row, 1969.

Upledger JE, Vredevoogd JD: *Craniosacral Therapy.* Chicago, Eastland Press, 1983.

Walton WJ: *Osteopathic Diagnosis and Technique Procedures.* ed 2, Colorado Springs, CO, American Academy of Osteopathy, 1970.

Ward RC, Sprafka S: Glossary of osteopathic terminology. *J Am Osteopath Assoc* 80:552–567,1981.

# Index

**343**